Immune C
Inflammation, and
Cardiovascular Diseases

Methods in Signal Transduction

Series Editors: Joseph Eichberg, Jr., Michael X. Zhu, and Harpreet Singh

The overall theme of this series continues to be the presentation of the wealth of up to date research methods applied to the many facets of signal transduction. Each volume is assembled by one or more editors who are pre-eminent in their specialty. In turn, the guiding principle for editors is to recruit chapter authors who will describe procedures and protocols with which they are intimately familiar in a reader-friendly format. The intent is to assure that each volume will be of maximum practical value to a broad audience, including students and researchers just entering an area, as well as seasoned investigators.

Immune cells, Inflammation, and Cardiovascular Diseases
Shyam S. Bansal

Nonclassical Ion Channels in the Nervous System
Tian-Le Xu, Long-Jun Wu

Neuron Signaling in Metabolic Regulation
Qingchun Tong

Ion and Molecule Transport in Lysosomes
Bruno Gasnier and Michael X. Zhu

New Techniques for Studying Biomembranes
Qiu-Xing Jiang

Polycystic Kidney Disease
Jinghua Hu and Yong Yu

Signal Transduction and Smooth Muscle
Mohamed Trebak and Scott Earley

Autophagy and Signaling
Esther Wong

Lipid-Mediated Signaling
Eric J. Murphy and Thad A. Rosenberger

TRP Channels
Michael X. Zhu

Immune Cells, Inflammation, and Cardiovascular Diseases

Edited by Shyam S. Bansal

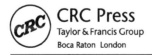

CRC Press
Taylor & Francis Group
Boca Raton London

CRC Press is an imprint of the
Taylor & Francis Group, an **informa** business

First edition published 2022
by CRC Press
6000 Broken Sound Parkway NW, Suite 300, Boca Raton, FL 33487–2742

and by CRC Press
4 Park Square, Milton Park, Abingdon, Oxon, OX14 4RN

CRC Press is an imprint of Taylor & Francis Group, LLC

© 2022 Taylor & Francis Group, LLC

Library of Congress Cataloging-in-Publication Data
Names: Bansal, Shyam S., editor.
Title: Immune cells, inflammation and cardiovascular diseases / edited by Shyam S. Bansal.
Description: First edition. | Boca Raton : CRC Press, 2022. | Series: Methods in signal transduction series | Includes bibliographical references and index. | Summary: "Inflammation, once considered a physiological response to foreign pathogens, is now recognized as a crucial pathological player in the initiation and progression of several chronic diseases including diabetes, obesity, cancer, Alzheimer's disease, Parkinson's diseases, and many others. Considering cardiovascular diseases are a leading cause of death in the United States and world-wide, identification of critical inflammatory processes is of utmost importance to devising new immune-based therapeutics that can be added to existing regimens. This book provides detailed information on aspects of inflammation, and the manner in which immune activation pathways affect the progression of cardiovascular diseases and the repair/regeneration mechanisms of underlying diseased tissues"—Provided by publisher.
Identifiers: LCCN 2021052182 (print) | LCCN 2021052183 (ebook) |
  ISBN 9780367459079 (hardback) | ISBN 9781032249247 (paperback) |
  ISBN 9781003280767 (ebook)
Subjects: LCSH: Cardiovascular system—Diseases—United States. | Inflammation. | Immunology.
Classification: LCC RC672 .I46 2022 (print) | LCC RC672 (ebook) |
  DDC 362.1961—dc23/eng/20211129
LC record available at https://lccn.loc.gov/2021052182
LC ebook record available at https://lccn.loc.gov/2021052183

ISBN: 978-0-367-45907-9 (hbk)
ISBN: 978-1-032-24924-7 (pbk)
ISBN: 978-1-003-28076-7 (ebk)

DOI: 10.1201/b22824

Typeset in Times New Roman
by Apex CoVantage, LLC

Contents

v

Chapter 9 Immune Responses Regulated by Exosomal Mechanisms in
Cardiovascular Disease

*Brooke Lee, Ioannis D. Kyriazis, Ruturaj Patil, Syed
Baseeruddin Alvi, Amit Kumar Rai, Mahmood Khan,
and Venkata Naga Srikanth Garikipati*

Chapter 10 Ion Channels in Immune Cells: Physiological and
Pathophysiological Roles

*Devasena Ponnalagu, Shridhar Sanghvi, Shyam S. Bansal,
and Harpreet Singh*

Editor Biography

Shyam S. Bansal is a cardiovascular immunologist with expertise in the immune-inflammatory pathways of myocardial infarction and heart failure. His research endeavors focus on the elucidation of innate (macrophages and dendritic cells) and adaptive (T-cells) immune responses during chronic heart failure (HF) and the roles of these immune cells in mediating pathological left-ventricular remodeling. He is particularly interested in deciphering the role of T-cell subsets and the time-dependent phenotypic changes that these cells undergo during chronic HF. He is also interested in identifying and developing novel therapeutic strategies to reverse pathological changes in the immune cells for their bench-to-bed transition. Shyam S. Bansal is an assistant professor in the Department of Physiology and Cell Biology at The Ohio State University, Columbus. He received a PhD from the Department of Pharmacology & Toxicology at the University of Louisville, Kentucky, in 2011. Bansal's first postdoctoral training was in the Department of Nanotechnology at the Methodist Hospital Research Institute, Houston, TX (09/2011–09/2012), followed by extensive postdoctoral training (09/2012–07/2018) studying the roles of helper T-cells and regulatory T-cells in mediating pathological left-ventricular remodeling and ischemic heart failure.

Contributors

Syed Baseeruddin Alvi, PhD
Departments of Emergency Medicine
  and Physiology and Cell Biology
The Dorothy M. Davis Heart & Lung
  Research Institute
The Ohio State University Wexner
  Medical Center
Columbus, OH

Shyam S. Bansal, PhD
Department of Physiology and
  Cell Biology
The Dorothy M. Davis Heart & Lung
  Research Institute and Division of
  Cardiovascular Medicine
Department of Internal Medicine
The Ohio State University Wexner
  Medical Center
Columbus, OH

Daniela Carnevale, PhD
Department of Angiocardioneurology
  and Translational Medicine
IRCCS Neuromed
Pozzilli, Italy
Department of Molecular Medicine
Sapienza University of Rome
Rome, Italy

Lorenzo Carnevale, PhD
Department of Angiocardioneurology
  and Translational Medicine
IRCCS Neuromed
Pozzilli, Italy

Nikolaos G. Frangogiannis, MD
The Wilf Family Cardiovascular
  Research Institute
Department of Medicine (Cardiology)
Albert Einstein College of Medicine
Bronx, NY

**Venkata Naga Srikanth Garikipati,
MSc, PhD**
Department of Emergency Medicine
The Dorothy M. Davis Heart & Lung
  Research Institute
The Ohio State University Wexner
  Medical Center
Columbus, OH

Sahil Gupta, BS
Department of Physiology and Cell
  Biology
The Dorothy M. Davis Heart & Lung
  Research Institute
The Ohio State University Wexner
  Medical Center
Columbus, OH

Claudio Humeres, PhD
The Wilf Family Cardiovascular
  Research Institute
Department of Medicine (Cardiology)
Albert Einstein College of Medicine
Bronx, NY

Mahmood Khan, PhD
Departments of Emergency Medicine
  and Physiology and Cell Biology
The Dorothy M. Davis Heart & Lung
  Research Institute
The Ohio State University Wexner
  Medical Center
Columbus, OH

Benjamin J. Kopecky, MD, PhD
Cardiovascular Division,
John T. Milliken Department of
  Internal Medicine
Washington University
St. Louis, MO

Vinay Kumar, PhD
Department of Physiology and Cell
  Biology
The Dorothy M. Davis Heart & Lung
  Research Institute
The Ohio State University Wexner
  Medical Center
Columbus, OH

Ioannis D. Kyriazis, PhD
Laboratory of Animal Physiology
Department of Biochemistry and
  Biotechnology
University of Thessaly
Larissa, Greece

Hind Lal, PhD
Division of Cardiovascular Disease
University of Alabama at Birmingham
Birmingham, AL

Kory J. Lavine, MD, PhD
Cardiovascular Division,
John T. Milliken Department of
  Internal Medicine
Washington University
St. Louis, MO

Brooke Lee, BS
Department of Emergency Medicine
The Dorothy M. Davis Heart & Lung
  Research Institute
The Ohio State University Wexner
  Medical Center
Columbus, OH

Giuseppe Lembo, PhD
Department of Angiocardioneurology
  and Translational Medicine
IRCCS Neuromed
Pozzilli, Italy
Department of Molecular Medicine
Sapienza University of Rome
Rome, Italy

Jacob T. Menzer, BS
Lewis Katz School of Medicine
Temple University
Philadelphia, PA

Sadia Mohsin, PhD
Independence Blue Cross
  Cardiovascular Research Center and
Department of Pharmacology
Lewis Katz School of Medicine
Temple University
Philadelphia, PA

Ruturaj Patil, MS
Rutgers Biomedical and Health Sciences
Rutgers University
Piscataway, NJ

Marialuisa Perrotta, PhD
Department of Molecular Medicine
Sapienza University of Rome
Rome, Italy

Devasena Ponnalagu, PhD
Department of Physiology and Cell Biology
The Dorothy M. Davis Heart & Lung
  Research Institute
The Ohio State University Wexner
  Medical Center
Columbus, OH

Stelios Psarras, PhD
Center of Basic Research, Biomedical
  Foundation of the Academy of
  Athens (BRFAA)
Athens, Greece

Amit Kumar Rai, PhD
Department of Emergency Medicine
The Dorothy M. Davis Heart & Lung
  Research Institute
The Ohio State University Wexner
  Medical Center
Columbus, OH

Rachel Rosenzweig, BS
Department of Physiology and Cell Biology
The Dorothy M. Davis Heart & Lung
  Research Institute
The Ohio State University Wexner
  Medical Center
Columbus, OH

Shridhar Sanghvi, PhD
Department of Physiology and Cell
  Biology
The Dorothy M. Davis Heart & Lung
  Research Institute
The Ohio State University Wexner
  Medical Center
Department of Molecular, Cellular and
  Developmental Biology
The Ohio State University
Columbus, OH

Danish Sayed, MBBS, PhD
Rutgers New Jersey Medical School
Rutgers University
Newark, NJ

Anand Prakash Singh, PhD
Division of Cardiovascular Disease,
  UAB
The University of Alabama at
  Birmingham
Birmingham, AL

Harpreet Singh, PhD
Department of Physiology and Cell
  Biology

The Dorothy M. Davis Heart & Lung
  Research Institute
The Ohio State University Wexner
  Medical Center and
Department of Molecular, Cellular and
  Developmental Biology
The Ohio State University
Columbus, OH

Sultan Tousif, PhD
Division of Cardiovascular Disease,
  UAB
The University of Alabama at
  Birmingham
Birmingham, AL

Prachi Umbarkar, PhD
Division of Cardiovascular Disease,
  UAB
The University of Alabama at
  Birmingham
Birmingham, AL

Marcus J. Wagner, PhD
Independence Blue Cross
  Cardiovascular Research Center
Lewis Katz School of Medicine
Temple University
Philadelphia, PA

Georgina Xanthou, PhD
Center of Basic Research, Biomedical
  Foundation of the Academy of
  Athens (BRFAA)
Athens, Greece

Introduction

Shyam S. Bansal

Inflammation is a vital factor in the initiation and progression of cardiovascular diseases (CVDs). Preclinical and clinical studies in the last two decades have identified several key inflammatory proteins that are significantly increased during CVDs and can predict future adverse cardiovascular events. Despite this understanding, very few therapies targeting inflammatory pathways have transitioned to the clinic. This is partly due to the fact that circulating inflammatory mediators do not provide any indication as to the source tissue or the cell types involved. For instance, C-reactive protein and serum amyloid-A are clinically recognized systemic biomarkers of acute cardiac injury. However, both of these proteins are produced by the liver remotely from the disease site and do not reflect underlying cellular and molecular processes at the site of injury. Another limitation of circulating factors is that they do not distinguish between the physiological activation pathways that are essential for healing and those that are pathological and could be targeted for therapeutic immune modulation. This is also evident from the fact that clinical trials aimed at antagonizing inflammatory cytokines failed to show clinical benefits and, paradoxically, enhanced morbidity and mortality. These findings underscored the importance of identifying cellular changes locally at the tissue level. In this regard, innate and adaptive immune cells, tissue-resident fibroblasts, and endothelial cells have garnered significant attention as they interdependently regulate and mediate wound healing, scar formation, and neovascularization to regain tissue homeostasis and function.

Cellular and vascular injury results in the release of intracellular damage-associated molecular patterns (DAMPs), cytokines, and chemokines, either as soluble molecules or entrapped as exosomal cargo. This triggers platelet activation and remodeling of the extracellular matrix to mediate leukocyte transmigration into the injured site. Innate immune cells such as neutrophils, monocytes/macrophages, and dendritic cells are the early responders to these injurious stimuli and aid in the clearance of dead and apoptotic cells by phagocytosing their cellular content. Neutrophilic degranulation and the production of proteases, cytokines, chemokines, and reactive oxygen species activate endothelial cells in a positive feedback loop to promote the expression of adhesion molecules, while loosening intercellular junctions to further aid immune cell transmigration into the tissues. Processing of antigenic proteins by the antigen-presenting cells and their presentation subsequently activate the adaptive immune cells such as B-cells and helper and cytotoxic T-cells. For clinically translatable immune-modulation therapies, it is critical to study all of these cell types to create their detailed phenotypic landscapes as they coexist during homeostasis and pathogenesis. Importantly, temporal changes in immune cell phenotypes need to be ascertained in detail to identify the precise window for

DOI: 10.1201/b22824-1

therapeutic immunomodulation that can be personalized according to disease severity and patient characteristics.

In this book, we highlight the roles of: (1) innate and adaptive immune activation mechanisms, neural control that regulates their release from the storage sites, and the role of ionic fluxes in regulating their activation mechanisms; (2) fibroblastic and myofibroblastic differentiation pathways; (3) glucocorticoid and checkpoint signaling in the development and pathogenesis of CVDs; (4) inflammatory pathways in regulating regeneration by the mesenchymal and induced pluripotent stem cells; and (5) exosomes as communication vehicles to activate immune cells and as potential therapeutics in CVDs. All of these research avenues have gained significant attention in the last two decades with the appreciation that targeting of these cells; pathways, and differentiation mechanisms can provide significant clinical benefits and has the potential to either blunt disease progression or, in some cases, reverse their pathogenesis.

1 Innate Immune System in Cardiovascular Diseases

Benjamin J. Kopecky and Kory J. Lavine

CONTENTS

INTRODUCTION TO INFLAMMATION IN CARDIOVASCULAR DISEASE

The immune system has been implicated in many cardiac disease pathologies, ranging from heart failure to coronary artery disease to myocarditis. In these disease states, markers of systemic inflammation are elevated and are associated with adverse outcomes. However, the cellular sources, mechanisms of activation, and temporal implications of the inflammatory cascade are poorly understood. Early clinical trials broadly targeting inflammation yielded underwhelming results, dampening enthusiasm for further drug development. Recently, there has been renewed interest in the field fueled by new studies identifying surprising heterogeneity within the innate immune cell repertoire. As such, we now understand that diverse populations of innate immune cells reside within the healthy as well as the diseased heart, each with unique origins, dynamics, functions, and potential therapeutic implications.

DOI: 10.1201/b22824-2

There are 12 times as many immune cells in the heart compared to skeletal muscle [1]. The immune response is divided into (1) the innate and (2) the humoral/adaptive responses. The innate immune system responds to molecular patterns found in pathogens (pathogen-associated molecular patterns, PAMPs) and to host proteins released following tissue injury (danger-associated molecular patterns, DAMPs). Following activation, innate immune cells express a diverse array of chemokines, cytokines, growth factors, lipid mediators, and oxidative products, with wide-ranging effects on tissue repair, inflammation, and adaptive immunity. During steady state, innate immunity restricts maladaptive activation of the adaptive immune system, but during disease, it activates and targets the adaptive response to the insult. In this chapter, we will focus on the role of the innate immune response and implications for health and cardiovascular disease.

INNATE IMMUNE CELL HETEROGENEITY

The innate immune system has a myriad of cells that can be distinguished by their ontological origin. Hematopoietic stem cells differentiate into common myeloid or lymphoid progenitors. Many innate immune cells originate from the common myeloid progenitor, which subsequently differentiates into the granulocytes (basophils, neutrophils, eosinophils, mast cells), monocytes, and dendritic cell precursors.

During steady-state conditions, granulocytes in the heart are rare. However, following injury, eosinophils, basophils, and mast cells infiltrate the heart. Following myocardial infarction, eosinophils are recruited to the heart in both clinical and experimental models [2, 3]. Genetic depletion of eosinophils in murine models resulted in a reduction of CD206 reparative macrophages (possibly through interleukin (IL)-4 signaling) and subsequent adverse remodeling [2, 3], implicating a role for eosinophils conferring protection following myocardial infarction. Opposingly, eosinophils are also associated with heart failure [3]. In a cohort of patients with symptomatic heart failure, Heat2, a long, noncoding RNA, was significantly upregulated [4]. Heat2 is expressed in both eosinophils and basophils and modulates the proliferation, adhesion, invasion, and transmigration of eosinophils and basophils into the heart in the setting of heart failure [4]. Mast cells, another granulocyte, release cytokines (such as tumor necrosis factor (TNF)) that promote myocardial fibrosis and lead to adverse cardiac remodeling after myocardial infarction [5–8]. Genetic depletion of mast cells or mast cell stabilization showed improved outcomes after myocardial injury [9]. Last, neutrophils respond to pro-inflammatory cytokines and chemokines and are recruited to the heart following injury. Heart-resident macrophages can promote recruitment of neutrophils [6]. In summary, the granulocytes are early innate immune response elements that play important roles in the pathogenesis of disease after cardiac injury. They play independent roles as well as integrative roles with other innate immune cells: the monocytes, macrophages, and dendritic cells. We will focus on these three cell populations for the remainder of the chapter.

MONOCYTES

Monocytes are produced in the bone marrow from hematopoietic precursors, most proximally from the common myeloid progenitor [10]. In mice, monocytes can be distinguished on the basis of their expression of Ly6C. Classical monocytes are iden-tified as Ly6c[high] CCR2[+] CX3CR1[low] CD62L[high] cells [10], while non-classical mono-cytes are defined as Ly6c[low] CCR2[−] CX3CR1[high] CD62L[low] cells [11, 12]. Classical (Ly6C[high]) monocytes can differentiate into macrophages or non-classical monocytes via Nr4a1 [13, 14]. In humans, classical monocytes are identified as CD14[+]CD16[−] cells, and nonclassical monocytes are defined as CD16[+]CD14[dim] cells [15]. Humans also contain intermediate monocytes (CD14[+]CD16[+]) that harbor functional and phe-notypic characteristics of both classical and non-classical monocyte populations. In steady state, mouse monocytes have a life span of 1–2 days, whereas human classical monocytes live for about 3 days [16].

During an inflammatory response, classical monocytes increase in abundance due to expanded myelopoiesis in the bone marrow and spleen through IL-1 signal-ing [17, 18]. Monocytes extravasate into the bloodstream through a C-C chemokine receptor 2 (CCR2) dependent mechanism [19]. Blood monocytes infiltrate into the heart and differentiate into macrophages or dendritic cell subtypes on the basis of instructive cues derived from the local microenvironment. The role of non-classical monocytes in response to inflammation is poorly understood. However, they are thought to act as intravascular macrophages, patrolling the vascular endo-thelium to maintain vascular integrity, and may also activate cells with the vascu-lar wall [12].

MACROPHAGES

Specialized macrophages exist in all tissues (liver: Kupfer cells; lung: alveolar mac-rophages; brain: microglia; bone: osteoclasts; lymph nodes: histiocytes) and play essential roles in embryonic development, homeostasis, disease, and wound healing [20, 21]. Tissue-resident macrophages perform housekeeping and sentinel activities [22–24]. Macrophages engulf pathogens, foreign bodies, and cell debris through phagocytosis to function as antigen-presenting cells to the adaptive immune system, but they are equally important as moderators of the innate immune system through expression of cytokines and chemokines. Paradigm shifting studies have demon-strated that specialized tissue macrophages have a developmental origin that is dis-tinct from that of monocytes and monocyte-derived macrophages that accumulate in infected and injured tissues. In mice, these cells are identified on the basis of lineage tracing and defined cell surface markers [13, 25–29].

Tissue-resident macrophages represent 6–8% of the non-cardiomyocyte popula-tion in mice [30] and are the largest immune population in the healthy heart. The majority of tissue-resident macrophages are derived from primitive (extraembryonic) hematopoietic progenitors found in the yolk sac and fetal liver. Primitive hematopoi-esis is differentiated from definitive hematopoiesis (intraembryonic, bone marrow) on the basis of lineage potential. Definitive hematopoiesis is MYB (myeloblastosis) protein dependent, and only definitive hematopoietic progenitors can give rise to lymphocytes [20, 24, 26]. In mice, FLT3 is uniquely expressed on definitive hemato-poietic progenitors, providing a methodology to distinguish cells derived from these hematopoietic lineages [31]. At steady state, the heart contains distinct macrophage populations with discrete origins, including primitive yolk sac-derived macrophages, fetal monocyte-derived macrophages, and adult monocyte-derived macrophages, which each enter the heart at different developmental time points [20, 24, 32]. Primitive (FLT3$^-$) and definitive (FLT3$^+$) macrophages co-exist [24]. Primitive or yolk sac-derived macrophages display a CX3CR1^{high} CD11b^{low} phenotype, whereas definitive macrophages transition through monocyte intermediates, express FLT3 as they differentiate [24, 33], and display a CX3CR1^{int} CD11b^{high} phenotype.

The adult mouse heart contains three macrophage subsets with the following cell surface phenotypes: (1) TIMD4$^+$ LYVE1$^+$ CCR2$^-$ MHC-II^{low}, (2) TIMD4$^-$ LYVE1$^-$ CCR2$^-$ MHC-II^{high}, and (3) TIMD4$^-$ LYVE1$^-$ CCR2$^+$ MHC-II^{high}. At steady state, TIMD4$^+$ LYVE1$^+$ CCR2$^-$ MHC-II^{low} macrophages participate in tissue repair and angiogenesis, as they express growth factors and extracellular matrix components that stimulate coronary angiogenesis and cardiomyocyte proliferation [33–35]. TIMD4$^+$ LYVE1$^+$ CCR2$^-$ MHC-II^{low} and TIMD4$^-$ LYVE1$^-$ CCR2$^-$ MHC-II^{high} (CCR2$^-$) macrophages are long lived, are derived from embryonic origins (yolk sac and fetal liver), and are maintained independent of monocyte input through local proliferation [20, 36, 37]. TIMD4$^-$ LYVE1$^-$ CCR2$^+$ MHC-II^{high} (CCR2$^+$) macrophages are derived from blood monocytes through a CCR2-dependent mechanism. CCR2$^+$ macrophages are enriched in pro-inflammatory genes, specifically the NLRP3 pathway leading to IL-1β signaling [33]. In the setting of injury, CCR2$^+$ macrophages are activated by DAMPs, including mitochondrial DNA, to secrete neutrophil and monocyte chemokines (CXCL2, CXCL5, CCL2, CCL7) and pro-inflammatory cytokines (IL-1β, IL-6, TNF) and trigger myocardial inflammation [38, 39]. The human heart contains conserved populations of CCR2$^-$ and CCR2$^+$ macrophages with analogous developmental origins, dynamics, and functions [40] and conserved markers, including TIMD4, LYVE1, and CCR2.

DENDRITIC CELLS

Compared to macrophages, dendritic cells are a rare innate immune cell population in the heart [23, 24, 41, 42]. Macrophages and dendritic cells share some cell surface markers (i.e., CD11c, MHC-II) with both sets of markers dynamically changing during an evolving immune response. Dendritic cells are composed of four subsets and can be distinguished from cardiac macrophages on the basis of the transcription factor ZBTB46 [43, 44]. Dendritic cells are classified as conventional/classical DC type 1 (cDC1), conventional/classical DC type 2 (cDC2), plasmacytoid DC (pDC), and monocyte-derived dendritic cells (mDCs). The latter subset shares features of macrophages and dendritic cells [45–47]. cDC1s and cDC2s require FLT3L signaling for their development. Committed precursor dendritic cells (CD103$^+$ and CD11b$^+$) migrate from the bone marrow to peripheral tissue, where they complete their differentiation into either cDC1s or cDC2s. cDC1s are dependent on IRF8, ID2, and BatF3 transcriptional activity, whereas cDC2s are dependent on IRF4, RelB, RBP-J, and IRF2 transcriptional activity [11, 48]. Under steady-state conditions, the heart contains cDC1s (Clec9a$^+$ CD103$^+$ CD24$^+$ XCR1$^+$) and cDC2s (CD11b$^+$ CD172a$^+$). As opposed to conventional DCs, which complete development in peripheral tissues, pDCs complete development in the bone marrow and express CD11c, CCR9, CD317, B220, and Siglec-H [46, 49]. pDCs have lower expression of MHC-II than do cDCs

TABLE 1.1
Origin, Phenotypic Markers and Functions of Different Innate Immune Cells in Mice and Humans

Name	Monocytes			Macrophages			Dendritic Cells			
	Classical	Non-Classical	Int.	CCR2$^-$		CCR2$^+$	cDC1	cDC2	pDC	moDC
Origin	Blood monocytes		N/A	Extraembryonic progenitors		Blood monocytes	Progenitor in the bone marrow			Blood Monocytes
Mouse markers	CD11b$^+$ Ly6G$^-$ CD64^{int} Ly6c^{high} CCR2$^+$	CD11b$^+$ Ly6G$^-$ NK1.1$^-$ SiglecF$^-$ CD64$^-$ Ly6c^{low} MHCII^{low}	N/A	CD64$^+$ CCR2$^-$ MHCII^{low} LYVE1 TIMD4	CD64$^+$ CCR2$^-$ MHCII^{high}	CD64$^+$ CD11b$^+$ CCR2$^+$ MHCII^{high}	CD103$^+$ MHCII^{high} Clec9a$^+$ XCR1$^+$	CD11b$^+$ MHCII^{high} CD172a$^+$	B220$^+$ Ly6c$^+$ Siglec-H$^+$ CD317$^+$	CD11b$^+$ CD14$^+$ CD172a$^+$ CD206$^+$
Human markers	CD14$^+$ CD16$^-$	CD14^{dim} CD16$^+$	CD14^{++} CD16$^+$	Same as mouse			CD141$^+$ XCR1$^+$ Clec9a$^+$	CD1c$^+$ CD11b$^+$ CD172a$^+$	CD123$^+$ CD304$^+$ CD303$^+$	CD1a$^+$ CD14$^+$ CD172a$^+$ CD206$^+$
General function	Differentiates into macrophages or dendritic cells	Patrols endothelium	Unknown	Coronary development, angiogenesis, tissue repair, suppress inflammation		Orchestrates leukocyte recruitment	Presents to T-cells to modulate T-cell reactivity and tolerance		Produces cytokines including type I IFN	

and less capacity for antigen presentation. pDCs are able to produce strong cytokine responses and influence T-regulatory cell development. Dendritic cells generally suppress self-reactive CD4[+] T-cells through modulation of T-regulatory cells [50], participate in viral clearance [51], and modulate left-ventricular (LV) remodeling [49]. Cardiac dendritic cells are short lived and are replenished from blood monocytes, and bone marrow-derived progenitors [52, 53].

Monocytes, macrophages, and dendritic cells are not homogeneously distributed throughout the heart. For example, during development, embryonically derived macrophages are located adjacent to the coronary vasculature and fetal-derived monocytes are near endocardial trabeculae. In adults, the aortic valve is densely enriched in dendritic cells, whereas the atrioventricular node contains numerous macrophages [54, 55].

INNATE IMMUNE PATHOGENESIS OF HEART FAILURE

Heart failure syndrome is a prime example of how the immune system impacts disease pathogenesis and progression. Heart failure is a systemic syndrome with insults not only to the heart (local inflammation) but also to skeletal muscle, liver, nervous system, and gastrointestinal tract (systemic inflammation) [56]. Heart failure syndrome is a continuous inflammatory cycle affecting the heart and peripheral tissues, creating a feed-forward pro-inflammatory state resulting in neurohormonal activation, systemic inflammation, progressive cardiac dysfunction, and peripheral organ dysfunction [56]. Initial myocardial insults (i.e., coronary ischemia, myocarditis, chemotoxicity) result in a local inflammatory response and resultant myocardial dysfunction that perpetuates systemic inflammation resulting from reduced systemic perfusion, vascular congestion, and tissue edema [57]. Activated inflammatory cells engage the systemic nervous and renin-angiotensin-aldosterone systems [58] and promote additional cardiomyocyte cell death and adverse cardiac remodeling through β1-adrenergic signaling and α-adrenergic-mediated vasoconstriction [59]. Sympathetic activation further stimulates innate immune cell recruitment and inflammatory signaling through β3-adrenergic mobilization of bone marrow monocytes [60]. Specifically, pro-inflammatory TNF, IL-1β, and IL-6 are secreted and are known to have negative inotropic effects on cardiomyocytes, leading to added myocardial dysfunction [61].

Confirming this local and systemic pro-inflammatory cycle in heart failure, patients with chronic heart failure had significant elevation of cytokines and chemokines, including TNF, IL-1β, IL-6, ST2, galectin-3, pentraxin-3, and IL-2 [62–66]. These inflammatory mediators are associated with worse heart failure outcomes [63, 64, 67]. They also illustrate a connection with the innate immune system and a pathway toward therapeutic intervention. Pentraxin-3 is produced by monocytes, macrophages, and dendritic cells in response to Toll-like receptor (TLR) engagement, and increased levels after myocardial infarction are associated with increased mortality [68]. Deletion of galectin-3 attenuates cardiac injury in a murine hypertension injury model [69] and is an FDA-approved biomarker for myocardial fibrosis and heart failure mortality [70]. In the Vesnarinon trial (VEST), TNF and IL-6 levels were elevated in heart failure and were predictive of increased mortality [63]. Medical treatment of heart failure reduced TNF and IL-6 levels [71].

While the preceding observations point to a pathological role of innate immunity and suggest that targeting of inflammatory pathways may be beneficial, early trials have yielded disappointing results. Immunomodulation with nonselective therapies such as prednisone [72] and methotrexate [73] have revealed modest benefit. TNF blockade (RENAISSANCE, RECOVER, RENEWAL, ATTACH) [74, 75] resulted in worse or unimproved clinical outcomes. It is unclear why this anti-inflammatory intervention had limited benefit given overwhelming evidence of the pathological role of inflammation in cardiovascular disease. It is plausible that targeting of individual cytokines (rather than their cellular source) is not sufficient or that treatment at later stages of disease has limited therapeutic potential. Future studies are underway to tease out these details and identify new targets for immunomodulatory therapy. In the meantime, it is prudent to gain a deeper understanding of the complexities among the cell types and the signaling pathways associated with the innate immune activation and to further identify the specific functions of cytokines and chemokines involved in cardiovascular disease.

INNATE IMMUNE RESPONSE TO INJURY

DAMPs/PAMPs

The cardiac innate immune cascade is initiated by myocardial injury. Myocardial injury and cell death are present across all forms of heart disease, including ischemic cardiomyopathy, nonischemic cardiomyopathies, and myocarditis, or after exposure to chemotherapeutic agents [76]. Programmed cell death and cardiac injury result in the release of alarmins and DAMPs, including various intracellular proteins, cytokines, mitochondrial DNA, and HMGB1 that are recognized by pattern recognition receptors (PRRs) to generate a profound inflammatory response [34, 77–82].

PRRs

PRRs are expressed on most cardiac cells (cardiomyocytes, leukocytes, endothelial cells, and fibroblasts) and include TLRs, NOD-like receptors (NLRs), RIG-I-like receptors, pentraxins, and C-type lectin receptors (CLRs). There are ten distinct TLRs [83], five NLRs [84], and two pentraxins (CRP and amyloid P), as well as RIG-I-like receptors and CLRs, expressed in the human heart [85]. TLR4 is upregulated in human heart failure with deletion of TLR2 and TLR4, halting the adverse remodeling and progression of heart failure in murine models of myocardial infarction [77, 80]. Cardiac macrophages encode PRRs that recognize alarmins and DAMPs, resulting in activation, proliferation, and chemokine and cytokine production [42, 86]. Together, myocardial insults result in the release of DAMPS that are recognized by the innate immune cell. Given the diversity of monocytes, macrophages, and dendritic cells, the specific cell type and the timing of its activation define the role it may play in disease prevention or progression.

INNATE IMMUNE SYSTEM IN HEART FAILURE ETIOLOGIES

ATHEROSCLEROSIS

The innate immune system is implicated in coronary development as well as in the progression and stabilization of atherosclerosis [18, 87]. CCR2⁻ macrophages are essential mediators of coronary development [35], and they aid in remodeling and maturation of the coronary vasculature through insulin-like growth factors 1 and 2 [35]. On the other hand, macrophages (CCR2⁺ predominantly) are essential to vascular inflammation and the progression of atherosclerosis [88]. Atherosclerosis is characterized by low-grade inflammation marked by macrophage-derived cytokines (IL-1β, IL-6, TNF) [88]. The Canakinumab Anti-Inflammatory Thrombosis Outcomes Study (CANTOS) trial enrolled patients with high-risk coronary artery disease to receive IL-1β blockade, and the results showed a significant reduction in ischemic and cardiovascular events [89].

Macrophages in atherosclerotic plaques are predominantly derived from circulating monocytes [90]. In murine models, hypercholesterolemia promotes selective expansion of classical monocytes through CSF1- and IL-3-dependent extramedullary hematopoiesis [90]. In humans, classical CD14^high CD16^low monocytes are increased in hypercholesterolemia [91]. Subendothelial retention of low-density lipoprotein (LDL) and local production of CCL2, CCL20, and sphingosine-1-phosphate recruit monocytes to the site of arterial inflammation [92, 93]. Suppression of monocyte recruitment led to plaque regression [94]. Myeloid-specific depletion of ATP-binding cassette transporters (ABCA1 and ABCG1), which are important in the efflux of LDL to high-density lipoprotein (HDL), led to increased atherosclerosis and monocytosis [95].

Upon infiltrating the vessel wall, monocytes differentiate into monocyte-derived macrophages and, after uptake of LDL, become foam cells [96]. Foam cells take on an inflammatory phenotype, whereas macrophages in a stable atherosclerotic plaque have a more anti-inflammatory phenotype, with high capacity for phagocytosis, but diminished capacity to handle cholesterol [97, 98]. Thus, macrophages participate in both lesion progression and lesion regression, potentially by reducing oxidative damage and necrotic core formation through negative regulation of the inflammasome [99].

Plasmacytoid dendritic cells (pDCs) have been implicated in atherosclerosis through cross talk with the adaptive immune system, specifically CD4⁺ T-cells [100, 101]. Activated CD4⁺ T-cells and Th17 cells produce cytokines and chemokines that recruit and polarize macrophages to an inflammatory phenotype [87, 92]. The innate immune cell composition of human atherosclerosis is less well defined and may differ from that of murine models. Advanced atherosclerotic plaques have higher percentages of moDCs and pDCs [102, 103]. The number of pDCs correlates with plaque instability [104].

HYPERTENSION

Atherosclerosis and hypertension are risk factors for myocardial infarction and heart failure. During hypertensive challenges, resident macrophage populations increase in number [24] and are joined by an influx of monocytes and monocyte-derived macrophages. In pressure overload models using trans-aortic constriction or angiotensin II infusion, monocyte-derived macrophages represent more than half of cardiac immune cells within the first week of injury. HMGB1 and ATP (DAMPs) are detected by TLR2 and TLR4 found on myeloid cells [105]. Treatment with TLR4 antagonist reduces hypertrophic changes in response to pressure overload, in part due to reduced monocyte infiltration [106, 107]. As the mouse transitions to chronic heart failure, additional monocyte-derived macrophages accumulate. Inhibition of CCR2+ signaling results in reduced monocyte-derived macrophage abundance and preserved systolic function [108].

MYOCARDIAL ISCHEMIA

Following myocardial infarction, macrophages are activated by mediators released from injured and dead cardiomyocytes, including alarmins, DAMPs, nucleic acids, and lipids [109]. Tissue-resident CCR2+ macrophages (~10–15% of the total resident macrophage population) are activated by products released by ferroptotic cardiomyocytes [110], and they signal through MYD88 (an adapter protein of TLR) to orchestrate monocyte and neutrophil recruitment through the expression of chemokines CXCL2, CXCL5, CCL2, and CCL7 and cytokines IL-1β, IL-6, and TNF [38, 39]. Mitochondrial and nuclear DNA are DAMPs recognized by TLR9 and stimulator of interferon genes (STING; expressed on resident macrophages) [38] and have been implicated in macrophage activation and heart failure [111, 112]. Myeloid-derived S100A8 and S100A9 also act as DAMPs following their release from dying immune cells and bind to receptors for advanced glycation endproducts (RAGE), resulting in NF-κβ signaling and amplification of a feed-forward loop driven by ongoing cytokine and DAMP release. These mediators contribute to accelerated myelopoiesis and mobilization of myeloid cells from hematopoietic tissues [113]. Recent studies have shown the ability of CCR2− macrophages to interrupt this feed-forward loop [114].

In some circumstances, CCR2− macrophages expand by local proliferation and suppress monocyte and neutrophil infiltration [34, 36, 39]. Depletion of CCR2− macrophages results in impaired tissue remodeling due to excessive inflammation and an inability to clear tissue debris, including necrotic cardiomyocytes [115]. When unable to sufficiently expand, tissue-resident macrophages (TIMD4− MHC-IIhi CCR2− and TIMD4+ MHC-IIlow CCR2−) are rapidly lost [42] and are largely replaced by infiltrating CCR2+ monocytes and CCR2+ monocyte-derived macrophages (TIMD4−). Genes associated with mature resident macrophages such as Lyve1, Timd4, Folr2, and Retnla are downregulated, but monocyte genes such as Spp1 and Ms4a7 were increased [36]. Early inflammatory responses to myocardial infarction involve the recruitment of neutrophils and inflammatory monocytes [116].

Stimulation of the sympathetic nervous system triggers the release of adrenaline and noradrenaline, which results in the maturation and emigration of myeloid cells, favors the production of CCR2+ precursors [34, 113, 117], and mobilizes monocytes to the spleen [118]. Classical monocytes are rapidly recruited to the infarct (~50% from a splenic reservoir) via MCP-1 [17, 119, 120]. Splenectomy post-myocardial infarction is protective and limits myocardial inflammation [121]. During this time, there are high levels of inflammatory cytokines such as TNF-α, IL-1β, and IL-6 [122] and proteases [123]. Blockade of monocyte recruitment improves outcomes in murine models of myocardial infarction [124, 125]. CCL2 and CCL7 deficiency inhibits monocyte recruitment post-myocardial infarction and attenuates adverse remodeling [119]. Loss of Nr4a1 (responsible for converting classical to non-classical monocytes) increases classical monocyte and pro-inflammatory macrophage abundance and results in worsening heart function [122]. It is believed that CCR2$^+$ macrophages, monocytes, and neutrophils impact collateral damage to the myocardium and accelerate adverse remodeling [110]. While there is a rapid influx of leukocytes, their persistence within the infarct is short lived (average is 20 hours). Most rapidly infiltrating innate immune cells undergo cell death, with a smaller number of cells exiting the heart and accumulating in the liver, lymph nodes, or spleen [116].

The local environment within the infarcted heart is dynamic. While initially inflammatory, there is a transition to a reparative milieu within 1 week following myocardial infarction [123]. This transition is marked by a phenotypic shift in macrophages that release IL-10, VEGF, TGF-β, and other mediators involved in extracellular matrix remodeling [123, 126]. Macrophages are implicated in the regeneration of vascular beds such that the depletion of macrophages following cardiac injury resulted in a reduction of VEGF-A and capillary density [127]. Based on recent single-cell RNA sequencing data [36, 39], at least seven distinct macrophage and three distinct dendritic cell subtypes exist within the myocardium after myocardial infarction. It is posited that monocyte fate is instructed by interactions with the local microenvironment [34]. Monocyte and macrophage determination may represent a target for therapy to reduce inflammatory macrophages and subsequent heart failure. Observational studies have shown that dendritic cell abundance correlates with cardiac rupture after myocardial infarction [128]. Similar to the heterogeneity evidenced in macrophages, dendritic cell subtypes may also have differing effects on cardiac remodeling and progression to heart failure after myocardial infarction [36]. pDCs and cDCs increase in response to myocardial ischemia. It has been postulated that, after endothelial damage, endothelial cells and macrophages produce GM-CSF, resulting in the maturation of cDC2s [49]. Genetic depletion of DCs reduces postischemic injury [49]. The lack of specific genetic models has impaired the ability to investigate DC subtypes. Future studies will identify relevant cell types and their respective functions.

MYOCARDITIS

Myocarditis originates from infectious (pathogens) or noninfectious (autoinflammatory) mechanisms. Infectious myocarditis may be caused by viruses, bacteria, parasites, or fungi [129]. In viral myocarditis, the hematological spread of viral particles results in direct infection of cardiomyocytes, cardiac fibroblasts, and/or endothelial cells, initiating cell damage and host immune responses. During the acute phase, tissue-resident innate immune cells are activated by various PAMPs and DAMPs, resulting in the production of interferons and pro-inflammatory cytokines (IL-12, IL-1β, TNF) with the resultant recruitment of neutrophils, monocytes, and dendritic cells. Not all PRRs are equivalent. TLR3-deficient mice have increased mortality, whereas TLR4-deficient mice have reduced inflammation [130]. In viral myocarditis models, there is a rapid loss of tissue-resident macrophages and a resulting influx of circulating monocytes [51, 131].

In the subacute phase, the combined innate and adaptive immune system effectively eliminates infected and dead cells but also contributes to myocardial damage. Removal of macrophages early in viral myocarditis resulted in early mortality, while removal in the chronic phase led to improved cardiac function and decreased adverse remodeling [132]. Deletion of CX3CL1 or its receptor (CX3CR1) worsens acute viral myocarditis [133]. Interference with monocyte recruitment by inhibiting CCL2 or CCL3 signaling reduced cardiac injury [134]. These data suggest that macrophages and monocytes may have distinct and temporally restricted functions in viral myocarditis. Consistent with this, tissue-resident macrophages secrete anti-inflammatory TGF-β and IL-10, promoting the resolution of inflammation and wound healing [135], an event essential to preventing autoimmune responses that perpetuate cardiac dysfunction. In experimental models of autoinflammatory myocarditis, the activation of monocytes and macrophages appears to promote chronic heart failure. Targeting of monocytes through blockade of the CCR2/CCL2 axis improves outcomes through a reduction of monocyte infiltration and differentiation into dendritic cells and monocyte-derived macrophages [131, 136].

Similarly, the depletion of dendritic cells leads to impaired cardiac dysfunction during viral myocarditis [51]. Dendritic cells have the strongest connection to the adaptive immune system in myocarditis. cDC1s (which are dependent on BATF3 for maturation) are implicated in CD8$^+$ T-cell activation. BATF3-deficient mice have reduced cDC1 populations, reduced antiviral CD8$^+$ T-cell response, and more severe viral myocarditis [51]. After viral convalescence, activated T-cells may drive autoinflammatory responses and ongoing myocarditis. Continued release of cytokines and DAMPs from dendritic cells may contribute to the generation of autoreactive CD4$^+$ T-cells [137]. Dendritic cells present antigen to T-cells, an activity necessary for inflammation and cardiac pathology [138]. However, dendritic cells can also render autoreactive T-cells anergic by converting naïve T-cells into regulatory T-cells [139, 140]. This represents an important function that could be harnessed to limit autoreactive responses. These observations suggest that cDC1s may play a bridging role in both viral and autoinflammatory myocarditis [52].

ARRHYTHMIAS

Inflammation is associated with cardiac arrhythmias. After myocardial infarction, electrical remodeling occurs, specifically in the infarct border zone where macrophages are observed. Macrophages may act as a substrate for ventricular arrhythmias by furthering fibrosis and contributing to conduction blocks [141]. Macrophages promote sympathetic innervation via nerve growth factor, resulting in sympathetic overactivity and ventricular arrhythmias. Substance P released by sympathetic fibers binds to neurokinin-1 receptors on macrophages to produce angiotensin II and norepinephrine [142]. Additionally, IL-1β, IL-6, and TNF-α produced in macrophages activate the sympathetic nervous system [141] and the mobilization of monocytes. The parasympathetic nervous system serves as a negative regulator of the pro-inflammatory innate response [60].

Outside of scar formation and hyperinnervation, macrophages secrete pro-inflammatory factors that directly affect myocardial electrophysiology, Cx43 expression, intracellular calcium, and potassium currents [143]. IL-1β is significantly elevated in patients with ventricular arrhythmias, and targeting of IL-1β reduced spontaneous ventricular arrhythmias [144, 145]. TNF-α is associated with ventricular arrhythmias, and experimental overexpression of TNF-α led to increased arrhythmias [146, 147]. Elevated IL-6 levels can lead to prolonged QT intervals and subsequent ventricular arrhythmias. Tocilizumab (IL-6 receptor antibody) has anti-arrhythmic properties [148]. Myocardial injury activates macrophages to secrete MMP-9 [141], which is linked to ventricular arrhythmias and sudden cardiac death by degrading Cx43 and leading to improper cell-cell electrical coupling [149].

Last, cardiac macrophages can directly induce changes in electrophysiology through the formation of gap junctions with cardiomyocytes [55]. Abundant populations of macrophages exist within both murine and human atrioventricular (AV) nodes. Within the node, tissue-resident macrophages directly interact with cardiomyocytes via gap junctions [20, 55]. Removal of tissue-resident macrophages impairs AV conduction and leads to heart block [55]. Intriguingly, individual macrophage populations can differentially influence cardiomyocyte action potential duration, a key electrophysiological property that influences arrhythmogenesis [141, 150].

CARDIO-ONCOLOGY

There remains limited knowledge on the role of macrophages in chemotherapy and radiation-induced heart disease. Macrophage production of IL-10 confers protection from doxorubicin cardiotoxicity [151]. Doxorubicin appears to increase HMGB1, and the pharmacologic inhibition of HMGB1 was protective [152]. TLRs sense damage by anthracyclines, and deletion of TLR2 partially preserved cardiac function in the setting of doxorubicin therapy [153]. Targeting of TLRs and downstream signaling reduced inflammatory activity after anthracycline challenge [154, 155]. There is increasing recognition that newer immunotherapies have cardiotoxicity. Monoclonal antibodies against immune checkpoint inhibitors can produce immune-related adverse events, including myocarditis and pericarditis [156]. Investigations are ongoing to evaluate the role of the innate immune system in checkpoint inhibitor myocarditis and related pathologies.

HEART TRANSPLANT

Heart transplant immunology is complex and beyond the scope of this chapter, but it is another example of innate and adaptive immunity playing complex and interconnected roles [157, 158]. Donor organs and the recipient immune systems must co-exist for the allograft to survive. Heart transplants undergo several insults, including ischemia-reperfusion injury and alloreactive responses. Ischemia-reperfusion injury and alloreactive T-cells each produces myocardial injury and DAMP release. DAMPs may signal through PRRs on donor and/or recipient innate immune cells [159]. Genetic depletion of TLR signaling results in improved allograft survival [160]. A host of DAMPs have all been implicated in heart transplant [157]. Monocyte, macrophage, and dendritic cell homeostasis is uniquely impacted by immunosuppression [161]. In the setting of experimental transplant tolerance, unique sets of tolerogenic monocytes and dendritic cells are generated with intriguing therapeutic potential [162–164].

CONCLUSION AND FUTURE DIRECTIONS

The innate immune system shapes the heart from embryogenesis to end-stage disease. Monocytes, macrophages, and dendritic cells are a heterogeneous array of gatekeepers between health and disease. Within each arm of the innate response, individual cells, identified by their origin, cell surface marker, and environmental niche, play unique roles in both health and disease. Only within the past decade have we begun to elucidate these heterogeneous populations, and future studies must further dissect their respective roles in the pathogenesis of disease.

The innate immune system interacts within itself as well as with the adaptive immune system. Innate immune cells can directly present antigen to T-cells [24] or secrete chemokines and cytokines that affect T-cell dynamics [39, 165]. At steady state, they patrol for disease and keep the adaptive immune system at bay. During disease, they rapidly neutralize the offending disease (virus, ischemia, etc.) and recruit the adaptive immune system to further defend against tissue harm. Explorations of T-cells and other adaptive immune response elements are described separately in this book.

BIBLIOGRAPHY

1. Ramos, G.C., et al., *Myocardial aging as a T-cell-mediated phenomenon.* Proc Natl Acad Sci U S A, 2017. **114**(12): p. E2420–E2429.
2. Toor, I.S., et al., *Eosinophil deficiency promotes aberrant repair and adverse remodeling following acute myocardial infarction.* JACC Basic Transl Sci, 2020. **5**(7): p. 665–681.
3. Lavine, K.J., *Eosinophils confer protection following myocardial infarction.* JACC Basic Transl Sci, 2020. **5**(7): p. 682–684.
4. Boeckel, J.N., et al., *Identification and regulation of the long non-coding RNA Heat2 in heart failure.* J Mol Cell Cardiol, 2019. **126**: p. 13–22.
5. Zhang, W., et al., *The development of myocardial fibrosis in transgenic mice with targeted overexpression of tumor necrosis factor requires mast cell-fibroblast interactions.* Circulation, 2011. **124**(19): p. 2106–2116.
6. Adamo, L., et al., *Reappraising the role of inflammation in heart failure.* Nat Rev Cardiol, 2020. **17**(5): p. 269–285.
7. Levick, S.P., et al., *Cardiac mast cells: the centrepiece in adverse myocardial remodelling.* Cardiovasc Res, 2011. **89**(1): p. 12–19.
8. Janicki, J.S., G.L. Brower, and S.P. Levick, *The emerging prominence of the cardiac mast cell as a potent mediator of adverse myocardial remodeling.* Methods Mol Biol, 2015. **1220**: p. 121–139.
9. Hara, M., et al., *Evidence for a role of mast cells in the evolution to congestive heart failure.* J Exp Med, 2002. **195**(3): p. 375–381.
10. Nahrendorf, M. and F.K. Swirski, *Monocyte and macrophage heterogeneity in the heart.* Circ Res, 2013. **112**(12): p. 1624–1633.

11. Geissmann, F., et al., *Development of monocytes, macrophages, and dendritic cells.* Science, 2010. **327**(5966): p. 656–661.

12. Carlin, L.M., et al., *Nr4a1-dependent Ly6C(low) monocytes monitor endothelial cells and orchestrate their disposal.* Cell, 2013. **153**(2): p. 362–375.

13. Yona, S., et al., *Fate mapping reveals origins and dynamics of monocytes and tissue macrophages under homeostasis.* Immunity, 2013. **38**(1): p. 79–91.

14. Hanna, R.N., et al., *The transcription factor NR4A1 (Nur77) controls bone marrow differentiation and the survival of Ly6C- monocytes.* Nat Immunol, 2011. **12**(8): p. 778–785.

15. Ingersoll, M.A., et al., *Comparison of gene expression profiles between human and mouse monocyte subsets.* Blood, 2010. **115**(3): p. e10–19.

16. Van Furth, R., M.C. Diesselhoff-den Dulk, and H. Mattie, *Quantitative study on the production and kinetics of mononuclear phagocytes during an acute inflammatory reaction.* J Exp Med, 1973. **138**(6): p. 1314–1330.

17. Swirski, F.K., et al., *Identification of splenic reservoir monocytes and their deployment to inflammatory sites.* Science, 2009. **325**(5940): p. 612–616.

18. Swirski, F.K. and M. Nahrendorf, *Leukocyte behavior in atherosclerosis, myocardial infarction, and heart failure.* Science, 2013. **339**(6116): p. 161–166.

19. Tsou, C.L., et al., *Critical roles for CCR2 and MCP-3 in monocyte mobilization from bone marrow and recruitment to inflammatory sites.* J Clin Invest, 2007. **117**(4): p. 902–909.

20. Lavine, K.J., et al., *The macrophage in cardiac homeostasis and disease: JACC macrophage in CVD series (Part 4).* J Am Coll Cardiol, 2018. **72**(18): p. 2213–2230.

21. Wynn, T.A., A. Chawla, and J.W. Pollard, *Macrophage biology in development, homeostasis and disease.* Nature, 2013. **496**(7446): p. 445–455.

22. Pinto, A.R., J.W. Godwin, and N.A. Rosenthal, *Macrophages in cardiac homeostasis, injury responses and progenitor cell mobilisation.* Stem Cell Res, 2014. **13**(3 Pt B): p. 705–714.

23. Pinto, A.R., et al., *An abundant tissue macrophage population in the adult murine heart with a distinct alternatively-activated macrophage profile.* PLoS One, 2012. **7**(5): p. e36814.

24. Epelman, S., et al., *Embryonic and adult-derived resident cardiac macrophages are maintained through distinct mechanisms at steady state and during inflammation.* Immunity, 2014. **40**(1): p. 91–104.

25. Ginhoux, F., et al., *Fate mapping analysis reveals that adult microglia derive from primitive macrophages.* Science, 2010. **330**(6005): p. 841–845.

26. Schulz, C., et al., *A lineage of myeloid cells independent of Myb and hematopoietic stem cells.* Science, 2012. **336**(6077): p. 86–90.

27. Hashimoto, D., et al., *Tissue-resident macrophages self-maintain locally throughout adult life with minimal contribution from circulating monocytes.* Immunity, 2013. **38**(4): p. 792–804.

28. Jakubzick, C., et al., *Minimal differentiation of classical monocytes as they survey steady-state tissues and transport antigen to lymph nodes.* Immunity, 2013. **39**(3): p. 599–610.

29. Guilliams, M., et al., *Alveolar macrophages develop from fetal monocytes that differentiate into long-lived cells in the first week of life via GM-CSF.* J Exp Med, 2013. **210**(10): p. 1977–1992.

30. Pinto, A.R., et al., *Revisiting cardiac cellular composition.* Circ Res, 2016. **118**(3): p. 400–409.

31. Orkin, S.H. and L.I. Zon, *Hematopoiesis: an evolving paradigm for stem cell biology.* Cell, 2008. **132**(4): p. 631–644.

32. Epelman, S., K.J. Lavine, and G.J. Randolph, *Origin and functions of tissue macrophages.* Immunity, 2014. **41**(1): p. 21–35.

33. Lavine, K.J., et al., *Distinct macrophage lineages contribute to disparate patterns of cardiac recovery and remodeling in the neonatal and adult heart.* Proc Natl Acad Sci U S A, 2014. **111**(45): p. 16029–16034.

34. Rhee, A.J. and K.J. Lavine, *New approaches to target inflammation in heart failure: harnessing insights from studies of immune cell diversity.* Annu Rev Physiol, 2020. **82**: p. 1–20.

35. Leid, J., et al., *Primitive embryonic macrophages are required for coronary development and maturation.* Circ Res, 2016. **118**(10): p. 1498–1511.

36. Dick, S.A., et al., *Self-renewing resident cardiac macrophages limit adverse remodeling following myocardial infarction.* Nat Immunol, 2019. **20**(1): p. 29–39.

37. Chakarov, S., et al., *Two distinct interstitial macrophage populations coexist across tissues in specific subtissular niches.* Science, 2019. **363**(6432).

38. Li, W., et al., *Heart-resident CCR2(+) macrophages promote neutrophil extravasation through TLR9/MyD88/CXCL5 signaling.* JCI Insight, 2016. **1**(12).

39. Bajpai, G., et al., *Tissue resident CCR2- and CCR2+ cardiac macrophages differentially orchestrate monocyte recruitment and fate specification following myocardial injury.* Circ Res, 2019. **124**(2): p. 263–278.

40. Bajpai, G., et al., *The human heart contains distinct macrophage subsets with divergent origins and functions.* Nat Med, 2018. **24**(8): p. 1234–1245.

41. Nahrendorf, M. and F.K. Swirski, *Innate immune cells in ischaemic heart disease: does myocardial infarction beget myocardial infarction?* Eur Heart J, 2016. **37**(11): p. 868–872.

42. Heidt, T., et al., *Differential contribution of monocytes to heart macrophages in steady-state and after myocardial infarction.* Circ Res, 2014. **115**(2): p. 284–295.

43. Meredith, M.M., et al., *Expression of the zinc finger transcription factor zDC (Zbtb46, Btbd4) defines the classical dendritic cell lineage.* J Exp Med, 2012. **209**(6): p. 1153–1165.

44. Satpathy, A.T., et al., *Zbtb46 expression distinguishes classical dendritic cells and their committed progenitors from other immune lineages.* J Exp Med, 2012. **209**(6): p. 1135–1152.

45. Guilliams, M., et al., *Dendritic cells, monocytes and macrophages: a unified nomenclature based on ontogeny.* Nat Rev Immunol, 2014. **14**(8): p. 571–578.

46. Merad, M., et al., *The dendritic cell lineage: ontogeny and function of dendritic cells and their subsets in the steady state and the inflamed setting.* Annu Rev Immunol, 2013. **31**: p. 563–604.

47. Wu, X., et al., *Mafb lineage tracing to distinguish macrophages from other immune lineages reveals dual identity of Langerhans cells.* J Exp Med, 2016. **213**(12): p. 2553–2565.

48. Hashimoto, D., J. Miller, and M. Merad, *Dendritic cell and macrophage heterogeneity in vivo.* Immunity, 2011. **35**(3): p. 323–335.

49. Lee, J.S., et al., *Conventional dendritic cells impair recovery after myocardial infarction.* J Immunol, 2018. **201**(6): p. 1784–1798.

50. Ganguly, D., et al., *The role of dendritic cells in autoimmunity.* Nat Rev Immunol, 2013. **13**(8): p. 566–577.

51. Clemente-Casares, X., et al., *A CD103(+) conventional dendritic cell surveillance system prevents development of overt heart failure during subclinical viral myocarditis.* Immunity, 2017. **47**(5): p. 974–989, e8.

52. Van der Borght, K. and B.N. Lambrecht, *Heart macrophages and dendritic cells in sickness and in health: a tale of a complicated marriage.* Cell Immunol, 2018. **330**: p. 105–113.

53. Hart, D.N. and J.W. Fabre, *Demonstration and characterization of Ia-positive dendritic cells in the interstitial connective tissues of rat heart and other tissues, but not brain.* J Exp Med, 1981. **154**(2): p. 347–361.

54. Maisch, B., *Cardio-immunology of myocarditis: focus on immune mechanisms and treatment options.* Front Cardiovasc Med, 2019. **6**: p. 48.

55. Hulsmans, M., et al., *Macrophages facilitate electrical conduction in the heart.* Cell, 2017. **169**(3): p. 510–522, e20.

56. Hartupee, J. and D.L. Mann, *Neurohormonal activation in heart failure with reduced ejection fraction.* Nat Rev Cardiol, 2017. **14**(1): p. 30–38.

57. Sullivan, M.J., et al., *Relation between central and peripheral hemodynamics during exercise in patients with chronic heart failure: muscle blood flow is reduced with maintenance of arterial perfusion pressure.* Circulation, 1989. **80**(4): p. 769–781.

58. Mentz, R.J. and C.M. O'Connor, *Pathophysiology and clinical evaluation of acute heart failure.* Nat Rev Cardiol, 2016. **13**(1): p. 28–35.

59. Nazare Nunes Alves, M.J., et al., *Mechanisms of blunted muscle vasodilation during peripheral chemoreceptor stimulation in heart failure patients.* Hypertension, 2012. **60**(3): p. 669–676.

60. Pereira, M.R. and P.E. Leite, *The involvement of parasympathetic and sympathetic nerve in the inflammatory reflex.* J Cell Physiol, 2016. **231**(9): p. 1862–1869.

61. Mann, D.L., *Inflammatory mediators and the failing heart: past, present, and the foreseeable future.* Circ Res, 2002. **91**(11): p. 988–998.

62. Cuoco, L., et al., *Skeletal muscle wastage in Crohn's disease: a pathway shared with heart failure?* Int J Cardiol, 2008. **127**(2): p. 219–227.

63. Deswal, A., et al., *Cytokines and cytokine receptors in advanced heart failure: an analysis of the cytokine database from the Vesnarinone trial (VEST).* Circulation, 2001. **103**(16): p. 2055–2059.

64. Torre-Amione, G., et al., *Proinflammatory cytokine levels in patients with depressed left ventricular ejection fraction: a report from the Studies of Left Ventricular Dysfunction (SOLVD).* J Am Coll Cardiol, 1996. **27**(5): p. 1201–1206.

65. Ferrari, R., et al., *Tumor necrosis factor soluble receptors in patients with various degrees of congestive heart failure.* Circulation, 1995. **92**(6): p. 1479–1486.

66. Levine, B., et al., *Elevated circulating levels of tumor necrosis factor in severe chronic heart failure.* N Engl J Med, 1990. **323**(4): p. 236–241.

67. Rehman, S.U., T. Mueller, and J.L. Januzzi, Jr., *Characteristics of the novel interleukin family biomarker ST2 in patients with acute heart failure.* J Am Coll Cardiol, 2008. **52**(18): p. 1458–1465.

68. Latini, R., et al., *Pentraxin-3 in chronic heart failure: the CORONA and GISSI-HF trials.* Eur J Heart Fail, 2012. **14**(9): p. 992–999.

69. Yu, L., et al., *Genetic and pharmacological inhibition of galectin-3 prevents cardiac remodeling by interfering with myocardial fibrogenesis.* Circ Heart Fail, 2013. **6**(1): p. 107–117.

70. Lok, D.J., et al., *Prognostic value of galectin-3, a novel marker of fibrosis, in patients with chronic heart failure: data from the DEAL-HF study.* Clin Res Cardiol, 2010. **99**(5): p. 323–328.

71. Vasan, R.S., et al., *Inflammatory markers and risk of heart failure in elderly subjects without prior myocardial infarction: the Framingham Heart Study.* Circulation, 2003. **107**(11): p. 1486–1491.

72. Parrillo, J.E., et al., *A prospective, randomized, controlled trial of prednisone for dilated cardiomyopathy.* N Engl J Med, 1989. **321**(16): p. 1061–1068.

73. Gong, K., et al., *The nonspecific anti-inflammatory therapy with methotrexate for patients with chronic heart failure.* Am Heart J, 2006. **151**(1): p. 62–68.
74. Mann, D.L., et al., *Targeted anticytokine therapy in patients with chronic heart failure: results of the Randomized Etanercept Worldwide Evaluation (RENEWAL).* Circulation, 2004. **109**(13): p. 1594–1602.
75. Chung, E.S., et al., *Randomized, double-blind, placebo-controlled, pilot trial of infliximab, a chimeric monoclonal antibody to tumor necrosis factor-alpha, in patients with moderate-to-severe heart failure: results of the anti-TNF Therapy Against Congestive Heart Failure (ATTACH) trial.* Circulation, 2003. **107**(25): p. 3133–3140.
76. Briasoulis, A., et al., *The role of inflammation and cell death in the pathogenesis, progression and treatment of heart failure.* Heart Fail Rev, 2016. **21**(2): p. 169–176.
77. Mann, D.L., et al., *Innate immunity in the adult mammalian heart: for whom the cell tolls.* Trans Am Clin Climatol Assoc, 2010. **121**: p. 34–50; discussion 50–51.
78. Mezzaroma, E., et al., *The inflammasome promotes adverse cardiac remodeling following acute myocardial infarction in the mouse.* Proc Natl Acad Sci U S A, 2011. **108**(49): p. 19725–19730.
79. Takeuchi, O. and S. Akira, *Pattern recognition receptors and inflammation.* Cell, 2010. **140**(6): p. 805–820.
80. Mann, D.L., *Innate immunity and the failing heart: the cytokine hypothesis revisited.* Circ Res, 2015. **116**(7): p. 1254–1268.
81. Chan, J.K., et al., *Alarmins: awaiting a clinical response.* J Clin Invest, 2012. **122**(8): p. 2711–2719.
82. Nakayama, H. and K. Otsu, *Mitochondrial DNA as an inflammatory mediator in cardiovascular diseases.* Biochem J, 2018. **475**(5): p. 839–852.
83. Nishimura, M. and S. Naito, *Tissue-specific mRNA expression profiles of human toll-like receptors and related genes.* Biol Pharm Bull, 2005. **28**(5): p. 886–892.
84. Yin, Y., et al., *Inflammasomes are differentially expressed in cardiovascular and other tissues.* Int J Immunopathol Pharmacol, 2009. **22**(2): p. 311–322.
85. Frantz, S., et al., *The innate immune system in chronic cardiomyopathy: a European Society of Cardiology (ESC) scientific statement from the Working Group on Myocardial Function of the ESC.* Eur J Heart Fail, 2018. **20**(3): p. 445–459.
86. Piccinini, A.M. and K.S. Midwood, *DAMPening inflammation by modulating TLR signalling.* Mediators Inflamm, 2010. **2010**.
87. Fredman, G. and M. Spite, *Recent advances in the role of immunity in atherosclerosis.* Circ Res, 2013. **113**(12): p. e111–114.
88. Moore, K.J., et al., *Macrophage trafficking, inflammatory resolution, and genomics in atherosclerosis: JACC macrophage in CVD series (part 2).* J Am Coll Cardiol, 2018. **72**(18): p. 2181–2197.
89. Ridker, P.M., et al., *Antiinflammatory therapy with canakinumab for atherosclerotic disease.* N Engl J Med, 2017. **377**(12): p. 1119–1131.
90. Robbins, C.S., et al., *Extramedullary hematopoiesis generates Ly-6C(high) monocytes that infiltrate atherosclerotic lesions.* Circulation, 2012. **125**(2): p. 364–374.
91. Berg, K.E., et al., *Elevated CD14++CD16- monocytes predict cardiovascular events.* Circ Cardiovasc Genet, 2012. **5**(1): p. 122–131.
92. Libby, P., A.H. Lichtman, and G.K. Hansson, *Immune effector mechanisms implicated in atherosclerosis: from mice to humans.* Immunity, 2013. **38**(6): p. 1092–1104.
93. Keul, P., et al., *Sphingosine-1-phosphate receptor 3 promotes recruitment of monocyte/macrophages in inflammation and atherosclerosis.* Circ Res, 2011. **108**(3): p. 314–323.

94. Potteaux, S., et al., *Suppressed monocyte recruitment drives macrophage removal from atherosclerotic plaques of Apoe-/- mice during disease regression.* J Clin Invest, 2011. **121**(5): p. 2025–2036.

95. Westerterp, M., et al., *Deficiency of ATP-binding cassette transporters A1 and G1 in macrophages increases inflammation and accelerates atherosclerosis in mice.* Circ Res, 2013. **112**(11): p. 1456–1465.

96. Moore, K.J. and I. Tabas, *Macrophages in the pathogenesis of atherosclerosis.* Cell, 2011. **145**(3): p. 341–355.

97. Hanna, R.N., et al., *NR4A1 (Nur77) deletion polarizes macrophages toward an inflammatory phenotype and increases atherosclerosis.* Circ Res, 2012. **110**(3): p. 416–427.

98. Chinetti-Gbaguidi, G., et al., *Human atherosclerotic plaque alternative macrophages display low cholesterol handling but high phagocytosis because of distinct activities of the PPARgamma and LXRalpha pathways.* Circ Res, 2011. **108**(8): p. 985–995.

99. Razani, B., et al., *Autophagy links inflammasomes to atherosclerotic progression.* Cell Metab, 2012. **15**(4): p. 534–544.

100. Daissormont, I.T., et al., *Plasmacytoid dendritic cells protect against atherosclerosis by tuning T-cell proliferation and activity.* Circ Res, 2011. **109**(12): p. 1387–1395.

101. Macritchie, N., et al., *Plasmacytoid dendritic cells play a key role in promoting atherosclerosis in apolipoprotein E-deficient mice.* Arterioscler Thromb Vasc Biol, 2012. **32**(11): p. 2569–2579.

102. Yilmaz, A., et al., *Emergence of dendritic cells in rupture-prone regions of vulnerable carotid plaques.* Atherosclerosis, 2004. **176**(1): p. 101–110.

103. Van Vre, E.A., et al., *Immunohistochemical characterisation of dendritic cells in human atherosclerotic lesions: possible pitfalls.* Pathology, 2011. **43**(3): p. 239–247.

104. Niessner, A., et al., *Pathogen-sensing plasmacytoid dendritic cells stimulate cytotoxic T-cell function in the atherosclerotic plaque through interferon-alpha.* Circulation, 2006. **114**(23): p. 2482–2489.

105. Chen, C.J., et al., *Identification of a key pathway required for the sterile inflammatory response triggered by dying cells.* Nat Med, 2007. **13**(7): p. 851–856.

106. Ehrentraut, H., et al., *The toll-like receptor 4-antagonist eritoran reduces murine cardiac hypertrophy.* Eur J Heart Fail, 2011. **13**(6): p. 602–610.

107. Matsuda, S., et al., *Angiotensin activates MCP-1 and induces cardiac hypertrophy and dysfunction via toll-like receptor 4.* J Atheroscler Thromb, 2015. **22**(8): p. 833–844.

108. Patel, B., et al., *CCR2(+) Monocyte-derived infiltrating macrophages are required for adverse cardiac remodeling during pressure overload.* JACC Basic Transl Sci, 2018. **3**(2): p. 230–244.

109. Dobaczewski, M., C. Gonzalez-Quesada, and N.G. Frangogiannis, *The extracellular matrix as a modulator of the inflammatory and reparative response following myocardial infarction.* J Mol Cell Cardiol, 2010. **48**(3): p. 504–511.

110. Li, W., et al., *Ferroptotic cell death and TLR4/Trif signaling initiate neutrophil recruitment after heart transplantation.* J Clin Invest, 2019. **129**(6): p. 2293–2304.

111. Oka, T., et al., *Mitochondrial DNA that escapes from autophagy causes inflammation and heart failure.* Nature, 2012. **485**(7397): p. 251–255.

112. King, K.R., et al., *IRF3 and type I interferons fuel a fatal response to myocardial infarction.* Nat Med, 2017. **23**(12): p. 1481–1487.

113. Sager, H.B., et al., *Proliferation and recruitment contribute to myocardial macrophage expansion in chronic heart failure.* Circ Res, 2016. **119**(7): p. 853–864.

114. Uderhardt, S., et al., *Resident macrophages cloak tissue microlesions to prevent neutrophil-driven inflammatory damage.* Cell, 2019. **177**(3): p. 541–555, e17.

115. Frantz, S., et al., *Monocytes/macrophages prevent healing defects and left ventricular thrombus formation after myocardial infarction*. FASEB J, 2013. **27**(3): p. 871–881.

116. Leuschner, F., et al., *Rapid monocyte kinetics in acute myocardial infarction are sustained by extramedullary monocytopoiesis*. J Exp Med, 2012. **209**(1): p. 123–137.

117. Dutta, P., et al., *Myocardial infarction activates CCR2(+) hematopoietic stem and progenitor cells*. Cell Stem Cell, 2015. **16**(5): p. 477–487.

118. Prabhu, S.D., *The cardiosplenic axis is essential for the pathogenesis of ischemic heart failure*. Trans Am Clin Climatol Assoc, 2018. **129**: p. 202–214.

119. Dewald, O., et al., *CCL2/Monocyte Chemoattractant Protein-1 regulates inflammatory responses critical to healing myocardial infarcts*. Circ Res, 2005. **96**(8): p. 881–889.

120. Leuschner, F., et al., *Angiotensin-converting enzyme inhibition prevents the release of monocytes from their splenic reservoir in mice with myocardial infarction*. Circ Res, 2010. **107**(11): p. 1364–1373.

121. Ismahil, M.A., et al., *Remodeling of the mononuclear phagocyte network underlies chronic inflammation and disease progression in heart failure: critical importance of the cardiosplenic axis*. Circ Res, 2014. **114**(2): p. 266–282.

122. Hilgendorf, I., et al., *Ly-6Chigh monocytes depend on Nr4a1 to balance both inflammatory and reparative phases in the infarcted myocardium*. Circ Res, 2014. **114**(10): p. 1611–1622.

123. Nahrendorf, M., et al., *The healing myocardium sequentially mobilizes two monocyte subsets with divergent and complementary functions*. J Exp Med, 2007. **204**(12): p. 3037–3047.

124. Hayasaki, T., et al., *CC chemokine receptor-2 deficiency attenuates oxidative stress and infarct size caused by myocardial ischemia-reperfusion in mice*. Circ J, 2006. **70**(3): p. 342–351.

125. Kaikita, K., et al., *Targeted deletion of CC chemokine receptor 2 attenuates left ventricular remodeling after experimental myocardial infarction*. Am J Pathol, 2004. **165**(2): p. 439–447.

126. Mouton, A.J., et al., *Mapping macrophage polarization over the myocardial infarction time continuum*. Basic Res Cardiol, 2018. **113**(4): p. 26.

127. van Amerongen, M.J., et al., *Macrophage depletion impairs wound healing and increases left ventricular remodeling after myocardial injury in mice*. Am J Pathol, 2007. **170**(3): p. 818–829.

128. Nagai, T., et al., *Decreased myocardial dendritic cells is associated with impaired reparative fibrosis and development of cardiac rupture after myocardial infarction in humans*. J Am Heart Assoc, 2014. **3**(3): p. e000839.

129. Caforio, A.L., et al., *Current state of knowledge on aetiology, diagnosis, management, and therapy of myocarditis: a position statement of the European Society of Cardiology Working Group on Myocardial and Pericardial Diseases*. Eur Heart J, 2013. **34**(33): p. 2636–2648, 2648a–2648d.

130. Abston, E.D., et al., *TLR3 deficiency induces chronic inflammatory cardiomyopathy in resistant mice following coxsackievirus B3 infection: role for IL-4*. Am J Physiol Regul Integr Comp Physiol, 2013. **304**(4): p. R267–277.

131. Leuschner, F., et al., *Silencing of CCR2 in myocarditis*. Eur Heart J, 2015. **36**(23): p. 1478–1488.

132. Wu, L., et al., *Cardiac fibroblasts mediate IL-17A-driven inflammatory dilated cardiomyopathy*. J Exp Med, 2014. **211**(7): p. 1449–1464.

133. Muller, I., et al., *CX3CR1 knockout aggravates Coxsackievirus B3-induced myocarditis*. PLoS One, 2017. **12**(8): p. e0182643.

134. Shen, Y., F.Q. Zhang, and X. Wei, *Truncated monocyte chemoattractant protein-1 can alleviate cardiac injury in mice with viral myocarditis via infiltration of mononuclear cells.* Microbiol Immunol, 2014. **58**(3): p. 195–201.

135. Papageorgiou, A.P. and S. Heymans, *Interactions between the extracellular matrix and inflammation during viral myocarditis.* Immunobiology, 2012. **217**(5): p. 503–510.

136. Goser, S., et al., *Critical role for monocyte chemoattractant protein-1 and macrophage inflammatory protein-1alpha in induction of experimental autoimmune myocarditis and effective anti-monocyte chemoattractant protein-1 gene therapy.* Circulation, 2005. **112**(22): p. 3400–3407.

137. Eriksson, U., et al., *Activation of dendritic cells through the interleukin 1 receptor 1 is critical for the induction of autoimmune myocarditis.* J Exp Med, 2003. **197**(3): p. 323–331.

138. Smith, S.C. and P.M. Allen, *Myosin-induced acute myocarditis is a T cell-mediated disease.* J Immunol, 1991. **147**(7): p. 2141–2147.

139. Kim, S.J. and B. Diamond, *Modulation of tolerogenic dendritic cells and autoimmunity.* Semin Cell Dev Biol, 2015. **41**: p. 49–58.

140. Van der Borght, K., et al., *Myocarditis elicits dendritic cell and monocyte infiltration in the heart and self-antigen presentation by conventional type 2 dendritic cells.* Front Immunol, 2018. **9**: p. 2714.

141. Chen, M., et al., *The role of cardiac macrophage and cytokines on ventricular arrhythmias.* Front Physiol, 2020. **11**: p. 1113.

142. Levick, S.P., et al., *Sympathetic nervous system modulation of inflammation and remodeling in the hypertensive heart.* Hypertension, 2010. **55**(2): p. 270–276.

143. Pinto, J.M. and P.A. Boyden, *Electrical remodeling in ischemia and infarction.* Cardiovasc Res, 1999. **42**(2): p. 284–297.

144. Monnerat, G., et al., *Macrophage-dependent IL-1beta production induces cardiac arrhythmias in diabetic mice.* Nat Commun, 2016. **7**: p. 13344.

145. De Jesus, N.M., et al., *Antiarrhythmic effects of interleukin 1 inhibition after myocardial infarction.* Heart Rhythm, 2017. **14**(5): p. 727–736.

146. Chen, Y., et al., *Effect of tumor necrosis factor-alpha on ventricular arrhythmias in rats with acute myocardial infarction in vivo.* World J Emerg Med, 2010. **1**(1): p. 53–58.

147. Petkova-Kirova, P.S., et al., *Electrical remodeling of cardiac myocytes from mice with heart failure due to the overexpression of tumor necrosis factor-alpha.* Am J Physiol Heart Circ Physiol, 2006. **290**(5): p. H2098–2107.

148. Lazzerini, P.E., et al., *Antiarrhythmic potential of anticytokine therapy in rheumatoid arthritis: tocilizumab reduces corrected QT interval by controlling systemic inflammation.* Arthritis Care Res (Hoboken), 2015. **67**(3): p. 332–339.

149. Mukherjee, R., et al., *Spatiotemporal induction of matrix metalloproteinase-9 transcription after discrete myocardial injury.* FASEB J, 2010. **24**(10): p. 3819–3828.

150. Fei, Y.D., et al., *Macrophages facilitate post myocardial infarction arrhythmias: roles of gap junction and KCa3.1.* Theranostics, 2019. **9**(22): p. 6396–6411.

151. Kobayashi, M., et al., *NLRP3 deficiency reduces macrophage interleukin-10 production and enhances the susceptibility to doxorubicin-induced cardiotoxicity.* Sci Rep, 2016. **6**: p. 26489.

152. Ma, Y., et al., *Toll-like receptor (TLR) 2 and TLR4 differentially regulate doxorubicin induced cardiomyopathy in mice.* PLoS One, 2012. **7**(7): p. e40763.

153. Nozaki, N., et al., *Modulation of doxorubicin-induced cardiac dysfunction in toll-like receptor-2-knockout mice.* Circulation, 2004. **110**(18): p. 2869–2874.

154. Riad, A., et al., *Toll-like receptor-4 deficiency attenuates doxorubicin-induced cardiomyopathy in mice.* Eur J Heart Fail, 2008. **10**(3): p. 233–243.

155. Krysko, D.V., et al., *TLR-2 and TLR-9 are sensors of apoptosis in a mouse model of doxorubicin-induced acute inflammation.* Cell Death Differ, 2011. **18**(8): p. 1316–1325.

156. Heinzerling, L., et al., *Cardiotoxicity associated with CTLA4 and PD1 blocking immunotherapy.* J Immunother Cancer, 2016. **4**: p. 50.

157. Todd, J.L. and S.M. Palmer, *Danger signals in regulating the immune response to solid organ transplantation.* J Clin Invest, 2017. **127**(7): p. 2464–2472.

158. Kim, I.K., et al., *Impact of innate and adaptive immunity on rejection and tolerance.* Transplantation, 2008. **86**(7): p. 889–894.

159. O'Neill, L.A., D. Golenbock, and A.G. Bowie, *The history of Toll-like receptors—redefining innate immunity.* Nat Rev Immunol, 2013. **13**(6): p. 453–460.

160. Tesar, B.M., et al., *TH1 immune responses to fully MHC mismatched allografts are diminished in the absence of MyD88, a toll-like receptor signal adaptor protein.* Am J Transplant, 2004. **4**(9): p. 1429–1439.

161. Kopecky, B.J., et al., *Role of donor macrophages after heart and lung transplantation.* Am J Transplant, 2020. **20**(5): p. 1225–1235.

162. Svajger, U. and P. Rozman, *Tolerogenic dendritic cells: molecular and cellular mechanisms in transplantation.* J Leukoc Biol, 2014. **95**(1): p. 53–69.

163. Moreau, A., et al., *Cell therapy using tolerogenic dendritic cells in transplantation.* Transplant Res, 2012. **1**(1): p. 13.

164. Dieterlen, M.T., et al., *Dendritic cells and their role in cardiovascular diseases: a view on human studies.* J Immunol Res, 2016. **2016**: p. 5946807.

165. Bajpai, G., et al., *The human heart contains distinct macrophage subsets with divergent origins and functions.* Nat Med, 2018. **24**(8): p. 1234–1245.

2 Helper T-Lymphocytes in Cardiovascular Diseases

*Vinay Kumar, Sahil Gupta, Rachel
Rosenzweig, and Shyam S. Bansal*

CONTENTS

INTRODUCTION

Cardiovascular disease (CVD) is the leading cause of morbidity and mortality in developed as well as developing countries[1]. CVD is a wide-ranging term, which includes cerebrovascular disease (disease of the blood vessels supplying the brain), congenital heart disease (malformations of the heart structure at birth), coronary heart disease (disease of the coronary blood vessels), hypertension, heart failure, peripheral vascular disease (disease of the blood vessels supplying the arms and legs), and rheumatic heart disease (damage to the heart muscle and heart valves from rheumatic fever, caused by pathogens)[2]. Preclinical and clinical studies over the last decade have clearly shown that an altered or insufficient immune response is one of the most significant contributors to the development and progression of CVDs.

Diminished blood flow, increased pre- or afterload, or damage to the vascular endothelium initiate a cascade of immune responses characterized by the activation and infiltration of innate and adaptive immune cells, as well as heightened inflammatory mediators such as cytokines and chemokines[3]. Such immune responses are physiologically necessary to initiate healing processes and/or

DOI: 10.1201/b22824-3

promote fibrotic scar formation. Early immune responses are associated predominantly with the activation of innate immune cells, as they do not require specific antigen-mediated activation mechanisms[4]. Once at the site of injury, they process neo-antigens consisting of altered or unaltered cytosolic or nuclear proteins that are released from the injured tissues, and they act as damage-associated molecular patterns (DAMPs) to interact with Toll-like receptors (TLRs) expressed on the surface of innate immune cells[5]. However, as the injury progresses (as in chronic disease) and inflammation is sustained, these antigens are further processed by the antigen-presenting cells (APCs) and, in conjunction with MHC-I or MHC-II, are presented to the adaptive immune cells such as cytotoxic CD8[+] or helper CD4[+] T-cells, respectively. Similar to nonsterile injury, recent evidence also suggests that sterile immune activation can also induce memory against self-antigens, as accumulation of memory T-cells has also been described in some CVDs[6-8], leading to autoimmune-like responses.

Lymphocyte progenitors originate in the bone marrow, differentiate into immunocompetent T-cells (i.e., helper T-cells, regulatory T-cells, cytotoxic T-cells, and memory T-cells) in the thymus, and then travel throughout the body via the circulatory system or the lymphatic system to encounter an infection, if any[9]. Diverse functions of CD4[+] helper T-cells could be assessed by their ability not only to help B-cells make antibodies but also to induce and/or recruit macrophages, neutrophils, eosinophils, and basophils to the sites of infection and inflammation[10]. T-cells recognize antigens through T-cell receptors (TCRs) expressed on their surface[11]. Immunologically, T-cell activation is a controlled cell-to-cell communication mechanism designed to prevent their activation against self-proteins, as T-cells lack the ability to recognize proteins by themselves, and they depend upon APCs such as macrophages and dendritic cells (DCs) to discern foreign peptides when presented in conjunction with MHC molecules and appropriate costimulatory signals[12].

Upon antigen binding and recognition by the TCR, naïve T-cells proliferate and polarize into distinct functional classes, depending upon the cytokine milieu encountered in the tissues[13] and the array of other signals received[10,14]. Different CD4[+] T-cell subsets have different transcription machineries and cytokine/chemokine specificities, and they regulate different responses to promote immunological healing while curbing overt autoimmune activation. Th1 cells (which produce mainly IFNγ, lymphotoxin α, and IL-2) mediate immune responses against intracellular pathogens[15], whereas Th2 cells (which produce mainly IL-4, IL-5, IL-9, IL-10, IL-13, IL-25, and amphiregulin) provide host defense from extracellular parasites[10,16]. Immune responses against extracellular bacteria and fungi are mediated by Th17 cells (which produce mainly IL-17a, IL-17f, IL-21, and IL-22)[17], and Treg cells (which produce mainly TGF-β, IL-10, and IL-35) play a central role in preserving self-tolerance and/or controlling immune responses[18] (Figure 2.1). Although there are several other T-cell subsets that have been identified in different immunological conditions, Th1, Th2, Th17, and Tregs are well studied with respect to CVDs and will be covered in subsequent sections.

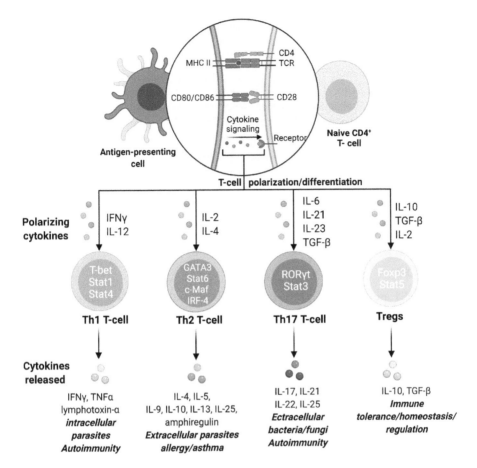

FIGURE 2.1 Activation, polarization, and differentiation of naïve CD4+ T-cells. Interaction of an antigen-presenting cell induces polarization/differentiation of a naïve CD4+ T-cell. Concerted action of various cytokines/chemokines and transcription factors in combination with environmental cues determines the eventual fate of a naïve T-cell to polarize to either a Th1, Th2, Th17, or regulatory T-cell (Tregs) phenotype. Different CD4+ T-cell subsets arbitrate disparate immune responses: Th1 T-cells deal with intracellular parasites and autoimmunity; Th2 T-cells regulate responses against extracellular parasites and allergy/asthma; Th17 T-cells protect against extracellular bacteria/fungi and autoimmunity; and Tregs mediate immune tolerance, homeostasis, and immune regulation. Abbreviations: MHC, major histocompatibility complex; TCR, T-cell receptor; T-bet, T-box expressed in T-cells; STAT, signal transducer and activator of transcription; GATA, recognizing the DNA consensus sequence (A/T)GATA(A/G); IRF-4, interferon regulatory factor-4; RORγt, retineic acid receptor–related orphan nuclear receptor gamma in Th17 cells; Foxp3, Forkhead box P3.

Source: Created with BioRender.com.

T-CELLS AND THEIR SUBSETS

TH1 T-CELLS

Th1 T-cells are characterized by the expression of pro-inflammatory cytokine IFNγ and transcription factor T-bet[19,20]. Differentiation of Th1 T-cells from naïve T-cells is induced by IL-12 produced by other pro-inflammatory immune cells such as neutrophils[21], Ly6C[hi] monocytes[22], and natural killer T-cells[23]. Additionally, while IL-18 cannot induce Th1 differentiation on its own, it can potently activate Th1 T-cells to produce IFNγ in the presence of IL-12[24]. Together with the innate immune system, Th1 T-cells promote the clearance of dead and apoptotic cells and are early responders in tissue injury. Considering that Th1 T-cells are known for and characterized by the production of several pro-inflammatory cytokines, as will be discussed in subsequent sections, Th1 T-cells are implicated in several inflammatory cardiovascular diseases.

TH2 T-CELLS

Th2 T-cells are classically defined as profibrotic and anti-inflammatory[25]. These cells regulate humoral immunity through the release of IL-4, IL-5, and IL-13 and are essential components of the immune response to bacterial infections and allergens, as they stimulate antibody production[25]. IL-4 is critical for the differentiation of naïve T-cells into Th2 T-cells through its activation of GATA3, in turn stimulating IL-5 and IL-13 production and further upregulating Th2 T-cell differentiation[25]. Due to their profibrotic and anti-inflammatory nature, Th2 T-cells can profoundly affect cardiovascular diseases such as atherosclerosis, myocarditis, hypertension, and heart failure, and they may have therapeutic potential in some of these conditions.

TH17 T-CELLS

The interleukin-17 (IL-17) family of cytokines and their ubiquitous receptors play a major role in host defense against pathogens. The IL-17 family (six known IL-17 family members: IL-17A–F) is characterized by a group of proteins with a highly conserved C-terminus domain comprising a cysteine-knot fold structure[26], and among the IL-17 family members, IL-17A is the most widely studied. T-helper 17 (Th17) cells are known for their expression of pro-inflammatory cytokine interleukin-17 (IL-17) under the control of transcription factor RORγt, and they regulate the functioning of stromal cells in many tissues[27]. IL-17A, IL-17F, and IL-22 are the signature cytokines released from Th17 cells, and by inducing anti-microbial peptides from epithelial cells, and also by recruiting neutrophils during inflammation, they act as essential regulators of the mucosal host defense against extracellular bacteria and fungi[28]. These vital effects of IL-17 on stromal cells result in not only the production of other inflammatory cytokines but also the recruitment of leukocytes, especially neutrophils, thereby orchestrating a link between the innate and the adaptive immune systems. Th17 cells also play a critical role in the pathogenesis of several autoimmune and chronic tissue inflammatory diseases and subsequent organ failure[29]. The critical role of IL-17 in regulating pro-inflammatory networks could also be gleaned from the fact that, in addition to Th17 cells, several other immune cells such as dendritic cells, macrophages, natural killer cells, natural killer T-cells, and γδT-cells have also been shown to secrete IL-17 during activation[30].

REGULATORY T-CELLS (TREGS)

Tregs constitute 5–10% of peripheral CD4+ T-cells[31]. Expression of Foxp3 transcription factor is characteristic of Tregs, at least in rodents, and is necessary for their differentiation and function[31]. While Foxp3 along with CD25 expression is specific to rodent Tregs, it is less specific in humans as effector T-cells also transiently express Foxp3 during activation. Because of this, Tregs in humans are defined as CD4+CD25+ cells with low CD127 expression[32]. Tregs that develop naturally in the thymus are called nTregs, whereas those that are derived in the periphery by the polarization of effector T-cells in conditions of chronic antigen stimulation and sustained TCR activation are termed peripheral Tregs (pTregs). Induced Tregs (iTregs) are derived from effector T-cells during *ex vivo* culture in the presence of cytokines such as IL-2 and TGFβ[33]. Recently, several tissues were identified that also retain specialized "tissue Tregs" that exhibit phenotypes more relevant to their host tissue. For example, Tregs residing in adipose tissues fine-tune metabolic indices of fat tissue[34], Tregs in muscles promote muscle repair[35], and those residing in the intestine maintain tolerance against the gut microbiome[36]. All of these Treg phenotypes exhibit highly potent immune-suppressive activities to prevent overt activation of immune responses and maintain immune tolerance either by contact-dependent inhibition of innate and adaptive immune responses, by secretion of anti-inflammatory cytokines such as IL-10, or by alteration of the metabolism of bystander cells[37]. Because Tregs are a highly specialized class of cells that are endowed with the most important function of maintaining immune and tissue homeostasis, they play a critical role in the pathophysiology of several inflammatory diseases, including cardiovascular ones.

T-CELLS IN ATHEROSCLEROSIS

Atherosclerosis involves the deposition of fatty plaques made up of cholesterol, fatty substances, cellular waste products, calcium, and fibrin in the intima of the arteries. This leads to thickening of the blood vessels and narrowing of the arterial lumen, decreasing the blood flow and the amount of oxygen and nutrients reaching the end organ[38]. Disturbed vascular flow also promotes the activation and infiltration of monocytes/macrophages and dendritic cells into the intima, where they encounter and process oxidized lipids or other antigens, resulting in their maturation. Subsequent antigen presentation to T-cells can take place either at the local site or in the secondary lymphoid organs to further aid T-cell recruitment[39]. Although the disease stage, lesion size, and location can modulate the prevalence of one T-cell subtype over another, activated T-lymphocytes are present in significant quantities at all stages of atherosclerosis, suggesting that they play an essential role in disease progression.

APCs infiltrated into the plaques produce IL-12 to activate Stat-4 and T-bet signaling to then upregulate IFNγ expression and polarization of effector T-cells into the Th1 phenotype[40]. IFNγ and IL-2 are present in the majority of plaques[41] and exert pro-atherogenic effects, as a deficiency of either IFNγ or its receptor blunts atherosclerotic lesions and improves plaque stability[42], while its exogenous administration promotes lesion development[21]. IFNγ has also been shown to inhibit the proliferation of vascular smooth muscle cells and their collagen content, resulting in the weakening of the fibrous cap[43]. Along similar lines, T-bet deficiency in mice results in reduced severity of atherosclerosis as naïve T-cells fail to differentiate into Th1 T-cells[44]. Atherosclerotic plaques also contain IL-18, which, in synergism with IL-12, promotes IFNγ expression in Th1 T-cells[45], and the inhibition of IL-18 either by IL-18 binding protein or by genetic deletion blunts lesion formation in ApoE[-/-] mice[46]. While IFNγ production is heavily implicated in lipid accumulation in atherosclerotic lesions, it has also been suggested that IFNγ can systemically inhibit the production of atheroprotective plasma lipoproteins such as apoA-IV[42]. Studies have also shown that the activation of T-bet transcription factor and expression of IFNγ in other differentiated T-cells, such as Tregs, are sufficient to alter their overall phenotype and function to turn them atherogenic from being protective[47]. These studies, in combination, suggest that, in addition to its local effects in the arterial endothelium, IFNγ has potentially wide-ranging effects during atherosclerosis (Figure 2.2).

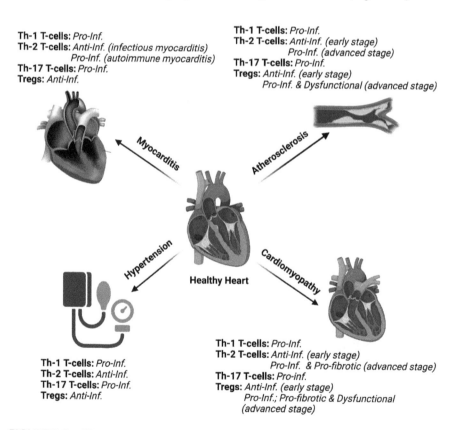

FIGURE 2.2   CD4+ T-cell subsets and their role in various CVDs.

Source: Created with BioRender.com.

Because Th1 T-cells are considered pro-atherogenic, Th2 T-cells were initially considered atheroprotective due to their potential to antagonize Th1 responses[48]. However, preclinical studies have shown that the site and the stage of the lesion can modulate the overall effects of Th2 T-cells. For example, overexpression of IL-4 results in a more significant reduction in lesion size when located in the aortic root than when located in the thoracic and abdominal aorta[48]. Similarly, in atherosclerosis-resistant BALB/c mice, IL-4 and Th2 T-cells reduce early fatty streak development[48]. Despite these well-documented protective responses, a deficiency in IL-4 has also been shown to decrease lesion formation, suggesting a pro-atherogenic role for IL-4 and, by extension, Th2 T-cells[48]. In contrast, other Th2 specific–cytokines such as IL-5 and IL-33 are known to confer atheroprotection. IL-5 stimulates humoral immunity and IgM-type anti-oxLDL antibodies, which, at high levels, are known to inhibit cholesterol uptake[49] and reduce lesion size[48]. IL-33 also acts on this pathway, as IL-33 overexpression causes a Th1 to Th2 shift, increasing IL-5 expression[48]. Thus, IL-5 and IL-33 may have anti-atherogenic effects due to their stimulation of protective antibodies[48]. Taken together, it appears that Th2 T-cells exert beneficial effects during the early stages of atherosclerosis but turn pathological and promote atherosclerosis during the advanced stage (Figure 2.2).

IL-17 is a potent regulator of atherosclerosis and mediates several signaling cascades in the vascular endothelial and smooth muscle cells[50]. Smith et al. have shown that the atherosclerotic pro-inflammatory milieu amplifies T-cell polarization into Th-17 cells and promotes their influx into the aortas of ApoE[-/-] mice[51]. An increase in Th17 cells further aids in the recruitment of monocytes and macrophages into the aortic wall, forming a pro-inflammatory, positive feedback loop[51]. The pro-atherogenic role of Th17 cells is also supported by the fact that blockade of IL-17A in ApoE[-/-] mice using adenovirus-produced IL-17 receptor-A reduced the plaque burden in Western diet–fed ApoE[-/-] mice[51]. In another study, the functional blockade of IL-17A was shown to decrease atherosclerotic lesion development and plaque vulnerability in ApoE[-/-] mice[52].

Atherosclerosis has also been shown to be associated with reduced Treg numbers along with their diminished immune-suppressive capacity[53]. In humans and rodents, there is a direct correlation between the reduced Treg levels and the accumulation of pro-inflammatory helper and cytotoxic T-cells in the plaques aiding disease progression[53,54]. Due to their ability to suppress the polarization of naïve T-cells into pro-atherogenic effector T-cells, several preclinical and clinical studies show an imbalance between the anti-inflammatory Tregs and pro-inflammatory Th1/Th17 T-cells during atherosclerosis[55,56]. Studies in rodents have shown that Treg depletion either by anti-CD25 neutralizing antibodies[57] or by genetic deletion of Foxp3-expressing cells[58] increases plasma cholesterol levels and alters hepatic lipid metabolism to augment plaque size and atherosclerotic lesions. This is further supported by the fact that adoptive transfer of nTregs potently inhibits immune accumulation and aortic plaque formation in ApoE[-/-] mice[53] (Figure 2.2).

In conjunction with reduced levels, atherosclerosis is also associated with diminished immune-suppressive potential of Tregs (Figure 2.2). Peripheral Tregs isolated from the PBMCs of acute coronary syndromes (ACS) patients are significantly immunocompromised and exhibit reduced potential to inhibit immune activation when compared with Tregs from control patients[54]. Similarly, Tregs from ApoE$^{-/-}$ mice demonstrate blunted inhibition of effector T-cells when compared with Tregs from WT C57BL/6 mice[53]. Studies have shown that Foxp3 expression in Tregs is directly associated with their competency to inhibit immune activation, and a reduction in its expression due to either increased methylation of its gene loci[59] or altered metabolism from oxidative to glycolytic[60] can directly modulate Treg activity. Recently, the activation of other transcription factors, such as T-bet, with increased expression of pro-inflammatory cytokines[47] or increased pro-apoptotic markers such as Bak has also been reported in Tregs[61]. These changes in the plasticity and phenotype of Tregs in the inflammatory milieu of atherosclerotic lesions due to the activation of T-bet gene locus and IFNγ expression ultimately result in their dysfunctional phenotype[47].

Tregs not only regulate adaptive immune cells but also check innate immune responses. Monocytes in the presence of Tregs exhibit polarization toward the tolerogenic anti-inflammatory phenotype associated with heightened phagocytic activity and expression of CD163 and CD206 with a concomitant reduction in pro-inflammatory cytokines such as IL-6 and TNFα[62]. Tregs can also downregulate the expression of scavenger receptors, such as SR-A, and chemotactic factors, such as MCP-1, to reduce lipid uptake and monocyte recruitment into the plaques[63]. Studies have also shown that direct binding of CTLA-4 expressed on Tregs can initiate trans-internalization of CD80/CD86 in innate immune cells, thus inhibiting APC maturation and blunting antigen presentation[64]. These findings suggest that nTregs are protective during atherosclerosis, and an increase in either their number or their immune competence could provide clinically translatable therapeutic benefits.

T-CELLS IN ISCHEMIC AND NONISCHEMIC CARDIOMYOPATHY

Ischemic and nonischemic cardiomyopathy is characterized by chronic, low-grade inflammation. Coronary artery blockade or increased afterload initiates an early innate immune response to engulf apoptotic cardiomyocytes and facilitate wound healing. Subsequent processing of cardiac antigens and their presentation in conjunction with MHC-II then lead to CD4$^+$ T-cell activation[65]. Studies have shown that T-cells undergo significant temporally regulated phenotypic changes to promote tissue clearance by pro-inflammatory subsets, followed by scar formation and neovascularization aided by anti-inflammatory subsets such as Tregs[66]. However, during chronic inflammation, as seen with cardiomyopathy and LV remodeling, CD4$^+$ T-cells undergo a pathological switch and play a critical role in disease pathophysiology[7] (Figure 2.2).

Th1 T-cells infiltrate the myocardium during the early phases of cardiac injury to amplify innate immune responses and to facilitate clearance of dead and apoptotic cells[66]. The production of IFNγ in the myocardium increases immediately after MI, and this upregulation is sustained for up to a month after ischemic insult, indicating a predominance of Th1 polarization post-MI. Th1 T-cells have also been found to be directly proportional to cardiac dysfunction post-injury, indicative of their critical role in regulating heart function[67]. IFNγ is known to regulate several wound-healing cascades, including TGF-β-mediated activation of cardiac fibroblasts, and it has been found that increased IFNγ leads to decreased expression of αSMA and collagens I and III. This in turn results in decreased myofibroblast differentiation and collagen deposition, thereby affecting scar formation and leading to cardiac rupture[68]. In the context of ischemic cardiac injury, such as coronary artery disease (CAD) or myocardial infarction (MI), the frequency of Th1 T-cells has been found to be directly associated with the disease severity[67,69], with Th1 to Th2 ratios significantly skewed toward Th1. Moreover, number of affected blood vessels, degree of coronary artery stenosis, and length of the coronary artery lesion are all significant contributing factors in promoting Th1 predominance in CAD[70]. Similarly, while IFNγ production results in decreased heart function, it is also necessary for CD25 expression on Tregs, which, in turn, suppresses pro-inflammatory functions of Th1 T-cells[71]. Based on these observations, it appears that the role of IFNγ in ischemic injury is likely more complex than can be gleaned from Th1 T-cell levels alone.

Pressure overload in rodents, mimicking increased afterload in humans, leads to nonischemic HF and is also associated with increased Th1 polarization[72] and infiltration[73]. Studies have shown that cardiac fibroblasts and CCR2+ macrophages produce CXCL10 and to a lesser extent CXCL9, which attracts CXCR3+ Th1 cells into the failing heart[25], suggesting a critical role of the CXCR3-CXCL9/CXCL10 pathway. T-cells in the fibrotic myocardium mainly produce IFNγ, suggesting that Th1 T-cells are the main drivers of cardiac fibrosis in nonischemic HF as well[73]. Through direct cell-cell contact with cardiac fibroblasts, Th1 T-cells induce TGF-β production and αSMA expression in cardiac fibroblasts to promote their transition into myofibroblasts[73]. Thus, both ischemic and nonischemic cardiomyopathies are associated with alterations in the ratio of Th1 to Th2 cells, with chronic HF leading to increased Th1 expression that is proportional to the severity of HF[74]. An increased ratio of Th1 to Th2 T-cells is also associated with increased production of IFNγ and TNFα in chronic HF[75,76].

Th2 T-cells are late responders in MI and, by releasing cytokines such as IL-4, IL-5, and IL-13, mediate anti-inflammatory and profibrotic responses to promote scar formation and immune resolution[7]. They work in conjunction with anti-inflammatory macrophages to promote their activity and aid in ECM remodeling and neovascularization[7]. Studies in rodents have shown that Th2 cell responses are sustained even during ischemic cardiomyopathy[7]. This chronic Th2 T-cell activation can cause pathological heart remodeling, which seems to be the case during HF. Thus, inhibition of the Th2 immune response may have therapeutic potential in reducing pathological LV remodeling and improving heart function post-MI, and it needs to be tested further.

IL-17 is augmented during acute myocardial infarction and, through its ability to mediate leukocyte activation, plays an important role in inflammatory cascades post-ischemic injury. Studies from Cheng et al. have shown that patients with acute coronary syndrome have a significant increase in peripheral Th17 cells, Th17-related cytokines (IL-17, IL-6, and IL-23), and RORγt levels with a concomitant decrease in Tregs and its associated cytokines, such as IL-10 and TGF-β[77]. It has been observed that IL-17 levels are significantly increased during ST-segment elevation myocardial infarction (STEMI) and post-STEMI, and they induce migration and activation of monocyte subsets through TLR4 and IL-6 secretion[78,79]. Additionally, Zhou et al. established the pathogenic role of IL-17A in the early and late stages of post-MI remodeling, and they reported that IL-17A stimulates murine cardiomyocyte apoptosis through the p38 MAPK-p53-Bax signaling pathway[80]. While blockade of the IL-23/IL-17A axis alleviates late LV remodeling[67], inhibition of IL-17 enhances myocardial connexin-43 levels and reduces the frequency of malignant arrhythmias post-MI[81].

Tregs are recruited to the heart within 24 h of ischemic injury and exhibit complex biphasic kinetics, with maximal levels seen at 3 d post-injury that decrease to baseline levels by 14 d[82]. However, due to sustained low-grade inflammation or to failure of complete resolution, Tregs levels increase again in hypertrophic hearts and are almost 10-fold higher than in controls during ischemic cardiomyopathy[82]. Treg activation and infiltration during MI are essential to curb excessive inflammation and promote resolution for efficient tissue clearance, wound healing, and scar formation[83]. While Treg depletion early after MI exacerbates cardiac inflammation and interferes with wound healing and fibrotic scar formation[84], adoptive transfer of competent Tregs[83] or their expansion during this period improves wound healing[85] by diminishing the infiltration of other immune cells (such as neutrophils, macrophages, and effector T-cells) and by reducing pro-inflammatory cytokines (such as TNFα and IL-1β)[85]. Similar inhibition of overt immune activation and disruption of pro-inflammatory cytokine networks by competent Tregs have also been reported in angiotensin-II-mediated cardiac hypertrophy[86]. In contrast to these protective effects, chronic inflammation during ischemic cardiomyopathy results in dysfunctional Treg phenotypes with loss of their immune-suppressive potential and increased levels of IFNγ and TNFα[82]. This pathological transition is temporal in nature, coincides with left-ventricular remodeling, and is critical for pathological cardiac hypertrophy, fibrosis, and progressive cardiac dysfunction, as Treg depletion from 4 to 8 weeks post-MI augments neovascularization, ameliorates LV remodeling, and improves cardiac function in rodents[82]. These studies suggest that promotion or expansion of Treg activity could provide therapeutic benefits immediately after MI, whereas resetting their pro-inflammatory phenotype back to normal or depleting pathologically altered cells could be a viable therapeutic strategy for ischemic cardiomyopathy.

T-CELLS IN HYPERTENSION

Increased vascular inflammation is a characteristic feature of hypertension and is a risk factor for several cardiovascular diseases, such as cardiomyopathy and pressure overload–induced nonischemic HF in humans and rodents. Activation of several immuno-inflammatory mechanisms by either increased Ang-II or increased redox levels plays a critical role in the initiation and progression of this disease, and in consequent vascular remodeling and end organ damage[87]. Upon encountering hypertensive stimuli such as angiotensin-II and high salt, T-cells turn pro-inflammatory and infiltrate into the heart, the kidney, and the brain. Moreover, a pro-inflammatory environment aggravates hypertensive responses, mediating both endothelial dysfunction and cardiac, renal, and neurodegenerative injury[88]. T-lymphocytes are one of the key players in the pathogenesis of hypertension, as Rag1$^{-/-}$ mice deficient in the adaptive immune response fail to develop high blood pressure upon administration of Ang-II or desoxycorticosterone acetate. Furthermore, adoptive transfer of

T-cells to Rag1$^{-/-}$ mice restores this hypertensive response[88], suggesting a prominent role of T-cells.

Angiotensin-II (Ang-II), commonly implicated in hypertension, can stimulate Th1 expansion during hypertension[89]. Increased Ang-II levels correlate to increased IFNγ expression, which in turn correlates to Ang-II-induced cardiac fibrosis and subsequent remodeling[89]. The frequency of Th1 cells is significantly increased in hypertensive patients, especially in those with non-dipper hypertension (those whose nocturnal blood pressure is within 10% of their daytime blood pressure) compared to those with dipper hypertension (those whose nocturnal blood pressure is at least 10% lower than their daytime blood pressure)[90]. The presence of carotid atherosclerotic plaques exacerbates this increase in Th1 levels[90]. Furthermore, increased expression of IFNγ and TNFα, which are typical of a Th1 effector response, is associated with increased vascular inflammation, dysfunction, and elevated blood pressure[91]. Levels of these cytokines are significantly increased in hypertensive patients[92], and the Th1 response is ameliorated by both IFNγ deficiency and administration of a TNFα antagonist, as indicated by reduced blood pressure in animal models of hypertension[93,94]. If Th1 effector responses are induced by external means, such as infection, hypertensive symptoms may also be exacerbated[91], suggesting an important link between the Th1 T-cells and the pathophysiology of this disease.

In addition to increased Th1 levels, hypertension is also associated with decreased Th2 levels and increased Th17 levels, as indicated by increased IFNγ, decreased IL-4, and increased IL-17 levels. These changes reflect a predominantly pro-inflammatory phenotype and skewed Th1/Th2 ratio (Figure 2.2). Th1, Th2, and Th17 levels are not affected by the administration of common hypertension medications, such as angiotensin-converting enzyme (ACE) inhibitors, angiotensin receptor blockers (ARBs), β-blockers, or calcium channel blockers (CCBs), but diuretic medications are associated with lower Th2 levels and higher Th17 levels[90]. It has been shown that the levels of circulating Th2 T-cells are lower in hypertensive patients than in non-hypertensive patients[90]. This effect is more pronounced in "non-dippers,"[90] significantly altering the overall Th1/Th2 T-cell balance in hypertensive patients[90]. However, the specific role that Th2 T-cells play in hypertension remains poorly understood. When we examine the effects of IL-4, the signature Th2 cytokine, on hypertension, we find a lot of conflicting evidence. Some clinical studies have found an increase in IL-4, while others have observed no change or significant decreases in IL-4 in hypertensive patients[90]. Studies with mouse models have also given indeterminate results. For example, Dicky et al. found that anti-IL-4 treatment of hypertensive mice resulted in decreased blood pressure[95]. However, another study, by Chatterjee et al., found that the administration of exogenous IL-4 resulted in reduced blood pressure[96]. Although increased IL-4 and Th2 T-cells have been shown to be protective against heart disease in healthy individuals, the conflicting evidence regarding IL-4 illustrates the need for detailed analysis of the effect of Th2 T-cells in different types of hypertension using more standardized protocols that closely mimic the pathophysiology of this disease in humans.

Pro-inflammatory cytokine IL-17 is one of the first known and best-characterized cytokines with respect to hypertension, and it plays an essential role in hypertensive autoimmune diseases and endothelial dysfunction[97]. Nguyen et al. showed that IL-17 promotes the development of systolic hypertension by increasing RhoA expression and eNOS Thr495 phosphorylation, thus decreasing aortic nitric oxide (NO)-dependent relaxation responses[97]. Guzik et al. demonstrated that the effects of angiotensin-II infusion and/or desoxycorticosterone acetate (DOCA) salt induced hypertension were diminished in RAG1[-/-] mice that lack T- and B-cells, whereas adoptive transfer of T- but not B-cells reinstated these effects[98]. Furthermore, to evaluate the effect of IL-17 on blood pressure and vascular function, Madhur et al. studied hypertensive response to angiotensin-II infusion in IL-17[-/-] mice[99]. Interestingly, the initial hypertensive response to angiotensin-II infusion was similar in IL-17[-/-] and C57BL/6J mice, but hypertension was not sustained in IL-17[-/-] mice, reaching levels 30 mmHg lower than those of wild-type mice by 4 weeks of angiotensin-II infusion. Moreover, vessels from IL-17[-/-] mice exhibited not only well-preserved vascular function and decreased superoxide production but also reduced aortic T-cell infiltration in response to angiotensin-II[99], suggesting an important pro-hypertensive role of IL-17 and Th17 T-cells.

Given the role of vascular inflammation in hypertension, Tregs play an important protective role in its pathogenesis. Studies in rodent models have shown that decreased Treg levels, as well as their dysfunction due to decreased Foxp3 expression, contribute to endothelial dysfunction and mediate vascular inflammation during hypertension[100]. Preclinical studies have also shown that adoptive transfer of immunocompetent Tregs to mice treated with either aldosterone[101] or Ang-II[102] attenuates progressive increase in BP and improves relaxation of the vascular endothelium. Some other studies have also suggested that adoptively transferred Tregs predominantly act by ameliorating LV remodeling (hypertrophy and fibrosis) and by improving electrical coupling without any direct effects on the SBP[86]. This is also consistent with the fact that depletion of Tregs from Ang-II-infused mice does not affect increased BP, suggesting that the protective effects of adoptively transferred Tregs in ameliorating hypertension are probably mediated through their effects on suppressing vascular inflammation and not BP[103]. Despite these discrepancies, it is clear that suppression of tissue inflammation by adoptive transfer of competent Tregs can blunt high BP-induced end organ damage and can provide significant clinical benefits in ameliorating renal damage[102].

T-CELLS IN MYOCARDITIS

Myocarditis is one of the principal reasons for HF in young patients and represents one of the most challenging clinical problems due to the absence of a precise diagnosis and effective therapy. It is characterized by the failure of tolerance against cardiac antigens and further signifies as a polymorphic, frequently infection-tripped, and immune-mediated inflammation of the heart[104]. Inflammation in the myocardium is one of the characteristic features and can be autoimmune in nature or caused by pathogens such as bacteria and viruses. While viral infection of the heart is considered a critical factor in acute myocarditis, chronic myocarditis often occurs after damage to cardiomyocytes and exposure of cardiac myosin, a potent autoantigen, and other cardiac proteins[104,105]. This exposure of cardiac myosin and other heart proteins alters the immune response in susceptible individuals and leads to autoimmunity[106–108]. However, autoimmune myocarditis has also been observed in patients with no evidence of viral infection. Loss of tolerance to α-myosin heavy-chain protein (αMyHC) has long been implicated in the progression of myocarditis. However, recent studies have shown that only a small amount (around 7%) of αMyHC is present in the human hearts[109], suggesting that the loss of this tolerance could be due to its decreased expression in the medullary thymic epithelial and lymphoid stromal cells[110]. This is further complicated by the fact that, during end-stage HF, cardiac αMyHC levels are known to decrease by ~15-fold[109] and are increased in systemic circulation during cell necrosis[111], suggesting its potential to antigenically activate CD4+ T-cells.

Whether myocarditis is autoimmune in nature or virally induced, Th1 T-cells have a significant role in its pathogenesis and progression to dilated cardiomyopathy[110]. T-cells that exhibit loss of tolerance to αMyHC predominantly secrete IFNγ and TNFα, suggesting that the loss of tolerance is mainly found in Th1 cells and that Th1 effector responses are primarily responsible for T-cell-mediated inflammatory cascades seen during autoimmune myocarditis. Although Th1 T-cells are involved in inflammation in myocarditis, not all Th1 cytokines exert the same effects during disease progression. For example, dilated cardiomyopathy (DCM) is associated with increased IL-2, IFNγ, and IL-12[112]; however, while IL-12 promotes disease progression, IFNγ has, interestingly, been found to be protective. IFNγ deficiency in animal models of autoimmune myocarditis leads to more severe cardiac dysfunction and progression to dilated cardiomyopathy and heart failure[71]. It has been shown that the IFNγ gene axis is essential for CD25 (part of the IL-2 receptor) expression[71], and a deficiency in IFNγ results in the expansion of antigenically activated CD4+CD44highCD25− T-cells and their transmigration into the heart[71]. Decreased expression of CD25 in T-cells also impairs apoptosis of activated T-cells, thus increasing the probability of progression to dilated cardiomyopathy[71].

Due to its anti-inflammatory nature and antagonism of Th1 responses, IL-4 deficiency results in the worsening of symptoms, suggesting a protective role of Th2 T-cells in the context of infectious myocarditis[113] (Figure 2.2). However, Th2 responses can lead to worse outcomes if the cause of inflammation is not mediated by pathogens. For example, in acute eosinophilic myocarditis, an anti-allergic Th2 cytokine inhibitor significantly reduced inflammation and ameliorated the disease[113] by blunting Th2-mediated eosinophilic expansion[113]. Due to these differences in disease etiologies, Th2 T-cells are considered protective during infectious myocarditis and pathological during autoimmune myocarditis.

While IFNγ is implicated in the initial stages of myocarditis, it has also been shown that the progression of myocarditis to dilated cardiomyopathy is more dependent upon IL-17 production; that is, disease initiation is dependent upon Th1 effector responses, but disease progression is dependent upon concurrent Th17 effector responses[114]. Studies by Yuan et al. in BALB/c mice infected with coxsackievirus B3 found a significant increase in splenic Th17 cells, serum IL-17, and cardiac IL-17 associated with viral replication and gradual cardiac damage[115]. In another study, Yan et al. studied the role of microRNA-155, a central regulator of the immune system, in experimental autoimmune myocarditis, which is characterized by cardiac inflammatory disease propelled by autoantigen-specific CD4+ T-cells[116]. They showed that miR-155 adversely affects experimental autoimmune myocarditis by driving a Th17/Treg imbalance in favor of Th17 cells and concluded that anti-miR-155 management can considerably ameliorate autoimmune response[116]. Studies in rodents have also shown that the therapeutic effects of bazedoxifene and valproic acid in myocarditis are partly derived by alteration of Th17 cells[117,118]. While bazedoxifene blunts Th17 polarization by inhibiting STAT3[117], valproic acid improves coxsackievirus B3–induced viral myocarditis by modulating Th17/Treg imbalance[118]. Largely, the immunopathogenesis role of Th17 cells in facilitating myocarditis has been investigated in recent studies, and the barricade of IL-17- and/or IL-17-stimulated pathways may provide a new therapeutic approach for its treatment.

Given the fact that Tregs exert effects opposite to those of Th17 T-cells, they exert significantly protective effects in both viral[119] and auto-immune myocarditis[120]. Preclinical studies in rodents have shown that Tregs restrain overt immune responses during viral[119] and autoimmune myocarditis[121] and promote cardiac antiviral immunity by the TGF-β receptor pathway[122]. This is also consistent with the findings showing aggravated myocarditis upon the administration of endothelin antagonists that reduce Tregs in the heart[123].

CONCLUSIONS

CD4+ T-cells are pivotal in several CVDs, and they directly or indirectly mediate autoimmune end organ damage and tissue remodeling. Through direct cell-cell interaction or through cytokines and chemokines, CD4+ T-cells have the potential to significantly alter the inflammatory milieu to promote both healing and blunt innate immune responses or to promote pathological tissue remodeling upon chronic activation. Undoubtedly, by using preclinical rodent models, we have learned a great deal regarding the role of CD4+ T-cells in CVDs; however, their translation into the clinic to understand the pathophysiology of human CVDs is still in its infancy. Despite this, it is clear that targeting of pathological T-cells could provide novel therapeutic avenues for several CVDs. It is, thus, critical to ascertain temporal phenotypic changes in T-cells to identify targetable signaling mechanisms, in order to blunt autoimmune T-cell activation while sparing tissue-protective responses.

ACKNOWLEDGMENTS

This work was supported by National Heart, Lung, and Blood Institute of the National Institutes of Health (NIH) grants (R00 HL132123 and R01HL153164) to SSB. VK and RR are supported (partly) by funds provided by the Drug Development Institute at The Ohio State University. Funding sources did not influence any part of this work.

ABBREVIATIONS

TCR: T-cell receptor; LV: left ventricle; MI: myocardial infarction; HF: heart failure; IFN: interferon; IL: interleukin; Treg: regulatory T-cell; APC: antigen-presenting cell; MHC: major histocompatibility complex; CVB3: coxsackievirus B3; STAT:

signal transducer and activator of transcription; ECM: extracellular matrix; DCM: dilated cardiomyopathy; TAC: transverse aortic constriction; EAM: experimental autoimmune myocarditis; MMP: matrix metalloproteinase; Ang-II: angiotensin-II; nTreg: natural regulatory T-cell; iTreg: induced regulatory T-cell; PD: programmed cell death; NK: natural killer; iNKT: invariant natural killer T-cell; ACE: angiotensin-converting enzyme; ApoE: apolipoprotein E gene; ARBs: angiotensin receptor blockers; BP: blood pressure; CAD: coronary artery disease; CCBs: calcium channel blockers; CD: cluster of differentiation; CVD: cardiovascular disease; DAMP: damage-associated molecular patterns; DC: dendritic cells; Foxp3: forkhead box P3; GATA: recognizing the DNA consensus sequence (A/T)GATA(A/G); IRF-4: interferon regulatory factor-4; PBMC: peripheral blood mononuclear cell; RAG1: recombination activating gene-1; RORγt: retineic acid receptor–related orphan nuclear receptor gamma in Th17-cells; STEMI: ST segment elevation myocardial infarction; T-bet: T-box expressed in T-cells; TGF-β: transforming growth factor-β.

BIBLIOGRAPHY

1. Goettsch C, Kjolby M, Aikawa E. Sortilin and its multiple roles in cardiovascular and metabolic diseases. *Arterioscler Thromb Vasc Biol.* 2018;38:19–25
2. Greenfield DM, Snowden JA. Cardiovascular diseases and metabolic syndrome. In: Carreras E, Dufour C, Mohty M, Kroger N, eds. *The EBMT handbook: Hematopoietic stem cell transplantation and cellular therapies.* Cham (CH); 2019:415–420
3. Nehra S, Gumina RJ, Bansal SS. Immune cell dilemma in ischemic cardiomyopathy: To heal or not to heal. *Curr Opin Physiol.* 2021;19:39–46
4. Rosenzweig R, Gupta S, Kumar V, Gumina RJ, Bansal SS. Estrogenic bias in t-lymphocyte biology: Implications for cardiovascular disease. *Pharmacol Res.* 2021;170:105606
5. Adamo L, Rocha-Resende C, Prabhu SD, Mann DL. Reappraising the role of inflammation in heart failure. *Nat Rev Cardiol.* 2020;17:269–285
6. Ngwenyama N, Kirabo A, Aronovitz M, Velazquez F, Carrillo-Salinas F, Salvador AM, Nevers T, Amarnath V, Tai A, Blanton RM, Harrison DG, Alcaide P. Isolevuglandin-modified cardiac proteins drive CD4+ T-cell activation in the heart and promote cardiac dysfunction. *Circulation.* 2021;143:1242–1255
7. Bansal SS, Ismahil MA, Goel M, Patel B, Hamid T, Rokosh G, Prabhu SD. Activated t lymphocytes are essential drivers of pathological remodeling in ischemic heart failure. *Circ Heart Fail.* 2017;10:e003688
8. Itani HA, McMaster WG, Jr., Saleh MA, Nazarewicz RR, Mikolajczyk TP, Kaszuba AM, Konior A, Prejbisz A, Januszewicz A, Norlander AE, Chen W, Bonami RH, Marshall AF, Poffenberger G, Weyand CM, Madhur MS, Moore DJ, Harrison DG, Guzik TJ. Activation of human T cells in hypertension: Studies of humanized mice and hypertensive humans. *Hypertension.* 2016;68:123–132
9. Wakim LM, Bevan MJ. From the thymus to longevity in the periphery. *Curr Opin Immunol.* 2010;22:274–278
10. Zhu J, Paul WE. CD4 T cells: Fates, functions, and faults. *Blood.* 2008;112:1557–1569
11. Huang J, Meyer C, Zhu C. T cell antigen recognition at the cell membrane. *Mol Immunol.* 2012;52:155–164
12. Kambayashi T, Laufer TM. Atypical mhc class ii-expressing antigen-presenting cells: Can anything replace a dendritic cell? *Nat Rev Immunol.* 2014;14:719–730
13. Pennock ND, White JT, Cross EW, Cheney EE, Tamburini BA, Kedl RM. T cell responses: Naive to memory and everything in between. *Adv Physiol Educ.* 2013;37:273–283

14. Raphael I, Nalawade S, Eagar TN, Forsthuber TG. T cell subsets and their signature cytokines in autoimmune and inflammatory diseases. *Cytokine*. 2015;74:5–17
15. Paul WE, Seder RA. Lymphocyte responses and cytokines. *Cell*. 1994;76:241–251
16. Mosmann TR, Coffman RL. Th1 and th2 cells: Different patterns of lymphokine secretion lead to different functional properties. *Annu Rev Immunol*. 1989;7:145–173
17. Weaver CT, Harrington LE, Mangan PR, Gavrieli M, Murphy KM. Th17: An effector CD4 T cell lineage with regulatory T cell ties. *Immunity*. 2006;24:677–688
18. Sakaguchi S. Naturally arising CD4+ regulatory T cells for immunologic self-tolerance and negative control of immune responses. *Annu Rev Immunol*. 2004;22:531–562
19. Cherwinski HM, Schumacher JH, Brown KD, Mosmann TR. Two types of mouse helper T cell clone. Iii. Further differences in lymphokine synthesis between th1 and th2 clones revealed by rna hybridization, functionally monospecific bioassays, and monoclonal antibodies. *J Exp Med*. 1987;166:1229–1244
20. Mosmann TR, Cherwinski H, Bond MW, Giedlin MA, Coffman RL. Two types of murine helper T cell clone. I. Definition according to profiles of lymphokine activities and secreted proteins. *J Immunol*. 1986;136:2348–2357
21. Whitman SC, Ravisankar P, Elam H, Daugherty A. Exogenous interferon-gamma enhances atherosclerosis in apolipoprotein e-/- mice. *Am J Pathol*. 2000;157:1819–1824
22. Casson CN, Doerner JL, Copenhaver AM, Ramirez J, Holmgren AM, Boyer MA, Siddarthan IJ, Rouhanifard SH, Raj A, Shin S. Neutrophils and ly6chi monocytes collaborate in generating an optimal cytokine response that protects against pulmonary legionella pneumophila infection. *PLoS Pathog*. 2017;13:e1006309
23. Manetti R, Parronchi P, Giudizi MG, Piccinni MP, Maggi E, Trinchieri G, Romagnani S. Natural killer cell stimulatory factor (interleukin 12 [il-12]) induces t helper type 1 (th1)-specific immune responses and inhibits the development of il-4-producing th cells. *J Exp Med*. 1993;177:1199–1204
24. Okamura H, Tsutsi H, Komatsu T, Yutsudo M, Hakura A, Tanimoto T, Torigoe K, Okura T, Nukada Y, Hattori K, et al. Cloning of a new cytokine that induces ifn-gamma production by T cells. *Nature*. 1995;378:88–91
25. Blanton RM, Carrillo-Salinas FJ, Alcaide P. T-cell recruitment to the heart: Friendly guests or unwelcome visitors? *Am J Physiol Heart Circ Physiol*. 2019;317: H124–H140
26. Weaver CT, Hatton RD, Mangan PR, Harrington LE. Il-17 family cytokines and the expanding diversity of effector T cell lineages. *Annu Rev Immunol*. 2007;25:821–852
27. Tesmer LA, Lundy SK, Sarkar S, Fox DA. Th17 cells in human disease. *Immunol Rev*. 2008;223:87–113
28. Littman DR, Rudensky AY. Th17 and regulatory T cells in mediating and restraining inflammation. *Cell*. 2010;140:845–858
29. Park H, Li Z, Yang XO, Chang SH, Nurieva R, Wang YH, Wang Y, Hood L, Zhu Z, Tian Q, Dong C. A distinct lineage of CD4 T cells regulates tissue inflammation by producing interleukin 17. *Nat Immunol*. 2005;6:1133–1141
30. Onishi RM, Gaffen SL. Interleukin-17 and its target genes: Mechanisms of interleukin-17 function in disease. *Immunology*. 2010;129:311–321
31. Romano M, Fanelli G, Albany CJ, Giganti G, Lombardi G. Past, present, and future of regulatory T cell therapy in transplantation and autoimmunity. *Front Immunol*. 2019;10:43
32. Rodriguez-Perea AL, Arcia ED, Rueda CM, Velilla PA. Phenotypical characterization of regulatory T cells in humans and rodents. *Clin Exp Immunol*. 2016;185:281–291
33. Vignali DA, Collison LW, Workman CJ. How regulatory T cells work. *Nat Rev Immunol*. 2008;8:523–532

34. Feuerer M, Herrero L, Cipolletta D, Naaz A, Wong J, Nayer A, Lee J, Goldfine AB, Benoist C, Shoelson S, Mathis D. Lean, but not obese, fat is enriched for a unique population of regulatory T cells that affect metabolic parameters. *Nat Med.* 2009;15:930–939

35. Burzyn D, Kuswanto W, Kolodin D, Shadrach JL, Cerletti M, Jang Y, Sefik E, Tan TG, Wagers AJ, Benoist C, Mathis D. A special population of regulatory T cells potentiates muscle repair. *Cell.* 2013;155:1282–1295

36. Hegazy AN, Powrie F. Microbiome. Microbiota rorgulates intestinal suppressor T cells. *Science.* 2015;349:929–930

37. Zhuang R, Feinberg MW. Regulatory T cells in ischemic cardiovascular injury and repair. *J Mol Cell Cardiol.* 2020;147:1–11

38. Taleb S, Tedgui A, Mallat Z. Interleukin-17: Friend or foe in atherosclerosis? *Curr Opin Lipidol.* 2010;21:404–408

39. Taleb S, Tedgui A, Mallat Z. Il-17 and th17 cells in atherosclerosis: Subtle and contextual roles. *Arterioscler Thromb Vasc Biol.* 2015;35:258–264

40. Davenport P, Tipping PG. The role of interleukin-4 and interleukin-12 in the progression of atherosclerosis in apolipoprotein e-deficient mice. *Am J Pathol.* 2003;163:1117–1125

41. Frostegard J, Ulfgren AK, Nyberg P, Hedin U, Swedenborg J, Andersson U, Hansson GK. Cytokine expression in advanced human atherosclerotic plaques: Dominance of pro-inflammatory (th1) and macrophage-stimulating cytokines. *Atherosclerosis.* 1999;145:33–43

42. Gupta S, Pablo AM, Jiang X, Wang N, Tall AR, Schindler C. Ifn-gamma potentiates atherosclerosis in apoe knock-out mice. *J Clin Invest.* 1997;99:2752–2761

43. Wang Y, Bai Y, Qin L, Zhang P, Yi T, Teesdale SA, Zhao L, Pober JS, Tellides G. Interferon-gamma induces human vascular smooth muscle cell proliferation and intimal expansion by phosphatidylinositol 3-kinase dependent mammalian target of rapamycin raptor complex 1 activation. *Circ Res.* 2007;101:560–569

44. Buono C, Binder CJ, Stavrakis G, Witztum JL, Glimcher LH, Lichtman AH. T-bet deficiency reduces atherosclerosis and alters plaque antigen-specific immune responses. *Proc Natl Acad Sci U S A.* 2005;102:1596–1601

45. Mallat Z, Corbaz A, Scoazec A, Besnard S, Leseche G, Chvatchko Y, Tedgui A. Expression of interleukin-18 in human atherosclerotic plaques and relation to plaque instability. *Circulation.* 2001;104:1598–1603

46. Elhage R, Jawien J, Rudling M, Ljunggren HG, Takeda K, Akira S, Bayard F, Hansson GK. Reduced atherosclerosis in interleukin-18 deficient apolipoprotein e-knockout mice. *Cardiovasc Res.* 2003;59:234–240

47. Butcher MJ, Filipowicz AR, Waseem TC, McGary CM, Crow KJ, Magilnick N, Boldin M, Lundberg PS, Galkina EV. Atherosclerosis-driven treg plasticity results in formation of a dysfunctional subset of plastic ifngamma+ th1/tregs. *Circ Res.* 2016;119:1190–1203

48. Mallat Z, Taleb S, Ait-Oufella H, Tedgui A. The role of adaptive T cell immunity in atherosclerosis. *J Lipid Res.* 2009;50 Suppl:S364–369

49. Chistiakov DA, Bobryshev YV, Orekhov AN. Macrophage-mediated cholesterol handling in atherosclerosis. *J Cell Mol Med.* 2016;20:17–28

50. Ramani K, Biswas PS. Interleukin-17: Friend or foe in organ fibrosis. *Cytokine.* 2019;120:282–288

51. Smith E, Prasad KM, Butcher M, Dobrian A, Kolls JK, Ley K, Galkina E. Blockade of interleukin-17a results in reduced atherosclerosis in apolipoprotein e-deficient mice. *Circulation.* 2010;121:1746–1755

52. Erbel C, Chen L, Bea F, Wangler S, Celik S, Lasitschka F, Wang Y, Bockler D, Katus HA, Dengler TJ. Inhibition of il-17a attenuates atherosclerotic lesion development in apoe-deficient mice. *J Immunol.* 2009;183:8167–8175

53. Mor A, Planer D, Luboshits G, Afek A, Metzger S, Chajek-Shaul T, Keren G, George J. Role of naturally occurring CD4+ CD25+ regulatory T cells in experimental atherosclerosis. *Arterioscler Thromb Vasc Biol.* 2007;27:893–900

54. Mor A, Luboshits G, Planer D, Keren G, George J. Altered status of CD4(+)CD25(+) regulatory T cells in patients with acute coronary syndromes. *Eur Heart J.* 2006;27:2530–2537

55. Liu ZD, Wang L, Lu FH, Pan H, Zhao YX, Wang SJ, Sun SW, Li CL, Hu XL. Increased th17 cell frequency concomitant with decreased foxp3+ treg cell frequency in the peripheral circulation of patients with carotid artery plaques. *Inflamm Res.* 2012;61:1155–1165

56. Han SF, Liu P, Zhang W, Bu L, Shen M, Li H, Fan YH, Cheng K, Cheng HX, Li CX, Jia GL. The opposite-direction modulation of CD4+CD25+ tregs and t helper 1 cells in acute coronary syndromes. *Clin Immunol.* 2007;124:90–97

57. Ait-Oufella H, Salomon BL, Potteaux S, Robertson AK, Gourdy P, Zoll J, Merval R, Esposito B, Cohen JL, Fisson S, Flavell RA, Hansson GK, Klatzmann D, Tedgui A, Mallat Z. Natural regulatory T cells control the development of atherosclerosis in mice. *Nat Med.* 2006;12:178–180

58. Klingenberg R, Gerdes N, Badeau RM, Gistera A, Strodthoff D, Ketelhuth DF, Lundberg AM, Rudling M, Nilsson SK, Olivecrona G, Zoller S, Lohmann C, Luscher TF, Jauhiainen M, Sparwasser T, Hansson GK. Depletion of foxp3+ regulatory T cells promotes hypercholesterolemia and atherosclerosis. *J Clin Invest.* 2013;123:1323–1334

59. Polansky JK, Kretschmer K, Freyer J, Floess S, Garbe A, Baron U, Olek S, Hamann A, von Boehmer H, Huehn J. DNA methylation controls foxp3 gene expression. *Eur J Immunol.* 2008;38:1654–1663

60. Onuora S. Immunology: Metabolic changes modify treg cell function. *Nat Rev Rheumatol.* 2016;12:621

61. Pierson W, Cauwe B, Policheni A, Schlenner SM, Franckaert D, Berges J, Humblet-Baron S, Schonefeldt S, Herold MJ, Hildeman D, Strasser A, Bouillet P, Lu LF, Matthys P, Freitas AA, Luther RJ, Weaver CT, Dooley J, Gray DH, Liston A. Antiapoptotic mcl-1 is critical for the survival and niche-filling capacity of foxp3(+) regulatory T cells. *Nat Immunol.* 2013;14:959–965

62. Tiemessen MM, Jagger AL, Evans HG, van Herwijnen MJ, John S, Taams LS. CD4+CD25+FOXP3+ regulatory T cells induce alternative activation of human monocytes/macrophages. *Proc Natl Acad Sci U S A.* 2007;104:19446–19451

63. Lin J, Li M, Wang Z, He S, Ma X, Li D. The role of CD4+CD25+ regulatory T cells in macrophage-derived foam-cell formation. *J Lipid Res.* 2010;51:1208–1217

64. Qureshi OS, Zheng Y, Nakamura K, Attridge K, Manzotti C, Schmidt EM, Baker J, Jeffery LE, Kaur S, Briggs Z, Hou TZ, Futter CE, Anderson G, Walker LS, Sansom DM. Trans-endocytosis of CD80 and CD86: A molecular basis for the cell-extrinsic function of CTLA-4. *Science.* 2011;332:600–603

65. Mora-Ruiz MD, Blanco-Favela F, Chavez Rueda AK, Legorreta-Haquet MV, Chavez-Sanchez L. Role of interleukin-17 in acute myocardial infarction. *Mol Immunol.* 2019;107:71–78

66. Hofmann U, Beyersdorf N, Weirather J, Podolskaya A, Bauersachs J, Ertl G, Kerkau T, Frantz S. Activation of CD4+ t lymphocytes improves wound healing and survival after experimental myocardial infarction in mice. *Circulation.* 2012;125:1652–1663

67. Yan X, Anzai A, Katsumata Y, Matsuhashi T, Ito K, Endo J, Yamamoto T, Takeshima A, Shinmura K, Shen W, Fukuda K, Sano M. Temporal dynamics of cardiac immune cell accumulation following acute myocardial infarction. *J Mol Cell Cardiol.* 2013;62:24–35

68. Yan X, Zhang H, Fan Q, Hu J, Tao R, Chen Q, Iwakura Y, Shen W, Lu L, Zhang Q, Zhang R. Dectin-2 deficiency modulates th1 differentiation and improves wound healing after myocardial infarction. *Circ Res.* 2017;120:1116–1129

69. Warren SG, Barnett JC. Guiding catheter exchange during coronary angioplasty. *Cathet Cardiovasc Diagn*. 1990;20:212–215
70. Li C, Zong W, Zhang M, Tu Y, Zhou Q, Ni M, Li Z, Liu H, Zhang J. Increased ratio of circulating t-helper 1 to t-helper 2 cells and severity of coronary artery disease in patients with acute myocardial infarction: A prospective observational study. *Med Sci Monit*. 2019;25:6034–6042
71. Afanasyeva M, Georgakopoulos D, Belardi DF, Bedja D, Fairweather D, Wang Y, Kaya Z, Gabrielson KL, Rodriguez ER, Caturegli P, Kass DA, Rose NR. Impaired up-regulation of CD25 on CD4+ T cells in ifn-gamma knockout mice is associated with progression of myocarditis to heart failure. *Proc Natl Acad Sci U S A*. 2005;102:180–185
72. Laroumanie F, Douin-Echinard V, Pozzo J, Lairez O, Tortosa F, Vinel C, Delage C, Calise D, Dutaur M, Parini A, Pizzinat N. CD4+ T cells promote the transition from hypertrophy to heart failure during chronic pressure overload. *Circulation*. 2014;129:2111–2124
73. Nevers T, Salvador AM, Velazquez F, Ngwenyama N, Carrillo-Salinas FJ, Aronovitz M, Blanton RM, Alcaide P. Th1 effector T cells selectively orchestrate cardiac fibrosis in nonischemic heart failure. *J Exp Med*. 2017;214:3311–3329
74. Cai YH, Ma ZJ, Lu XY, He EL, You MY. Study on the effect and mechanism of the dysfunction of CD4(+) T cells in the disease process of chronic cardiac failure. *Asian Pac J Trop Med*. 2016;9:682–687
75. Fukunaga T, Soejima H, Irie A, Sugamura K, Oe Y, Tanaka T, Kojima S, Sakamoto T, Yoshimura M, Nishimura Y, Ogawa H. Expression of interferon-gamma and interleukin-4 production in CD4+ T cells in patients with chronic heart failure. *Heart Vessels*. 2007;22:178–183
76. Satoh S, Oyama J, Suematsu N, Kadokami T, Shimoyama N, Okutsu M, Inoue T, Sugano M, Makino N. Increased productivity of tumor necrosis factor-alpha in helper T cells in patients with systolic heart failure. *Int J Cardiol*. 2006;111:405–412
77. Cheng X, Yu X, Ding YJ, Fu QQ, Xie JJ, Tang TT, Yao R, Chen Y, Liao YH. The th17/treg imbalance in patients with acute coronary syndrome. *Clin Immunol*. 2008;127:89–97
78. Garza-Reyes MG, Mora-Ruiz MD, Chavez-Sanchez L, Madrid-Miller A, Cabrera-Quintero AJ, Maravillas-Montero JL, Zentella-Dehesa A, Moreno-Ruiz L, Pastor-Salgado S, Ramirez-Arias E, Perez-Velazquez N, Chavez-Rueda AK, Blanco-Favela F, Vazquez-Gonzalez WG, Contreras-Rodriguez A. Effect of interleukin-17 in the activation of monocyte subsets in patients with st-segment elevation myocardial infarction. *J Immunol Res*. 2020;2020:5692829
79. Simon T, Taleb S, Danchin N, Laurans L, Rousseau B, Cattan S, Montely JM, Dubourg O, Tedgui A, Kotti S, Mallat Z. Circulating levels of interleukin-17 and cardiovascular outcomes in patients with acute myocardial infarction. *Eur Heart J*. 2013;34:570–577
80. Zhou SF, Yuan J, Liao MY, Xia N, Tang TT, Li JJ, Jiao J, Dong WY, Nie SF, Zhu ZF, Zhang WC, Lv BJ, Xiao H, Wang Q, Tu X, Liao YH, Shi GP, Cheng X. Il-17a promotes ventricular remodeling after myocardial infarction. *J Mol Med (Berl)*. 2014;92:1105–1116
81. Chang HY, Li X, Tian Y. Telmisartan reduces arrhythmias through increasing cardiac connexin43 by inhibiting il-17 after myocardial infarction in rats. *Eur Rev Med Pharmacol Sci*. 2017;21:5283–5289
82. Bansal SS, Ismahil MA, Goel M, Zhou G, Rokosh G, Hamid T, Prabhu SD. Dysfunctional and proinflammatory regulatory t-lymphocytes are essential for adverse cardiac remodeling in ischemic cardiomyopathy. *Circulation*. 2019;139:206–221
83. Saxena A, Dobaczewski M, Rai V, Haque Z, Chen W, Li N, Frangogiannis NG. Regulatory T cells are recruited in the infarcted mouse myocardium and may modulate fibroblast phenotype and function. *Am J Physiol Heart Circ Physiol*. 2014;307:H1233–1242

84. Weirather J, Hofmann UD, Beyersdorf N, Ramos GC, Vogel B, Frey A, Ertl G, Kerkau T, Frantz S. Foxp3+ CD4+ T cells improve healing after myocardial infarction by modulating monocyte/macrophage differentiation. *Circ Res.* 2014;115:55–67

85. Zeng Z, Yu K, Chen L, Li W, Xiao H, Huang Z. Interleukin-2/anti-interleukin-2 immune complex attenuates cardiac remodeling after myocardial infarction through expansion of regulatory T cells. *J Immunol Res.* 2016;2016:8493767

86. Kvakan H, Kleinewietfeld M, Qadri F, Park JK, Fischer R, Schwarz I, Rahn HP, Plehm R, Wellner M, Elitok S, Gratze P, Dechend R, Luft FC, Muller DN. Regulatory T cells ameliorate angiotensin ii-induced cardiac damage. *Circulation.* 2009;119:2904–2912

87. Ren J, Crowley SD. Role of t-cell activation in salt-sensitive hypertension. *Am J Physiol Heart Circ Physiol.* 2019;316:H1345-H1353

88. Mikolajczyk TP, Guzik TJ. Adaptive immunity in hypertension. *Curr Hypertens Rep.* 2019;21:68

89. Han YL, Li YL, Jia LX, Cheng JZ, Qi YF, Zhang HJ, Du J. Reciprocal interaction between macrophages and T cells stimulates ifn-gamma and mcp-1 production in ang ii-induced cardiac inflammation and fibrosis. *PLoS One.* 2012;7:e35506

90. Ji Q, Cheng G, Ma N, Huang Y, Lin Y, Zhou Q, Que B, Dong J, Zhou Y, Nie S. Circulating th1, th2, and th17 levels in hypertensive patients. *Dis Markers.* 2017;2017:7146290

91. Czesnikiewicz-Guzik M, Nosalski R, Mikolajczyk TP, Vidler F, Dohnal T, Dembowska E, Graham D, Harrison DG, Guzik TJ. Th1-type immune responses to porphyromonas gingivalis antigens exacerbate angiotensin ii-dependent hypertension and vascular dysfunction. *Br J Pharmacol.* 2019;176:1922–1931

92. Mirhafez SR, Mohebati M, Feiz Disfani M, Saberi Karimian M, Ebrahimi M, Avan A, Eslami S, Pasdar A, Rooki H, Esmaeili H, Ferns GA, Ghayour-Mobarhan M. An imbalance in serum concentrations of inflammatory and anti-inflammatory cytokines in hypertension. *J Am Soc Hypertens.* 2014;8:614–623

93. Kamat NV, Thabet SR, Xiao L, Saleh MA, Kirabo A, Madhur MS, Delpire E, Harrison DG, McDonough AA. Renal transporter activation during angiotensin-ii hypertension is blunted in interferon-gamma-/- and interleukin-17a-/- mice. *Hypertension.* 2015;65:569–576

94. Elmarakby AA, Quigley JE, Pollock DM, Imig JD. Tumor necrosis factor alpha blockade increases renal cyp2c23 expression and slows the progression of renal damage in salt-sensitive hypertension. *Hypertension.* 2006;47:557–562

95. van Heuven-Nolsen D, De Kimpe SJ, Muis T, van Ark I, Savelkoul H, Beems RB, van Oosterhout AJ, Nijkamp FP. Opposite role of interferon-gamma and interleukin-4 on the regulation of blood pressure in mice. *Biochem Biophys Res Commun.* 1999;254:816–820

96. Chatterjee P, Chiasson VL, Seerangan G, Tobin RP, Kopriva SE, Newell-Rogers MK, Mitchell BM. Cotreatment with interleukin 4 and interleukin 10 modulates immune cells and prevents hypertension in pregnant mice. *Am J Hypertens.* 2015;28:135–142

97. Nguyen H, Chiasson VL, Chatterjee P, Kopriva SE, Young KJ, Mitchell BM. Interleukin-17 causes rho-kinase-mediated endothelial dysfunction and hypertension. *Cardiovasc Res.* 2013;97:696–704

98. Guzik TJ, Hoch NE, Brown KA, McCann LA, Rahman A, Dikalov S, Goronzy J, Weyand C, Harrison DG. Role of the T cell in the genesis of angiotensin ii induced hypertension and vascular dysfunction. *J Exp Med.* 2007;204:2449–2460

99. Madhur MS, Lob HE, McCann LA, Iwakura Y, Blinder Y, Guzik TJ, Harrison DG. Interleukin 17 promotes angiotensin ii-induced hypertension and vascular dysfunction. *Hypertension.* 2010;55:500–507

100. Meng X, Yang J, Dong M, Zhang K, Tu E, Gao Q, Chen W, Zhang C, Zhang Y. Regulatory T cells in cardiovascular diseases. *Nat Rev Cardiol.* 2016;13:167–179

101. Kasal DA, Barhoumi T, Li MW, Yamamoto N, Zdanovich E, Rehman A, Neves MF, Laurant P, Paradis P, Schiffrin EL. T regulatory lymphocytes prevent aldosterone-induced vascular injury. *Hypertension*. 2012;59:324–330

102. Barhoumi T, Kasal DA, Li MW, Shbat L, Laurant P, Neves MF, Paradis P, Schiffrin EL. T regulatory lymphocytes prevent angiotensin ii-induced hypertension and vascular injury. *Hypertension*. 2011;57:469–476

103. Ait-Oufella H, Wang Y, Herbin O, Bourcier S, Potteaux S, Joffre J, Loyer X, Ponnuswamy P, Esposito B, Dalloz M, Laurans L, Tedgui A, Mallat Z. Natural regulatory T cells limit angiotensin ii-induced aneurysm formation and rupture in mice. *Arterioscler Thromb Vasc Biol*. 2013;33:2374–2379

104. Myers JM, Cooper LT, Kem DC, Stavrakis S, Kosanke SD, Shevach EM, Fairweather D, Stoner JA, Cox CJ, Cunningham MW. Cardiac myosin-th17 responses promote heart failure in human myocarditis. *JCI Insight*. 2016;1

105. Huber SA, Gauntt CJ, Sakkinen P. Enteroviruses and myocarditis: Viral pathogenesis through replication, cytokine induction, and immunopathogenicity. *Adv Virus Res*. 1998;51:35–80

106. Zhang P, Cox CJ, Alvarez KM, Cunningham MW. Cutting edge: Cardiac myosin activates innate immune responses through tlrs. *J Immunol*. 2009;183:27–31

107. Mascaro-Blanco A, Alvarez K, Yu X, Lindenfeld J, Olansky L, Lyons T, Duvall D, Heuser JS, Gosmanova A, Rubenstein CJ, Cooper LT, Kem DC, Cunningham MW. Consequences of unlocking the cardiac myosin molecule in human myocarditis and cardiomyopathies. *Autoimmunity*. 2008;41:442–453

108. Caforio AL, Mahon NG, McKenna WJ. Clinical implications of anti-cardiac immunity in dilated cardiomyopathy. *Ernst Schering Res Found Workshop*. 2006:169–193

109. Miyata S, Minobe W, Bristow MR, Leinwand LA. Myosin heavy chain isoform expression in the failing and nonfailing human heart. *Circ Res*. 2000;86:386–390

110. Lv H, Havari E, Pinto S, Gottumukkala RV, Cornivelli L, Raddassi K, Matsui T, Rosenzweig A, Bronson RT, Smith R, Fletcher AL, Turley SJ, Wucherpfennig K, Kyewski B, Lipes MA. Impaired thymic tolerance to alpha-myosin directs autoimmunity to the heart in mice and humans. *J Clin Invest*. 2011;121:1561–1573

111. Danielsson T, Schreyer H, Woksepp H, Johansson T, Bergman P, Mansson A, Carlsson J. Two-peaked increase of serum myosin heavy chain-alpha after triathlon suggests heart muscle cell death. *BMJ Open Sport Exerc Med*. 2019;5:e000486

112. Efthimiadis I, Skendros P, Sarantopoulos A, Boura P. CD4+/CD25+ t-lymphocytes and th1/th2 regulation in dilated cardiomyopathy. *Hippokratia*. 2011;15:335–342

113. Wang J, Han B. Dysregulated CD4+ T cells and micrornas in myocarditis. *Front Immunol*. 2020;11:539

114. Nindl V, Maier R, Ratering D, De Giuli R, Zust R, Thiel V, Scandella E, Di Padova F, Kopf M, Rudin M, Rulicke T, Ludewig B. Cooperation of th1 and th17 cells determines transition from autoimmune myocarditis to dilated cardiomyopathy. *Eur J Immunol*. 2012;42:2311–2321

115. Yuan J, Yu M, Lin QW, Cao AL, Yu X, Dong JH, Wang JP, Zhang JH, Wang M, Guo HP, Cheng X, Liao YH. Th17 cells contribute to viral replication in coxsackievirus b3-induced acute viral myocarditis. *J Immunol*. 2010;185:4004–4010

116. Yan L, Hu F, Yan X, Wei Y, Ma W, Wang Y, Lu S, Wang Z. Inhibition of microrna-155 ameliorates experimental autoimmune myocarditis by modulating th17/treg immune response. *J Mol Med (Berl)*. 2016;94:1063–1079

117. Wang J, Liu T, Chen X, Jin Q, Chen Y, Zhang L, Han Z, Chen D, Li Y, Lv Q, Xie M. Bazedoxifene regulates th17 immune response to ameliorate experimental autoimmune myocarditis via inhibition of stat3 activation. *Front Pharmacol*. 2020;11:613160

118. Jin H, Guo X. Valproic acid ameliorates coxsackievirus-b3-induced viral myocarditis by modulating th17/treg imbalance. *Virol J.* 2016;13:168
119. Rouse BT, Sarangi PP, Suvas S. Regulatory T cells in virus infections. *Immunol Rev.* 2006;212:272–286
120. Chen P, Baldeviano GC, Ligons DL, Talor MV, Barin JG, Rose NR, Cihakova D. Susceptibility to autoimmune myocarditis is associated with intrinsic differences in CD4(+) T cells. *Clin Exp Immunol.* 2012;169:79–88
121. Ono M, Shimizu J, Miyachi Y, Sakaguchi S. Control of autoimmune myocarditis and multiorgan inflammation by glucocorticoid-induced tnf receptor family-related protein(high), foxp3-expressing CD25+ and CD25- regulatory T cells. *J Immunol.* 2006;176:4748–4756
122. Shi Y, Fukuoka M, Li G, Liu Y, Chen M, Konviser M, Chen X, Opavsky MA, Liu PP. Regulatory T cells protect mice against coxsackievirus-induced myocarditis through the transforming growth factor beta-coxsackie-adenovirus receptor pathway. *Circulation.* 2010;121:2624–2634
123. Tajiri K, Sakai S, Kimura T, Machino-Ohtsuka T, Murakoshi N, Xu D, Wang Z, Sato A, Miyauchi T, Aonuma K. Endothelin receptor antagonist exacerbates autoimmune myocarditis in mice. *Life Sci.* 2014;118:288–296

3 Glucocorticoid Signaling in the Heart

Danish Sayed

CONTENTS

INTRODUCTION

Glucocorticoids are steroid hormones released from the adrenal cortex, under the control of the hypothalamus–pituitary–adrenal axis, to maintain homeostasis during physiological variations (e.g., circadian rhythms) and in response to stress. Glucocorticoids (cortisol in humans and corticosteroids in rodents) have been so dubbed due their role in glucose metabolism and cellular bioenergetic homeostasis. Secretion of glucocorticoids from the adrenal glands is controlled by the corticotrophin-release hormone (CRH) released from the hypothalamus. CRH regulates the production and secretion of adrenocorticotrophic hormone (ACTH) from the pituitary, which in turn activates cortisol release in a melanocyte type-2 receptor (MC2R) dependent manner (1) (2). In circulation, cortisol could be in "free" form, where it can diffuse into cells and activate cytosolic glucocorticoid receptors, or it can be bound to corticosteroid binding globulin (CBG) or albumin, depending on the circulating levels (3) (4). Synthetic glucocorticoids, which are structurally related to cortisol and corticosteroids, are one of the most frequently used drugs in clinical settings for their anti-inflammatory and immune regulatory actions in acute and chronic conditions like asthma and rheumatoid arthritis, respectively. These are available in moderate-acting (e.g., prednisolone, methylprednisolone; biological half-life 12–36 hours) to long-acting versions (e.g., dexamethasone and betamethasone; biological half-life 36–72 hours), with varying potency and affinity for glucocorticoid receptor (GR), and they can be administered in diverse formulations such as oral, intramuscular, intravenous, inhaled, intraarticular, and topical (4) (5). High levels of circulating glucocorticoids due to increased secretion (endogenous) or prolonged administration

DOI: 10.1201/b22824-4

(synthetic) could result in the development of Cushing's syndrome (hypercorti-solism), which presents with hypertension, obesity, diabetes mellitus, weak muscles, and other manifestations (6). On the other hand, adrenal insufficiency or Addison's disease (hypocortisolism) results in a decrease in circulating steroids, presenting with various associated signs and symptoms including low blood pressure, fatigue, muscle weakness, and weight loss (7). In this chapter, we review the effects of gluco-corticoid signaling in cardiac development, physiology, and pathogenesis.

GLUCOCORTICOID RECEPTOR

Endogenous and synthetic glucocorticoid downstream function is mostly mediated by activation of nuclear receptor subfamily 3, group C, member 1 (Nr3c1) or gluco-corticoid receptor (GR) (8) (9). GR encoded by the Nr3c1 gene is a ligand-activated transcription factor and part of the nuclear receptor superfamily with canonical structure, including highly variable N-terminal activation domain, conserved DNA-binding domain, and C-terminal ligand-binding domain (10) (11). Several receptor isoforms have been identified for GR. Spliced variant GR-α, the classical nuclear receptor, has been linked with most of the downstream glucocorticoid-mediated transcriptional regulation. Interestingly, spliced variant GR-β, generated as a result of splicing between exon 8 and exon 9, has no affinity for glucocorticoids and shows nuclear localization even under unstimulated conditions. This variant, through com-petitive inhibition, restricts GR-α mediated genomic effects of glucocorticoids (12). In addition, at least eight isoforms of GR-α have been identified, as a result of alter-native initiation sites in the GR-α transcript. These isoforms can lead to a differential regulatory influence of glucocorticoid on dependent gene transcription. GR associates with the genome at GR response element (GRE), which is an imperfect palindromic sequence comprising two hexamer half sites linked by three nucleotides. GR associ-ates with the consensus sequence GGAACAnnnTGTTCT as a homodimer and has been shown mostly to be involved in gene activation. On the other hand, studies have also identified a negative GRE with consensus sequence $CTCC(n)_{0-2}GGAGA$, which is associated with gene repression and involves binding of GR monomers (13) (14). Recently, an additional regulatory step has been identified in human cells, before the nuclear GR associates with its response element (GRE) on the DNA. Growth arrest specific 5 (Gas5), a long noncoding RNA, has been shown to encompass decoy GRE in its stem-loop and competes for GR binding, thus preventing its genomic associa-tion and downstream regulatory influence on gene transcription (15).

Under unstimulated conditions, GR is located in the cytosolic fraction of the cel-lular compartment bound to a large, multiprotein chaperone complex, which includes heat-shock protein (HSP) 90, HSP70, and HSP40 and several other co-chaperones (16) (17). Binding of glucocorticoid to GR results in conformational change, exposing the nuclear localization signal and resulting in its nuclear translocation (18). Genomic and non-genomic effects of GR have been identified and implicated in downstream signaling and change in cardiac phenotype (19). Several underlying mechanisms have been identified, through which activated GR can impart anti-inflammatory effects (20). Direct targets of GR include the induction of anti-inflammatory genes like mitogen-activated protein kinase phosphatase-1 (MKP-1) (21) or the inhibition of inflammatory genes like nuclear factor-kB (NF-kb) and activated protein-1 (AP-1) (22). Activated GR can recruit histone deacetylases (HDACs) at inflammatory genes, thus resulting in gene repression (23). Further, by regulating the expression of genes involved in mRNA destabilization, glucocorticoids have also been shown to promote the rapid degradation of pro-inflammatory transcripts, like TNF-α, thus regulating the protein levels of these genes (24) (25). Because glucocorticoid signaling is mediated predominantly by GR activation, it presents as the best target to study the downstream cellular effects of glucocorticoids.

GLUCOCORTICOIDS IN CARDIAC DEVELOPMENT

Glucocorticoid levels increase in late gestation and are required for fetal organ maturation, most importantly the lungs (26). Glucocorticoids are administered antenatally in preterm deliveries as a measure to promote fetal development and preparedness for postnatal challenges (27). GR expression, although seen as early as 12 weeks and E9.5–10.5 day of gestation in human and mouse hearts, respectively, is not activated until the late gestational period, which coincides with a surge in endogenous glucocorticoid levels (E15.5–E17.5 day in mice) (28) (29). Global GR knockout mice show perinatal lethality – those that survive at birth die within a few hours due to respiratory failure, which is attributed to immature lungs. In addition, these mice show altered liver and adrenal function, resulting in impaired glucose metabolism and adrenaline synthesis, respectively (30). Conditional GR knockout under SM22a promoter shows impaired fetal heart function. Structural and biochemical analyses of these hearts confirm immature, short, and disorganized myofibrils associated with inhibited expression of contractile and metabolic genes. Further characterization of these immature cardiomyocytes identified PGC-1α as a critical downstream target of GR that contributes to cardiomyocyte maturity, along with other targets including transcription regulators (29) (31). However, while GR signaling is essential for postnatal survival, studies have implicated excessive prenatal endogenous or exogenous glucocorticoids as a risk factor for development of adult cardiovascular disease (32) (33) (34).

Increases in endogenous glucocorticoids linked to changes in maternal nutritional status or stress levels, as well as to antenatal corticosteroid therapy, are associated with changes in fetal hemodynamics and a higher risk of developing chronic heart disease (CHD) in adult life (35) (36) (37) (38) (39). On the other hand, while there are limited conclusive data showing adverse effects of antenatal administration of synthetic glucocorticoids in humans, *in vivo* studies in other vertebrates have shown fetal heart enlargement and increases in blood pressure in adult progeny, which possibly could contribute to cardiovascular pathogenesis (40) (41) (42) (43). Neonatal rats injected with dexamethasone in the first 3 days after birth develop dyslipidemia along with structural cardiac mitochondrial abnormalities as adults. In addition, at 24 weeks these rats, when subjected to ischemia reperfusion, show increase in infarct size and impaired cardiac recovery (44). However, it should be noted that the underlying conditions – preterm vs normal, maternal nutritional status, active HPA axis regulating endogenous glucocorticoid levels, timing (gestational age), and the number of doses administered – could result in varying responses and outcomes in prenatal, postnatal, and adult life. An additional confounding factor is the high affinity of the mineralocorticoid receptor (MR) for glucocorticoids, although two commonly used synthetic glucocorticoids in antenatal clinics, betamethasone and dexamethasone (Dex), have been shown to poorly activate MR (5). Therefore, although with caution, it can be presumed that the benefits of antenatal glucocorticoid administration in preterm pregnancies in humans outweigh the potential detrimental effects later in life until we have new conclusive data from adults who were born preterm and present with higher incidence of CHD or other related illnesses.

GLUCOCORTICOID IN CARDIAC HYPERTROPHY AND FAILURE

Cardiac-specific knockout (KO) of GR generated by mating αMHC-Cre to Floxed GR mice showed no obvious difference compared to wild-type (Wt) littermates at birth or early in life. However, these mice developed spontaneous progressive pathological cardiac hypertrophy by 3 months with associated left-ventricular dysfunction, but no interstitial fibrosis. Loss of GR function results in increased mortality by 5 months of age due to heart failure. Microarray analysis on hearts from 1-month- and 2-month-old mice show increases in the expression of genes involved in inflammation and immune response, which are further dysregulated by 3 months of age contributing to cardiac dysfunction. In addition, a decrease in cardiac-enriched and functional genes like calcium handling gene RyR2 and transcriptional regulator Klf15 is observed. Ingenuity pathway analysis characterized these dysregulated genes as those involved in "cardiovascular diseases" (45). A similar hypertrophic phenotype is observed after 6 months in mice subjected to adrenalectomy at 1 month of age. Transcriptome analysis in these hearts reveals the dysregulation of genes involved in cardiac hypertrophy and arrythmias. Interestingly, supplementation with exogenous corticosterone reverses left-ventricular dysfunction and hypertrophic phenotype; however, the EKG changes of prolonged QT and QTc observed in adrenalectomized mice persist, which are reversible with aldosterone treatment (46). Characterization of cardiac-specific double knockout of GR and MR (cGRMRdKO) in comparison with GR (cGRKO) and MR (cMRKO) knockouts alone reveals the critical role of GR in cardiac physiology. On the other hand, activated MR signaling is seen as detrimental for cardiac function. Although the cGRMRdKO mice displayed altered gene regulation, as seen in cGRKO, these mice did not develop spontaneous cardiac pathology. Similarly, no obvious cardiac phenotype is observed in cMRKO mice. Genome-wide microarray analysis of transcriptome in these KO models shows the differential regulation of genes that could be contributing to the cardiac pathogenesis in cGRKO mice and include genes involved in Ca^{2+} handling, oxidative stress, and cell death. In addition, cGRMRdKO mice also showed an increase in cardioprotective genes like Ccnd2, Hdac4, and Ankrd23, accompanied by a decrease in Agt (47). These genes have been shown to be involved in regulating cardiac hypertrophy and survival and, thus, were restricting cardiac enlargement and dysfunction in cGRMRdKO compared to cGRKO (47). Work overload, in the form of excessive exercise or transverse aortic constriction (TAC) induced pressure overload, results in a decrease in GR expression and dependent gene transcription. This decrease is associated with the development of pathological cardiac hypertrophy and dysfunction (48) (49).

Interestingly, in contrast to the phenotype observed in *in vivo* KO models, Dex-mediated GR activation in the embryonic H9C2 cell line, isolated primary myocytes, and neonatal rat hearts results in the development of cardiomyocyte hypertrophy (50) (51) (52). In rat ventricular neonatal myocytes (NRVM), GR nuclear translocation is seen as early as 1 hour after Dex treatment, with induced cardiomyocyte hypertrophy by 24 hours. Integration of high resolution of GR-ChIP-Seq at 1 hour and RNAseq at 1 and 24 hours of Dex treatments identified direct and indirect targets of activated GR signaling. Data reveal that after 1 hour of Dex treatment, 69.38% of genes that show significant differential regulation (>twofold) are associated with genomic GR binding. Conversely, after 24 hours, only 45.31% of differentially regulated genes are associated with genomic GR binding, while the majority (54.69%) are not associated with GR, and most likely are indirect targets or secondary to hypertrophy development. Early direct targets of GR include regulators of RNA polymerase II–dependent gene expression, genes involved in cell death, and mechanical or insulin stimulus. These early factors mostly include transcription factors like Per1, from the Klf family, which could be working as feed-forward mediators of GR signaling. On the other hand, at 24 hours most of the differentially regulated genes include those of growth-related pathways involved in cardiomyopathy. Ingenuity pathway analysis of genes suggests early regulation of genes that favored the transactivation of transcriptome, while genes dysregulated at 24 hours are involved in cardiac hypertrophy and failure. Notably, 12 members of the Klf family are associated with genomic GR binding after 1 hour, five of which show significant changes in expression at 1 and 24 hours of Dex treatment as measured by RNAseq in cardiomyocytes (52).

GLUCOCORTICOIDS AND CARDIAC ISCHEMIA

Myocardial inflammation is one of the major contributing factors to cardiac remodeling, dysfunction, and development of chronic heart failure (CHF) (53) (54). A surge in inflammatory cytokines from the myocardium and mononuclear cells recruited to the heart in response to cardiac injury, like myocardial infarction (MI), promote cardiac remodeling and progression of failure. TNF-α, interleukin (IL-1), and IL-6 are a few of the major players in immune activation and have been shown to be involved in cardiomyocyte apoptosis, ventricular dysfunction, and remodeling (55) (56) (57). Activation of systemic inflammatory response, as seen in sepsis or lipopolysaccharide (LPS) administration, leads to the release of NFκB-dependent TNF-α release, which can precipitate myocardial inflammation and failure (58) (59). Thus, glucocorticoids, due to potent anti-inflammatory actions, present as a good therapeutic approach to restrict the progression of failure.

Glucocorticoids have been shown to inhibit LPS-induced inflammation and attenuate cardiac dysfunction in mice (60). Methylprednisolone injections before or after the induction of acute or chronic microembolization of the coronary artery inhibit leukocyte infiltration and prevent associated cardiac dysfunction (61). However, there have been conflicting reports with respect to the role of supplementary exogenous glucocorticoids during an acute myocardial infarction episode. An early study in dogs showed that injecting cortisone (1–2 mg/kg) for 2–3 weeks post-MI reduced residual fibrosis, decreased infarct size, and increased coronary anastomoses (62).

This was followed by several studies that showed no beneficial effects of cortisone injections during acute myocardial infarction (63) (64) (65). Thus, to settle the issue, using ST elevation and change in creatinine phosphokinase (CPK) activity as measures of cardiac damage, as opposed to measuring infarct size alone, hydrocortisone injections in dogs post-MI were shown to reduce infarct size with reversal in ST elevation. These changes were attributed to hydrocortisone-mediated inhibition of ischemia-induced cardiomyocyte necrosis (66). Similar studies in cats using dexamethasone showed normalization of ST elevation and an increase in CPK activity after acute MI, along with the preservation of lysosomal enzymes and function that was predicted to prevent the spread of the infarct in the ischemic myocardium (67). Ischemia reperfusion (IR) injury in rats with high corticosterone levels results in an increase in infarct size, along with an increase in mean arterial pressure (68). Similarly, dexamethasone administration in rats subjected to IR results in increased apoptosis and infarct size. These effects are reversed by spironolactone injections, suggesting the activation of MR receptors in these hearts (69). In contrast, acute administration of methylprednisolone during IR injury in rats showed improved coronary circulation and prevented ventricular dysfunction during reperfusion, with reduced infarct size (70).

In addition to cardiomyocytes, the infiltration of immune cells in the heart also contributes to ischemic stress–induced remodeling and scar formation (71). Mice with macrophage-specific (bone marrow-derived) GR knockout showed a 56% increase in mortality, worsened cardiac function, and ventricular remodeling within 7 days post-MI. This was associated with impaired scar formation due to inhibited differentiation of monocyte-derived macrophages, resulting in scar rupture. Further, GR activation in these macrophages was shown to be involved in myofibroblast differentiation, which could play an essential role in infarct healing (72).

A double-blinded clinical study examining the effects of methylprednisolone (30 mg/kg, IV, every 6 hours, 4 doses) in 42 individuals with acute myocardial infarction showed no beneficial effects of glucocorticoids on outcome with respect to infarct size, dysfunction, or occurrence of arrhythmias 2 weeks post-MI (73). Similar results were observed in a randomized, double-blinded study in which patients were given 2 g of methylprednisolone at admission and an additional IV infusion after 3 hours. No difference was observed in the rate of mortality, occurrence of arrythmias, infarct size, ST elevation, or other parameters in methylprednisolone-treated vs placebo groups at discharge or at a 6-month follow-up in surviving patients (74). On the other hand, a retrospective study using autopsy data from patients who sustained left-ventricular rupture after acute MI showed direct correlation between the administration of anti-inflammatory agents, like corticosteroids, and rupture due to delayed and hampered healing post-injury (75). Corticosteroids along with their anti-inflammatory actions inhibit fibroblast proliferation, collagen production, and angiogenesis, resulting in the thinning of scar formation at the injury site (76) (77). A dose-dependent examination of corticosteroid therapy during acute MI in dogs showed that a high dose of methylprednisolone (50 mg/kg, IV, multiple injections at 15 minutes and 3, 24, and 48 hours post-MI) was associated with scar thinning and regional dysfunction, while a low dose (30 mg/kg, IV, 15 minutes post-MI) of methylprednisolone did not show any different effects compared to controls (78).

GLUCOCORTICOIDS AND HEART BLOCK

Corticotrophin or ACTH and corticosteroids restore sinus rhythm in acute and chronic heart block, secondary to coronary artery disease, rheumatic heart disease, or unknown etiology (79) (80) (81) (82). Complete heart block due to incomplete infarction near the septum could be due to inflammation of the atrioventricular (AV) node and not due to myocardium damage, which could explain the beneficial actions of the steroid therapy under these stress conditions (83). Further, cases with AV block without coronary artery disease present with foci of myocardial fibrosis with lymphocytic infiltration (84). In addition, corticoids can also directly influence and facilitate AV conduction (85). An independent study examining the effects of prednisolone on grade 1, partial, complete but intermittent, and complete with permanent AV block showed moderate effects with the last group. The improvements in the other three groups were attributed to the effects of corticosteroids on edema surrounding AV node due to the underlying pathology (86).

GLUCOCORTICOIDS AND ATHEROSCLEROSIS

Atherosclerosis, although a vascular disease, is one of the leading contributors of cardiac pathogenesis. Characterized by arterial blockage due to lipid deposition, it involves the infiltration of leukocytes, including macrophages that form foam cells, inflammation, endothelial dysfunction, and smooth muscle proliferation (87). Several studies looking at data from individuals with adrenal insufficiency who were on glucocorticoid replacement therapy, including children and adults, showed an increased risk of ischemic cardiovascular disease compared to healthy individuals. These risks were mostly linked to incorrect levels of circulating corticosteroids due to replacement therapy, in which excess or insufficient glucocorticoid levels, especially during underlying illness or stress condition, could trigger systemic disturbances, for example, metabolic or endothelial dysfunction (88) (89) (90) (91). Similar increases in risk and mortality due to cardiac failure have been reported in patients with Cushing's disease and were attributed to increased atherosclerotic plaque formation and a higher incidence of vascular disease due to hypercortisolemia, compared to healthy individuals (92) (93) (94).

In contrast to clinical data, there are conflicting and variable reports from rabbit and mice studies. Administration of exogenous glucocorticoids via the oral or intramuscular route in rabbits reduced high cholesterol diet–induced plaque formation. These effects were attributed to the anti-inflammatory actions of glucocorticoids, where reduction in macrophage and lymphocyte recruitment was observed at lesion (95) (96) (97). Further, glucocorticoids were shown to prevent aortic cholesterol uptake and, thus, can inhibit the formation of atherosclerotic plaques (98). On the other hand, studies in mice showed glucocorticoids to be pro-atherogenic (99) (100) (101). However, a reduction in endogenous glucocorticoid activity via GR disruption or bilateral adrenalectomy showed no effect on the atherosclerotic plaque formation in LDLR or ApoE mouse models (102) (103).

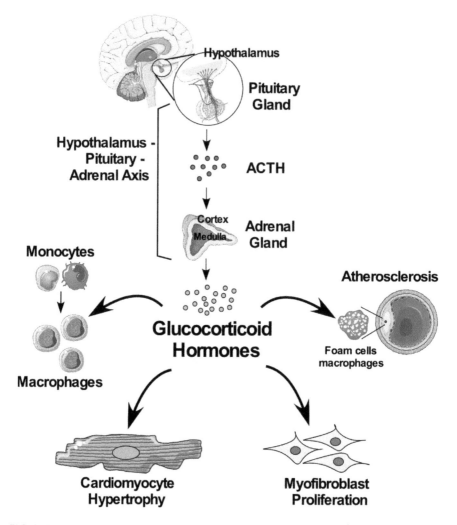

FIGURE 3.1   Glucocorticoid actions on cardiac cells, including myocyte and non-myocyte cell population, and during atherosclerosis.

Source: Figure was made by using images from Servier Medical Art (SMART).

CONCLUDING REMARKS

Glucocorticoid or "stress hormone" is secreted as an adaptive response to maintain homeostasis during physiological variations or to accommodate the demands during "flight or fight" situations. Classical glucocorticoid signaling includes activation of the cytoplasmic GR, which then mediates the downstream genomic effects. Due to ubiquitous GR expression, glucocorticoids can influence all cells and their cellular function. Glucocorticoid signaling has an essential role in the heart, with respect to cardiac development, physiology, or pathogenesis. Synthetic glucocorticoids, due to their anti-inflammatory and immunosuppressive actions, are one of the most commonly used drugs for acute and chronic conditions. However, on the basis of conflicting research data and case studies, the therapeutic potential of glucocorticoid administration during myocardial ischemia and failure is still debatable, and may be assessed on a case-by-case basis.

With the advancement of high-throughput techniques, more research work should focus on the GR genomic targeting and change in the overall transcriptome on a cellular level. Infiltration of cytokine-induced immune cells during acute ischemic insult or the chronic inflammation seen during failure or aging contributes to the underlying pathology and phenotype. Thus, using cell-specific knockout models, the role of these immune cells in cardiac pathogenesis needs to be thoroughly examined. Glucocorticoid levels are highly regulated and fluctuate with circadian rhythms; thus, data outcomes with supplementation of synthetic glucocorticoids should consider diurnal vs nocturnal administration and its impact on the circulating levels and the systemic downstream actions.

BIBLIOGRAPHY

1. Cone RD, Mountjoy KG. Molecular genetics of the ACTH and melanocyte-stimulating hormone receptors. *Trends Endocrinol Metabolism: TEM*. 1993;4(7):242–247.
2. Raff H, Sharma ST, Nieman LK. Physiological basis for the etiology, diagnosis, and treatment of adrenal disorders: Cushing's syndrome, adrenal insufficiency, and congenital adrenal hyperplasia. *Compr Physiol*. 2014;4(2):739–769.
3. Lin HY, Muller YA, Hammond GL. Molecular and structural basis of steroid hormone binding and release from corticosteroid-binding globulin. *Mol Cell Endocrinol*. 2010;316(1):3–12.
4. Perogamvros I, Ray DW, Trainer PJ. Regulation of cortisol bioavailability—effects on hormone measurement and action. *Nat Rev Endocrinol*. 2012;8(12):717–727.
5. Karssen AM, de Kloet ER. Synthetic Glucocorticoids*. In: Fink G, ed. *Encyclopedia of Stress* (Second Edition). New York: Academic Press; 2007:704–708.
6. Orth DN. Cushing's syndrome. *N Engl J Med*. 1995;332(12):791–803.
7. Burke CW. Adrenocortical insufficiency. *Clin Endocrinol Metab*. 1985;14(4):947–976.
8. Wrange O, Carlstedt-Duke J, Gustafsson JA. Stoichiometric analysis of the specific interaction of the glucocorticoid receptor with DNA. *J Biol Chem*. 1986;261(25):11770–11778.
9. Carlstedt-Duke J, Gustafsson JA. Structure and function of the glucocorticoid receptor. *J Steroid Biochem*. 1987;27(1–3):99–104.
10. Beato M. Gene regulation by steroid hormones. *Cell*. 1989;56(3):335–344.
11. Robinson-Rechavi M, Escriva Garcia H, Laudet V. The nuclear receptor superfamily. *J Cell Sci*. 2003;116(Pt 4):585–586.
12. Kino T, Su YA, Chrousos GP. Human glucocorticoid receptor isoform beta: recent understanding of its potential implications in physiology and pathophysiology. *Cell Mol Life Sci: CMLS*. 2009;66(21):3435–3448.
13. Hudson WH, Youn C, Ortlund EA. The structural basis of direct glucocorticoid-mediated transrepression. *Nat Struct Mol Biol*. 2013;20(1):53–58.
14. Liu B, Zhang TN, Knight JK, Goodwin JE. The glucocorticoid receptor in cardiovascular health and disease. *Cells*. 2019;8(10).
15. Kino T, Hurt DE, Ichijo T, Nader N, Chrousos GP. Noncoding RNA gas5 is a growth arrest- and starvation-associated repressor of the glucocorticoid receptor. *Sci Signal*. 2010;3(107):2000568.

16. Grad I, Picard D. The glucocorticoid responses are shaped by molecular chaperones. *Mol Cell Endocrinol.* 2007;275(1–2):2–12.
17. Echeverria PC, Picard D. Molecular chaperones, essential partners of steroid hormone receptors for activity and mobility. *Biochim Biophys Acta.* 2010;1803(6):641–649.
18. Freedman ND, Yamamoto KR. Importin 7 and importin alpha/importin beta are nuclear import receptors for the glucocorticoid receptor. *Mol Biol Cell.* 2004;15(5):2276–2286.
19. Lee SR, Kim HK, Youm JB, Dizon LA, Song IS, Jeong SH, Seo DY, Ko KS, Rhee BD, Kim N, Han J. Non-genomic effect of glucocorticoids on cardiovascular system. *Pflug Arch: Eur J Physiol.* 2012;464(6):549–559.
20. Barnes PJ. Mechanisms and resistance in glucocorticoid control of inflammation. *J Steroid Biochem Mol Biol.* 2010;120(2–3):76–85.
21. Clark AR. MAP kinase phosphatase 1: a novel mediator of biological effects of glucocorticoids? *J Endocrinol.* 2003;178(1):5–12.
22. Barnes PJ, Adcock IM. How do corticosteroids work in asthma? *Ann Intern Med.* 2003;139(5 Pt 1):359–370.
23. Ito K, Barnes PJ, Adcock IM. Glucocorticoid receptor recruitment of histone deacetylase 2 inhibits interleukin-1beta-induced histone H4 acetylation on lysines 8 and 12. *Mol Cell Biol.* 2000;20(18):6891–6903.
24. Bergmann MW, Staples KJ, Smith SJ, Barnes PJ, Newton R. Glucocorticoid inhibition of granulocyte macrophage-colony-stimulating factor from T cells is independent of control by nuclear factor-kappaB and conserved lymphokine element 0. *Am J Respir Cell Mol Biol.* 2004;30(4):555–563.
25. Smoak K, Cidlowski JA. Glucocorticoids regulate tristetraprolin synthesis and posttranscriptionally regulate tumor necrosis factor alpha inflammatory signaling. *Mol Cell Biol.* 2006;26(23):9126–9135.
26. Fowden AL, Li J, Forhead AJ. Glucocorticoids and the preparation for life after birth: are there long-term consequences of the life insurance? *Proc Nutr Soc.* 1998;57(1):113–122.
27. Roberts D, Dalziel S. Antenatal corticosteroids for accelerating fetal lung maturation for women at risk of preterm birth. *Cochrane Database Syst Rev.* 2006;(3):Cd004454.
28. Ballard PL, Ballard RA. Cytoplasmic receptor for glucocorticoids in lung of the human fetus and neonate. *J Clin Invest.* 1974;53(2):477–486.
29. Rog-Zielinska EA, Thomson A, Kenyon CJ, Brownstein DG, Moran CM, Szumska D, Michailidou Z, Richardson J, Owen E, Watt A, Morrison H, Forrester LM, Bhattacharya S, Holmes MC, Chapman KE. Glucocorticoid receptor is required for foetal heart maturation. *Hum Mol Genet.* 2013;22(16):3269–3282.
30. Cole TJ, Blendy JA, Monaghan AP, Krieglstein K, Schmid W, Aguzzi A, Fantuzzi G, Hummler E, Unsicker K, Schütz G. Targeted disruption of the glucocorticoid receptor gene blocks adrenergic chromaffin cell development and severely retards lung maturation. *Genes Dev.* 1995;9(13):1608–1621.
31. Rog-Zielinska EA, Craig MA, Manning JR, Richardson RV, Gowans GJ, Dunbar DR, Gharbi K, Kenyon CJ, Holmes MC, Hardie DG, Smith GL, Chapman KE. Glucocorticoids promote structural and functional maturation of foetal cardiomyocytes: a role for PGC-1α. *Cell Death Differ.* 2015;22(7):1106–1116.
32. Benediktsson R, Lindsay RS, Noble J, Seckl JR, Edwards CR. Glucocorticoid exposure in utero: new model for adult hypertension. *Lancet.* 1993;341(8841):339–341.
33. Barker DJ, Fall CH. Fetal and infant origins of cardiovascular disease. *Arch Dis Child.* 1993;68(6):797–799.
34. Rog-Zielinska EA, Richardson RV, Denvir MA, Chapman KE. Glucocorticoids and foetal heart maturation; implications for prematurity and foetal programming. *J Mol Endocrinol.* 2014;52(2):R125–135.

35. Langley-Evans SC, Gardner DS, Welham SJ. Intrauterine programming of cardiovascular disease by maternal nutritional status. *Nutrition.* 1998;14(1):39–47.
36. Gardner DS, Jackson AA, Langley-Evans SC. The effect of prenatal diet and glucocorticoids on growth and systolic blood pressure in the rat. *Proc Nutr Soc.* 1998;57(2):235–240.
37. Langley-Evans SC, Nwagwu M. Impaired growth and increased glucocorticoid-sensitive enzyme activities in tissues of rat fetuses exposed to maternal low protein diets. *Life Sci.* 1998;63(7):605–615.
38. Seckl JR, Holmes MC. Mechanisms of disease: glucocorticoids, their placental metabolism and fetal 'programming' of adult pathophysiology. *Nat Clin Pract Endocrinol Metab.* 2007;3(6):479–488.
39. Mulder EJ, de Heus R, Visser GH. Antenatal corticosteroid therapy: short-term effects on fetal behaviour and haemodynamics. *Semin Fetal Neonatal Med.* 2009;14(3):151–156.
40. Slotkin TA, Seidler FJ, Kavlock RJ, Bartolome JV. Fetal dexamethasone exposure impairs cellular development in neonatal rat heart and kidney: effects on DNA and protein in whole tissues. *Teratology.* 1991;43(4):301–306.
41. Dodic M, Moritz K, Wintour EM. Prenatal exposure to glucocorticoids and adult disease. *Arch Physiol Biochem.* 2003;111(1):61–69.
42. Jensen EC, Gallaher BW, Breier BH, Harding JE. The effect of a chronic maternal cortisol infusion on the late-gestation fetal sheep. *J Endocrinol.* 2002;174(1):27–36.
43. de Vries A, Holmes MC, Heijnis A, Seier JV, Heerden J, Louw J, Wolfe-Coote S, Meaney MJ, Levitt NS, Seckl JR. Prenatal dexamethasone exposure induces changes in nonhuman primate offspring cardiometabolic and hypothalamic-pituitary-adrenal axis function. *J Clin Invest.* 2007;117(4):1058–1067.
44. Jiang X, Ma H, Li C, Cao Y, Wang Y, Zhang Y, Liu Y. Effects of neonatal dexamethasone administration on cardiac recovery ability under ischemia-reperfusion in 24-wk-old rats. *Pediatric Res.* 2016;80(1):128–135.
45. Oakley RH, Ren R, Cruz-Topete D, Bird GS, Myers PH, Boyle MC, Schneider MD, Willis MS, Cidlowski JA. Essential role of stress hormone signaling in cardiomyocytes for the prevention of heart disease. *Proc Natl Acad Sci U S A.* 2013;110(42):17035–17040.
46. Cruz-Topete D, Myers PH, Foley JF, Willis MS, Cidlowski JA. Corticosteroids are essential for maintaining cardiovascular function in male mice. *Endocrinology.* 2016;157(7):2759–2771.
47. Oakley RH, Cruz-Topete D, He B, Foley JF, Myers PH, Xu X, Gomez-Sanchez CE, Chambon P, Willis MS, Cidlowski JA. Cardiomyocyte glucocorticoid and mineralocorticoid receptors directly and antagonistically regulate heart disease in mice. *Sci Signal.* 2019;12(577).
48. da Rocha AL, Teixeira GR, Pinto AP, de Morais GP, Oliveira LDC, de Vicente LG, da Silva L, Pauli JR, Cintra DE, Ropelle ER, de Moura LP, Mekary RA, de Freitas EC, da Silva ASR. Excessive training induces molecular signs of pathologic cardiac hypertrophy. *J Cell Physiol.* 2018;233(11):8850–8861.
49. Matsuhashi T, Endo J, Katsumata Y, Yamamoto T, Shimizu N, Yoshikawa N, Kataoka M, Isobe S, Moriyama H, Goto S, Fukuda K, Tanaka H, Sano M. Pressure overload inhibits glucocorticoid receptor transcriptional activity in cardiomyocytes and promotes pathological cardiac hypertrophy. *J Mol Cell Cardiol.* 2019;130:122–130.
50. La Mear NS, MacGilvray SS, Myers TF. Dexamethasone-induced myocardial hypertrophy in neonatal rats. *Biol Neonate.* 1997;72(3):175–180.
51. Ren R, Oakley RH, Cruz-Topete D, Cidlowski JA. Dual role for glucocorticoids in cardiomyocyte hypertrophy and apoptosis. *Endocrinology.* 2012;153(11):5346–5360.
52. Severinova E, Alikunju S, Deng W, Dhawan P, Sayed N, Sayed D. Glucocorticoid receptor-binding and transcriptome signature in cardiomyocytes. *J Am Heart Assoc.* 2019;8(6):e011484.

53. Mann DL, Young JB. Basic mechanisms in congestive heart failure. Recognizing the role of proinflammatory cytokines. *Chest.* 1994;105(3):897–904.
54. Kan H, Finkel MS. Interactions between cytokines and neurohormonal systems in the failing heart. *Heart Fail Rev.* 2001;6(2):119–127.
55. Ono K, Matsumori A, Shioi T, Furukawa Y, Sasayama S. Cytokine gene expression after myocardial infarction in rat hearts: possible implication in left ventricular remodeling. *Circulation.* 1998;98(2):149–156.
56. Irwin MW, Mak S, Mann DL, Qu R, Penninger JM, Yan A, Dawood F, Wen WH, Shou Z, Liu P. Tissue expression and immunolocalization of tumor necrosis factor-alpha in postinfarction dysfunctional myocardium. *Circulation.* 1999;99(11):1492–1498.
57. Deten A, Volz HC, Briest W, Zimmer HG. Cardiac cytokine expression is upregulated in the acute phase after myocardial infarction. Experimental studies in rats. *Cardiovasc Res.* 2002;55(2):329–340.
58. Feldman AM, Combes A, Wagner D, Kadakomi T, Kubota T, Li YY, McTiernan C. The role of tumor necrosis factor in the pathophysiology of heart failure. *J Am College Cardiol.* 2000;35(3):537–544.
59. Ahn J, Kim J. Mechanisms and consequences of inflammatory signaling in the myocardium. *Curr Hypertens Rep.* 2012;14(6):510–516.
60. Zhang HN, He YH, Zhang GS, Luo MS, Huang Y, Wu XQ, Liu SM, Luo JD, Chen MS. Endogenous glucocorticoids inhibit myocardial inflammation induced by lipopolysaccharide: involvement of regulation of histone deacetylation. *J Cardiovasc Pharmacol.* 2012;60(1):33–41.
61. Skyschally A, Haude M, Dörge H, Thielmann M, Duschin A, van de Sand A, Konietzka I, Büchert A, Aker S, Massoudy P, Schulz R, Erbel R, Heusch G. Glucocorticoid treatment prevents progressive myocardial dysfunction resulting from experimental coronary microembolization. *Circulation.* 2004;109(19):2337–2342.
62. Johnson AS, Gerisch RA, Girton FW, Scheinberg SR, Saltzstein HC. Effect of cortisone on the size of experimentally produced myocardial infarcts. *J Mich State Med Soc.* 1953;52(12):1298–1299; passim 1305.
63. Opdyke DF, Lambert A, Stoerk HC, Zanetti ME, Kuna S. Failure to reduce the size of experimentally produced myocardial infarcts by cortisone treatment. *Circulation.* 1953;8(4):544–548.
64. Hepper NG, Pruitt RD, Donald DE, Edwards JE. The effect of cortisone on experimentally produced myocardial infarcts. *Circulation.* 1955;11(5):742–748.
65. Hoover MP, Manning GW. The effects of cortisone and ACTH on artificially induced cardiac infarction in the dog. *Am Heart J.* 1954;47(3):343–347.
66. Libby P, Maroko PR, Bloor CM, Sobel BE, Braunwald E. Reduction of experimental myocardial infarct size by corticosteroid administration. *J Clin Invest.* 1973;52(3):599–607.
67. Spath JA, Lefer AM. Effects of dexamethasone on myocardial cells in the early phase of acute myocardial infarction. *Am Heart J.* 1975;90(1):50–55.
68. Scheuer DA, Mifflin SW. Chronic corticosterone treatment increases myocardial infarct size in rats with ischemia-reperfusion injury. *Am J Physiol.* 1997;272(6 Pt 2):R2017–2024.
69. Mihailidou AS, Loan Le TY, Mardini M, Funder JW. Glucocorticoids activate cardiac mineralocorticoid receptors during experimental myocardial infarction. *Hypertension.* 2009;54(6):1306–1312.
70. Valen G, Kawakami T, Tähepôld P, Dumitrescu A, Löwbeer C, Vaage J. Glucocorticoid pretreatment protects cardiac function and induces cardiac heat shock protein 72. *Am J Physiol Heart Circ Physiol.* 2000;279(2):H836–843.
71. Pluijmert NJ, Atsma DE, Quax PHA. Post-ischemic myocardial inflammatory response: a complex and dynamic process susceptible to immunomodulatory therapies. *Front Cardiovasc Med.* 2021;8:647785.

72. Galuppo P, Vettorazzi S, Hövelmann J, Scholz CJ, Tuckermann JP, Bauersachs J, Fraccarollo D. The glucocorticoid receptor in monocyte-derived macrophages is critical for cardiac infarct repair and remodeling. *FASEB J.* 2017;31(11):5122–5132.

73. Bush CA, Renner W, Boudoulas H. Corticosteroids in acute myocardial infarction. *Angiology.* 1980;31(10):710–714.

74. Madias JE, Hood WB, Jr. Effects of methylprednisolone on the ischemic damage in patients with acute myocardial infarction. *Circulation.* 1982;65(6):1106–1113.

75. Silverman HS, Pfeifer MP. Relation between use of anti-inflammatory agents and left ventricular free wall rupture during acute myocardial infarction. *Am J Cardiol.* 1987;59(4):363–364.

76. Sandberg N. Time relationship between administration of cortisone and wound healing in rats. *Acta Chir Scand.* 1964;127:446–455.

77. Bulkley BH, Roberts WC. Steroid therapy during acute myocardial infarction. A cause of delayed healing and of ventricular aneurysm. *Am J Med.* 1974;56(2):244–250.

78. Hammerman H, Kloner RA, Hale S, Schoen FJ, Braunwald E. Dose-dependent effects of short-term methylprednisolone on myocardial infarct extent, scar formation, and ventricular function. *Circulation.* 1983;68(2):446–452.

79. Lindsay JD, Jr., Phelps MD, Jr. Cortisone in Stokes-Adams disease secondary to myocardial infarction; report of a case. *N Engl J Med.* 1957;256(5):204–208.

80. Litchfield JW, Manley KA, Polak A. Stokes-Adams attacks treated with corticotrophin. *Lancet.* 1958;1(7027):935–938.

81. Aber CP, Jones EW. Complete heart block treated with corticostrophin and corticosteroid. *Br Heart J.* 1960;22(5):723–728.

82. Aber CP, Jones EW. Corticotrophin and corticosteroids in the management of acute and chronic heart block. *Br Heart J.* 1965;27(6):916–925.

83. Prinzmetal M, Kennamer R. Emergency treatment of cardiac arrhythmias. *J Am Med Assoc.* 1954;154(13):1049–1054.

84. Zoob M, Smith KS. The aetiology of complete heart-block. *Br Med J.* 1963;2(5366):1149–1153.

85. Lown B, Arons WL, Ganong WF, Vazifdar JP, Levine SA. Adrenal steroids and auriculoventricular conduction. *Am Heart J.* 1955;50(5):760–769.

86. Caramelli Z, Tellini RR. Treatment of atrioventricular block with prednisone. *Am J Cardiol.* 1960;5:263–265.

87. Ross R. The pathogenesis of atherosclerosis—an update. *N Engl J Med.* 1986;314(8):488–500.

88. Tamhane S, Rodriguez-Gutierrez R, Iqbal AM, Prokop LJ, Bancos I, Speiser PW, Murad MH. Cardiovascular and metabolic outcomes in congenital adrenal hyperplasia: a systematic review and meta-analysis. *J Clin Endocrinol Metab.* 2018;103(11):4097–4103.

89. Akyürek N, Atabek ME, Eklioğlu BS, Alp H. Ambulatory blood pressure and subclinical cardiovascular disease in patients with congenital adrenal hyperplasia: a preliminary report. *J Clin Res Pediatr Endocrinol.* 2015;7(1):13–18.

90. Bergthorsdottir R, Leonsson-Zachrisson M, Odén A, Johannsson G. Premature mortality in patients with Addison's disease: a population-based study. *J Clin Endocrinol Metab.* 2006;91(12):4849–4853.

91. Skov J, Sundström A, Ludvigsson JF, Kämpe O, Bensing S. Sex-specific risk of cardiovascular disease in autoimmune addison disease: a population-based cohort study. *J Clin Endocrinol Metab.* 2019;104(6):2031–2040.

92. Etxabe J, Vazquez JA. Morbidity and mortality in Cushing's disease: an epidemiological approach. *Clin Endocrinol (Oxf).* 1994;40(4):479–484.

93. Di Dalmazi G, Vicennati V, Garelli S, Casadio E, Rinaldi E, Giampalma E, Mosconi C, Golfieri R, Paccapelo A, Pagotto U, Pasquali R. Cardiovascular events and mortality in patients with adrenal incidentalomas that are either non-secreting or associated with intermediate phenotype or subclinical Cushing's syndrome: a 15-year retrospective study. *Lancet Diabetes Endocrinol.* 2014;2(5):396–405.

94. Lupoli R, Ambrosino P, Tortora A, Barba L, Lupoli GA, Di Minno MN. Markers of atherosclerosis in patients with Cushing's syndrome: a meta-analysis of literature studies. *Ann Med.* 2017;49(3):206–216.

95. Bailey JM, Butler J. Anti-inflammatory drugs in experimental atherosclerosis. I. Relative potencies for inhibiting plaque formation. *Atherosclerosis.* 1973;17(3):515–522.

96. Asai K, Funaki C, Hayashi T, Yamada K, Naito M, Kuzuya M, Yoshida F, Yoshimine N, Kuzuya F. Dexamethasone-induced suppression of aortic atherosclerosis in cholesterol-fed rabbits. Possible mechanisms. *Arterioscler Thromb.* 1993;13(6):892–899.

97. Poon M, Gertz SD, Fallon JT, Wiegman P, Berman JW, Sarembock IJ, Taubman MB. Dexamethasone inhibits macrophage accumulation after balloon arterial injury in cholesterol fed rabbits. *Atherosclerosis.* 2001;155(2):371–380.

98. Tvedegaard E, Szpirt W, Nielsen M. Effect of chronic renal failure and methylprednisolone treatment on the uptake of labelled plasma cholesterol into the aorta of normocholesterolemic rabbits. *Atherosclerosis.* 1983;47(2):199–209.

99. Hermanowski-Vosatka A, Balkovec JM, Cheng K, Chen HY, Hernandez M, Koo GC, Le Grand CB, Li Z, Metzger JM, Mundt SS, Noonan H, Nunes CN, Olson SH, Pikounis B, Ren N, Robertson N, Schaeffer JM, Shah K, Springer MS, Strack AM, Strowski M, Wu K, Wu T, Xiao J, Zhang BB, Wright SD, Thieringer R. 11beta-HSD1 inhibition ameliorates metabolic syndrome and prevents progression of atherosclerosis in mice. *J Exp Med.* 2005;202(4):517–527.

100. van der Valk FM, Schulte DM, Meiler S, Tang J, Zheng KH, Van den Bossche J, Seijkens T, Laudes M, de Winther M, Lutgens E, Alaarg A, Metselaar JM, Dallinga-Thie GM, Mulder WJ, Stroes ES, Hamers AA. Liposomal prednisolone promotes macrophage lipotoxicity in experimental atherosclerosis. *Nanomedicine.* 2016;12(6):1463–1470.

101. van der Sluis RJ, Hoekstra M. Glucocorticoids are active players and therapeutic targets in atherosclerotic cardiovascular disease. *Mol Cell Endocrinol.* 2020;504:110728.

102. Preusch MR, Rattazzi M, Albrecht C, Merle U, Tuckermann J, Schütz G, Blessing E, Zoppellaro G, Pauletto P, Krempien R, Rosenfeld ME, Katus HA, Bea F. Critical role of macrophages in glucocorticoid driven vascular calcification in a mouse-model of atherosclerosis. *Arterioscler Thromb Vasc Biol.* 2008;28(12):2158–2164.

103. Hoekstra M, Frodermann V, van den Aardweg T, van der Sluis RJ, Kuiper J. Leukocytosis and enhanced susceptibility to endotoxemia but not atherosclerosis in adrenalectomized APOE knockout mice. *PLoS One.* 2013;8(11):e80441.

4 Transforming Growth Factor-β/Smad Signaling in Myocardial Disease

Claudio Humeres and Nikolaos G. Frangogiannis

CONTENTS

INTRODUCTION

The three transforming growth factor-β (TGF-β) isoforms are critically involved in the regulation of cell survival, differentiation, phenotype, and function, and they have been implicated in organ development and in the pathogenesis of many pathologic conditions. Tissue injury is associated with rapid activation of latent TGF-β stores and de novo synthesis of TGF-β isoforms, resulting in marked increases in TGF-β activity. Active TGF-βs bind to the ubiquitously expressed TGF-β receptors and modulate cell phenotype and function, signaling through activation of a family of intracellular effectors, the Smads. In addition to Smad-dependent signaling, TGF-βs also transduce Smad-independent signals involving a wide range of intracellular pathways, including p38 mitogen-activated protein kinase (MAPK), Erk

DOI: 10.1201/b22824-5

MAPK, transforming growth factor-β–activated kinase 1 (TAK1), phosphoinositide 3-kinase (PI-3K), and Rho kinase cascades.

A large body of evidence suggests an important role for TGF-β signaling in cardiac pathology. TGF-β is a central mediator in the pathophysiology of myocardial infarction and chronic heart failure and in the cardiomyopathies associated with metabolic diseases and aging. Smad cascades are rapidly activated in injured and remodeling hearts and are prominently involved in modulating cellular phenotype and regulating cardiac function. This chapter reviews the role of Smad-dependent signaling in the pathogenesis of myocardial diseases. We discuss the cell-specific actions of Smad cascades in cardiac pathophysiology, the molecular mechanisms responsible for Smad-dependent actions, and the involvement of TGF-β/Smad-dependent signaling in common myocardial diseases. Despite its complexity and context-specific actions, the TGF-β/Smad cascade may be a promising therapeutic target for patients with myocardial diseases.

THE TGF-β SIGNALING CASCADE

Most tissues contain latent stores of TGF-β that can be activated following injury. It has been suggested that activation of a small fraction of the preexisting latent TGF-β stores is sufficient to trigger a maximal cellular response[1]. Following activation, TGF-βs bind to their receptors, initiating signaling. All members of the TGF-β superfamily signal through characteristic combinations of type I and type II TGF-β receptors (TβRs)[2,3]. In humans, there are seven type I TβRs [also known as activin-like receptor kinase (ALK) 1–7] and five type II TβRs (TβRII, ActRII, ActRIIB, AMHRII, and BMPRII)[4]. Activins typically signal through ALK4 or ALK7 after binding to ActRII or ActRIIB. The bone morphogenetic protein (BMP) family signals through a number of combinations, including one of the type I receptors ALK1, ALK2, ALK3, and ALK6 and one of the ActRII, ActRIIB, and BMPRII type II TβRs[5,6]. All three TGF-β isoforms (TGF-β1, -β2, and -β3) act through a single type II receptor (TβRII). In most cells, TGF-β isoforms signal through ALK5-TβRII activation[7]; however, in endothelial cells, TGF-β is known to transduce key signals though the ALK1/TβRII pathway[8,9]. Although some studies have suggested that the TGF-β/ALK1 cascade can also be activated in non–endothelial cell types, including fibroblasts[10] and macrophages[11], the pathophysiological role of these pathways is unclear.

Binding of TGF-βs to the constitutively active TβRII promotes recruitment of the type I receptor (ALK5 or ALK1) and formation of a stable, heterotetrameric complex composed of two TβRI-TβRII dimers (Figure 4.1). Stable proximity induces receptor complex rotation and subsequent TβRII transphosphorylation of serine residues at the conserved glycine-serine-rich domain (GS domain) within TβRI. Subsequently, TβRI interacts with and phosphorylates a series of intracellular effectors, called Smads, activating downstream signaling pathways broadly termed as Smad-dependent (canonical) pathways.

On a functional basis, the Smads are classified into three groups: (1) the receptor-activated Smads (R-Smads: Smad1, Smad2, Smad3, Smad5, and Smad8); (2) the common Smad (Co-Smad: Smad4); and (3) the inhibitory Smads (I-Smads: Smad6 and Smad7)[12]. Upon TGFβ-induced ALK5 activation, the R-Smads Smad2 and Smad3 are recruited to the TGF-β complex by the auxiliary adaptor protein SARA (SMAD anchor for receptor activation), which facilitates the interaction of the

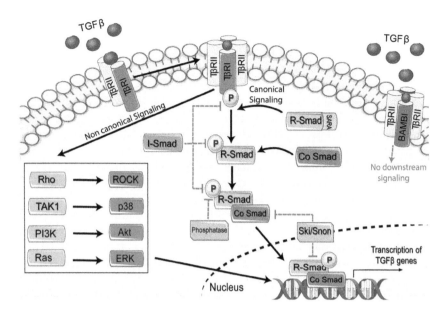

FIGURE 4.1 Schematic cartoon illustrating the TGF-β signaling cascade. Active TGF-β binds to the constitutively active type II receptor (TβRII), recruiting a type I receptor (TβRI, ALK5, or ALK1) and forming a stable heterotetrameric complex composed of two TβRI-TβRII dimers. Subsequent transphosphorylation of serine residues within TβRI leads to interaction of the catalytic region of TβRI with the carboxyl MH2 domain of receptor-activated Smads (R-Smads). Activated R-Smads associate with the common Smad (Co-Smad), Smad4. The R-Smad/Smad4 complex translocates to the nucleus, where it binds to Smad-binding elements or GC-rich sequences in the promoter regions of TGFβ effector genes, regulating the transcription of target genes. Smad-dependent pathways are negatively regulated through several different mechanisms: (1) at the receptor level, expression of the cell surface pseudo-receptor BAMBI (BMP and activin membrane-bound inhibitor) that competes with TβRII for ligand binding suppresses TGF-β/Smad responses; (2) the inhibitory Smads (I-Smads), Smad6/7, are induced and compete with R-Smads for their binding to activated TβRI or Smad4; (3) protein phosphatases dephosphorylate R-Smads; and (4) nuclear co-repressors, like Ski and SnoN, bind to the translocated R-Smad/Co-Smad complex, promoting its degradation or directly preventing the transcription of Smad target genes through recruitment of histone deacetylases. In addition to its Smad-mediated actions, TGF-β also activates noncanonical signaling pathways, including MAPKs, TAK1, Rho GTPases, and FAK.

catalytic region of TβRI with the carboxyl MH2 domain of the R-Smads, leading to R-Smad phosphorylation in the C-terminal SXSS motif[13]. R-Smad phosphorylation induces a conformational change in the MH2 domain, enabling its dissociation from TβRI/SARA and subsequent association with Smad4[14]. Finally, nuclear localization signal (NLS) motifs in the amino-terminal MH1 domain of the R-Smad/Smad4 complex allow its translocation to the nucleus, where it binds to Smad-binding elements or GC-rich sequences in the promoter regions of TGFβ effector genes, regulating the transcription of target genes[15]. Typically, ALK5 signaling triggers Smad2 and Smad3 activation, whereas ALK1 signaling activates Smad1/5; these two cascades have been suggested to play antagonistic roles in certain cell types[16,17].

The balance between downstream activation of the ALK5-Smad2/3 and ALK1-Smad1/5 cascades is regulated through interactions between TGF-β receptors and "accessory receptors"[3]. Endoglin acts as an accessory protein for TGF-β signaling predominantly in endothelial cells and in activated fibroblasts, negatively regulating ALK5-Smad2/3 responses while enhancing ALK1-Smad1/5/8 signaling[18,19,20]. Betaglycan, a transmembrane glycoprotein that serves as a co-receptor, can either activate or inhibit TGF-β signaling responses, depending on its expression levels, and on contextual factors[21,22]. Although betaglycan and endoglin are the best-studied TGF-β co-receptors, a growing list of other transmembrane molecules (such as CD44 and neuropilin-1)[23,24,25] may also modulate TGF-β responses. In most cases, these co-receptors are promiscuous and interact with many other growth factors; thus, their role in modulating TGF-β responses in vivo remains unclear.

The canonical pathway is tightly regulated through negative feedback-regulatory mechanisms at several different levels. First, at the receptor level, increased expression of the cell surface pseudo-receptor BAMBI (BMP and activin membrane-bound inhibitor) that competes with TβRII for ligand binding[26,27] suppresses TGF-β/Smad responses. Second, the I-Smads Smad6 and Smad7 compete with R-Smads for their binding to activated TβRI or Smad4 and may also mediate TβRI degradation by recruitment of Smurf ubiquitin ligases[28]. Third, protein phosphatases dephosphorylate the R-Smad/Smad4 complex[29]. Fourth, nuclear co-repressors, like Ski and SnoN, bind to the translocated R-Smad/Co-Smad complex, promoting its degradation via Smurf2 or directly preventing transcription of Smad target genes by recruiting histone deacetylases[30].

In addition to the effects mediated by Smad signaling pathways, TGF-βs activate noncanonical signaling pathways, including MAPK family responses, TAK1, Rho GTPase pathways, PI-3K/AKT, and focal adhesion kinases (FAK)[31,32,33]. Cross-talk interactions between canonical and noncanonical pathways[34,35,36] and cooperation between TGF-β signaling pathways and other cascades [such as nuclear factor-κB (NF-κB), Wnt/β-catenin, and notch signaling][37,38,39] provide additional layers of complexity that contribute to the wide range of context-dependent effects of TGF-βs

THE EFFECTS OF TGF-β/SMAD CASCADES ON MYOCARDIAL CELLS

Although cardiomyocytes occupy most of the volume of the heart, the adult myocardium also contains large numbers of non-cardiomyocytes (predominantly endothelial cells, fibroblasts, macrophages, lymphocytes, dendritic cells, mast cells, vascular smooth muscle cells, and pericytes)[40] that can become activated following injury and play an important role in cardiac repair. Although TGF-βs are known to exert a wide range of actions on all myocardial cell types, the relative significance of Smad-dependent signaling in mediating these actions remains poorly understood. In some cases, contrasting actions of various TGF-β superfamily ligands are attributed to the same Smad-dependent molecular pathway, illustrating the challenges to understanding how mediators with similar pathway activation profiles in vitro can have very different in vivo actions.

SMAD-DEPENDENT SIGNALING PATHWAYS IN CARDIOMYOCYTES

Cardiomyocytes express R-Smads that can be activated upon stimulation with TGF-β superfamily members. Angiotensin II stimulation also activates Smad2/3 in cardiomyocytes[41], presumably through TGF-β-dependent actions. In vitro studies have implicated the gap junction protein connexin43 (Cx43) in the regulation of the subcellular localization of R-Smads in cardiomyocytes. Cx43 promotes the release of Smad2 and Smad3 from microtubules, increasing phosphorylation and facilitating subsequent nuclear accumulation[42].

In vitro, TGF-βs have profound effects on cardiomyocyte phenotype and function, stimulating hypertrophic responses and inducing fetal patterns of contractile protein gene expression[43,44,45]. However, to what extent these responses are mediated through R-Smad signaling remains unknown. Moreover, attempts to explain the anti-hypertrophic effects of other members of the TGF-β superfamily by attributing them to Smad activation have produced contradictory conclusions. Some studies have implicated the activation of Smad2 and Smad3 pathways in the pathogenesis of cardiomyocyte hypertrophy[46]. This is consistent with experimental findings showing a crucial role for Smad3 signaling in mediating glucose-induced cellular hypertrophy[47]. By contrast, in other studies Smad2 and Smad3 have been implicated as mediators of anti-hypertrophic effects. In skeletal muscle, Smad2 and Smad-3 have been suggested to induce an atrophy program in response to myostatin[48], another member of the TGF-β superfamily. In cardiomyocytes, Smad2 overexpression attenuated hypertrophic responses[49,50], and Smad3 was found to mediate Pak-1-induced inhibition of hypertrophy[51]. Other investigations have suggested neutral effects of Smad2 and Smad3 in cardiomyocyte hypertrophy. In rat ventricular cardiomyocytes, angiotensin II–induced hypertrophy was dependent on TAK1 and not on Smad2/3 signaling[41]. In addition to hypertrophy, other cardiomyocyte responses may also involve R-Smad activation. Experiments in cardiomyocyte-specific Smad3 knockout mice suggested that Smad3 may mediate the apoptosis of cardiomyocytes in the remodeling heart[52]. Whether these findings are due to direct effects of Smad3 on cardiomyocyte survival under conditions of stress or reflect changes secondary to adverse remodeling and increased ventricular pressures remains unknown. Cardiomyocyte Smad3 may also regulate the metabolic function of cardiomyocytes. In isolated cardiomyocytes, Smad3 overexpression suppressed cardiac fatty acid beta oxidation[53], suggesting potentially significant effects of R-Smad signaling on substrate utilization. Experiments in zebrafish suggested that TGF-β/Smad3 signaling may be critically involved in cardiac regeneration[54]. However, the relevance of these observations in mammalian cell biology remains unclear.

Smad1, on the other hand, has been implicated in the inhibition of cardiomyocyte apoptosis[55], and cardiomyocyte Smad1 overexpression was found to protect from myocardial ischemia/reperfusion injury[56]. However, the relative role of the Smad1 cascade in mediating effects of TGF-βs in cardiomyocytes is unknown. BMPs are also rapidly induced in ischemic and remodeling hearts[57] and may be the predominant activators of Smad1 signaling in stressed cardiomyocytes.

THE ROLE OF SMAD SIGNALING CASCADES IN FIBROBLASTS

Fibroblasts rapidly activate Smad2 and Smad3 signaling in response to TGF-βs, both in vitro and in vivo, in a wide range of cardiac pathophysiologic conditions[58,59,60]. In vitro, TGF-β/Smad3 activation has robust and highly reproducible activating effects on cardiac fibroblasts[61], inducing a myofibroblast phenotype, stimulating the transcription of structural and matricellular extracellular matrix protein genes[62], and promoting a matrix-preserving phenotype characterized by the suppressed synthesis of matrix metalloproteinases (MMPs) and the induction of anti-proteases, such as tissue inhibitor of metalloproteinase-1 (TIMP-1) and plasminogen activator inhibitor-1 (PAI-1)[58,63]. Moreover, Smad3 stimulates fibroblast expression of integrins, facilitating interactions between the fibroblasts and the extracellular matrix and promoting the formation of an organized scar[52]. Smad3 has anti-proliferative effects on cardiac fibroblasts[62], suggesting that Smad3-dependent myofibroblast activation is accompanied by tight regulation of the expanding fibroblast population.

Although some studies have attributed the profibrotic actions of TGF-βs to the stimulation of Smad2 signaling[64], the direct in vivo evidence implicating Smad2 in fibroblast activation is limited. In vitro, Smad2 has been implicated in cardiac fibroblast to myofibroblast conversion; however, in vivo, myofibroblast-specific activation of Smad2 was not involved in the activation of reparative fibroblasts following myocardial infarction[60]. Smad3, but not Smad2, was involved in fibroblast integrin synthesis. These findings contrast the essential activating effects of Smad3 on fibroblast-driven repair of the infarcted heart[60]. The contrasting effects of these closely related R-Smads may be due to distinct patterns of activation or nuclear translocation or to differences in their transcriptional actions.

Very little is known regarding the potential role of Smad1 signaling in the regulation of fibroblast phenotype in response to TGF-β. Surprisingly, in a mouse model of scleroderma-like fibrosis due to forced expression of ALK5, activation of a fibrogenic transcriptional program was found to be dependent on Smad1 and Erk1/2, and not on Smad2/3[65], suggesting that an ALK1/Smad1 pathway may be critically involved in certain fibrotic conditions. However, the role of Smad1 signaling in the activation of cardiac fibroblasts remains unknown.

SMAD SIGNALING CASCADES IN MONOCYTES AND MACROPHAGES

TGF-β is a central regulator of leukocyte phenotype and function. Its effects on monocytes and macrophages can be either stimulatory or inhibitory, depending on the cytokine milieu and the state of differentiation of the cells[66]. TGF-β is a potent chemotactic mediator for monocytes, acting in femtomolar concentrations[67]. Moreover, picomolar concentrations of TGF-β have been suggested to stimulate monocyte synthesis of cytokines, chemokines, growth factors, and integrins[67,68]. In contrast to its activating effects on monocytes, TGF-β exerts predominantly suppressive actions on mature macrophages, attenuating cytokine and chemokine secretion[69]. In infarcted hearts, Smad3 is rapidly activated in macrophages infiltrating the ischemic zone. Smad3 activation in infarct macrophages not only may involve the effects of TGF-βs but may also be directly triggered by phagocytosis (Figure 4.2) through an as-yet-unidentified mechanism[70]. Smad3 was found to activate a phagocytic program in macrophages by inducing the expression of milk fat globule-epidermal growth factor-factor VIII (Mfge8). Moreover, macrophage Smad3 has been implicated in the anti-inflammatory transition of macrophages[70] and in TGF-β-mediated suppression of a matrix-degrading program[71]. The role of Smad2 in the regulation of macrophage phenotype and function remains unknown. Moreover, in vitro studies have suggested that TGF-β may also modulate macrophage phenotype

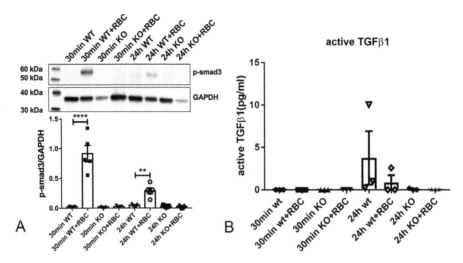

FIGURE 4.2 Phagocytosis activates Smad3 in macrophages in the absence of TGF-β release. This figure shows an intriguing mechanism of R-Smad activation that may not involve TGF-βs. When incubated with bone marrow (BM) macrophages, aged sheep red blood cells (RBCs) are rapidly phagocytosed. (A) After 30 minutes of incubation with RBCs, wild-type (WT) BM macrophages exhibited markedly increased expression of p-Smad3 (****p < 0.0001 vs. control cells). BM macrophages harvested from Smad3 knockout mice (KO) served as a negative control, exhibiting no Smad3 activation. After 24 hours of incubation with RBCs, WT BM macrophages exhibited persistent activation of Smad3 (**p < 0.01 vs. corresponding control). (B) In order to examine whether the rapid activation of Smad3 signaling is due to release of TGF-β upon RBC phagocytosis, we assessed the levels of TGF-β1 in the supernatant. No active TGF-β1 was detected after 30 minutes of incubation with RBCs. After 24 hours of incubation, the supernatant from control WT cells and from cells incubated with RBCs had low levels of active TGF-β1. The findings are consistent with the phagocytosis-mediated activation of Smad3 signaling in macrophages that occurs in the absence of TGF-β and may be ligand independent. Thus, in healing infarcts, macrophage Smad3 may be activated both by TGF-βs and in response to phagocytosis of dead cells.

Source: Reproduced with permission from Chen et al.[70].

by activating Smad1[11]. However, in vivo studies examining the role of macrophage Smad1 actions have not been performed.

R-SMADS IN REGULATION OF LYMPHOCYTE PHENOTYPE

TGF-β is a critical regulator of lymphocyte phenotype in homeostasis and in disease[72,73,74]. Lymphocyte subpopulations have been implicated in the regulation of inflammatory and fibrotic responses following myocardial infarction. Regulatory T cells are recruited in healing infarcts and have been suggested to act as suppressors of the post-infarction inflammatory response[75,76,77]. In contrast, in chronic heart failure, dysregulation of Treg function may be involved in adverse remodeling[78]. CD4+ T lymphocytes have been implicated in the repair of the infarcted heart[79], whereas Th1 effector T cells have been involved in the pathogenesis of cardiac fibrotic responses following pressure overload[80]. The effects of TGF-β on lymphocyte phenotype and function may involve both Smad2/3-dependent signaling and non-Smad cascades[81]. Unfortunately, the patterns of activation and the effects of Smad signaling pathways in lymphocytes infiltrating the injured and remodeling myocardium have not been investigated.

Smad Cascades in Vascular Endothelial Cells

TGF-βs play a critical role in the regulation of endothelial cell, pericyte, and vascular smooth muscle cell phenotype and function in homeostasis and disease[82], exerting a wide range of context-dependent actions[82,83,84]. Both angiogenic and angiostatic effects of TGF-β have been reported, depending on the experimental context and the type of assay used[82]. The relative role of R-Smads in mediating the effects of TGF-β superfamily members on the vasculature remains poorly understood. In vitro studies have identified Smad2 as a critical regulator of autophagy in endothelial cells, suggesting that Smad2 actions may inhibit angiogenesis[85]. It has also been suggested that TGF-β-mediated endothelial activation of Smad3 may be responsible for endothelial to mesenchymal transition, contributing to fibrosis in the heart and in other organs[86,87].

TGF-β/SMAD SIGNALING IN MYOCARDIAL HOMEOSTASIS AND DISEASE

Smad-Dependent Signaling in Homeostasis of the Adult Heart

Although the role of TGF-β/Smad-dependent signaling in cardiac development is well established[88], whether these pathways play a role in homeostasis of the adult heart is unknown. Adult mouse hearts express significant amounts of Smad2 and Smad3; however, the level of baseline R-Smad activation is low[89]. The absence of significant baseline defects in adult cardiomyocyte-specific Smad3 knockout mice[52] suggests that the pathway does not play a critical role in cardiomyocyte homeostasis. Fibroblasts are abundant in normal adult mouse hearts and may maintain the integrity of the cardiac extracellular matrix network. In vivo studies showed that inducible fibroblast-specific Smad3 loss modestly but significantly attenuated collagen levels in young adult mouse hearts, without affecting cardiac function and ventricular geometry, suggesting a role of baseline Smad3 activity in cardiac matrix homeostasis[89]. In contrast, fibroblast Smad2 loss had no significant effect on collagen levels. Whether Smad-dependent pathways are involved in the regulation of phenotype and function of vascular and immune cells in normal adult hearts remains unknown.

Smad-Dependent Signaling in Injury, Repair, and Remodeling Following Myocardial Infarction

In the infarcted myocardium, release of active TGF-β rapidly stimulates Smad2 and Smad3 signaling in border zone cardiomyocytes, infarct fibroblasts, and macrophages[58,60,70]. In vivo studies using cell-specific loss-of-function models have suggested an important role for Smad3 in the regulation of cellular phenotype and function in infarcted and remodeling hearts (Table 4.1). Cardiomyocyte Smad3 is involved in the pathogenesis of adverse remodeling and dysfunction following reperfused myocardial

TABLE 4.1
Experimental Evidence on the Role of Smad2/3 Signaling in Myocardial Disease

Condition/Model	Intervention	Major Findings	Reference
Mouse/reperfused and non-reperfused MI	Myofibroblast-specific loss of Smad3	Activation of Smad3 in infarct myofibroblasts induces synthesis of integrins, triggering an α5 integrin-NOX2 axis and promoting formation of organized scars containing aligned myofibroblasts. Formation of an organized scar protects from rupture (in non-reperfused infarcts) and from adverse remodeling.	52
Mouse/reperfused MI	Cardiomyocyte-specific loss of Smad3	Cardiomyocyte-specific Smad3 accentuates NOX2 expression/nitrosative stress–promoting cell apoptosis and augments MMP2-dependent degradation of matrix in the non-infarcted remote remodeling myocardium, leading to systolic dysfunction.	52
Mouse/non-reperfused MI	Myeloid cell–specific loss of Smad3	Myeloid cell–specific Smad3 signaling promotes macrophage-mediated phagocytosis and anti-inflammatory transition, contributing to repair of the infarcted heart.	70
Mouse/non-reperfused infarction	Myofibroblast-specific Smad2 loss Myofibroblast-specific Smad3 loss	Smad2 activation in myofibroblasts does not play a major role in repair and fibrosis of the infarcted heart. Smad3 (but not Smad2) induces an increase in fibroblast integrins α2 and α5 and RhoA GTPase (mediator of planar cell polarity pathways) expression, regulating fibroblast activation and organization into well-arranged fibers in the healing infarct.	60
Mouse/obese diabetic db/db mice	Obese diabetic leptin-resistant db/db with partial or complete Smad3 loss	Smad3 mediates fibrosis and promotes diastolic dysfunction in obese diabetic mice, at least in part through suppression of MMP2 and MMP9 activity and through attenuation of oxidative/nitrosative stress.	

(Continued)

TABLE 4.1
(Continued)

Condition/Model	Intervention	Major Findings	Reference
		However, Smad3-mediated suppression of MMPs is important for matrix preservation, preventing chamber dilation. Complete loss of Smad3 in diabetic mice decreased collagen synthesis and increased MMP expression in the aorta, leading to aortic dilation.	106
Mouse/reperfused MI	Global Smad3 null mice	Smad3 critically regulated TGF-β1-mediated extracellular matrix synthesis (collagen III and tenascin-C) as well as the expression of TIMP1-2.	58
Mouse/reperfused MI	Global Smad3 null mice	Smad3 mediates several of TGFβ1 actions of fibroblasts in infarct such as anti-proliferative, pro-migratory, and pro-contractile effects, promoting extracellular matrix synthesis and fibrosis-associated and -inducing CCN2 gene expression.	62
Mouse/cardiomyopathy induced through infusion of angiotensin II	Global Smad3 null mice	Smad3 mediates cardiac fibrosis and dysfunction in a model of angiotensin II infusion.	94
Mouse/-pressure overload induced through TAC	Global Smad3 null mice	Smad3 protected from death and mediated fibrosis, but attenuated hypertrophy after TAC.	95
Mouse/pressure overload induced through TAC	Myofibroblast-specific Smad3 KO mice	Myofibroblast Smad3 protected the pressure-overloaded hearts from systolic dysfunction by preserving the matrix (through downmodulation of collagenases) and by reducing release of matrix fragments with pro-inflammatory and pro-apoptotic properties.	63
Mouse/pressure overload induced through TAC	Conditional fibroblast- and myofibroblast-specific TGFβR1, TGFβR2, Smad2, Smad3, and Smad2/3 knockout mice	Smad2/Smad3 signaling mediated fibroblast activation, inducing Col1a1, Col1a2, Col3a1, fibronectin, α-SMA, Lox12, Adam12, Adam30, Sparc, and integrins α2, α8, and β3.	100

Condition/Model	Intervention	Major Findings	Reference
Mouse/pressure overload induced through aortic constriction	Oral administration of TGFβ1 receptor type 1 (ALK5) small molecule inhibitor (SM16)	Inhibition of ALK5 improved systolic (increased fractional shortening) and diastolic function (decreased mitral flow deceleration). Protective effects were attributed to Smad2 inhibition (despite the lack of specificity of the approach). Protection was associated with attenuated collagen (I, III, VIII, XV) expression and improved calcium handling through prevention of SERCA2 intracellular depletion.	98
Rat/non-reperfused MI	Oral administration of TGFβ1 receptor type 1 (ALK5) inhibitor (GW788388)	ALK5 inhibition attenuated myofibroblast accumulation, collagen deposition, and cardiomyocyte hypertrophy, leading to an improvement in systolic function after infarction.	97
Mouse/pressure overload induced through aortic constriction	Oral administration of TGFβ1 receptor type 1 (ALK5) small molecule inhibitor (SM16)	ALK5 inhibition reduced fibrosis (collagen deposition and cross-linking) following aortic banding, improved diastolic function, and reduced pulmonary congestion. Protective actions were attributed to inhibition of Smad2 and subsequent reduction in expression of TGFβ1-induced fibrotic and collagen cross-linking genes, such as Col1a2, LOX, SPARC, and osteopontin.	96

infarction through effects on the apoptosis of cardiomyocytes in the remodeling non-infarcted myocardium[52]. Smad3-mediated cardiomyocyte apoptosis may involve the activation of oxidative stress. Moreover, cardiomyocyte Smad3 was implicated in the induction and activation of MMP2 that may mediate matrix degradation, accentuating adverse dilative remodeling[52]. The role of cardiomyocyte Smad2 in myocardial infarction remains unknown. On the other hand, cardiomyocyte Smad1 overexpression was found to protect ischemic cardiomyocytes from apoptosis[55]. The anti-apoptotic signals activated by Smad1 in cardiomyocytes remain unknown.

In infarct myofibroblasts, Smad3 was found to be critically involved in the regulation of fibroblast:matrix interactions by inducing the synthesis of integrins, the molecular signals that link the cells to the extracellular matrix[52]. Myofibroblast-specific Smad3 loss attenuated the expression of α2, α5, and β3 integrins, disrupting fibroblast:matrix interactions critical for fibroblast function. Smad-dependent integrin synthesis in fibroblasts was critical for the activation of an oxidative response and for the formation of an organized scar containing aligned myofibroblasts. Thus, following myocardial infarction, myofibroblast Smad3 plays a critical reparative role, protecting the infarcted ventricle from rupture and reducing adverse remodeling. In contrast, myofibroblast Smad2 did not play a significant role in the activation of reparative fibroblasts in vivo[60].

Interestingly, in senescent mice, impaired infarct healing and accentuated adverse remodeling are associated with perturbed activation of TGF-β/R-Smad pathways in fibroblasts[90]. These observations support the intriguing hypothesis that aging-associated impairment in repair following myocardial infarction may be related to attenuated TGF-β/Smad3 activation. Perturbed Smad3 signaling in senescent fibroblasts may indicate a reduced reparative reserve, which may be responsible for the formation of a disorganized scar, reduced tensile strength of the infarct, and accentuated adverse remodeling in senescent subjects that survive acute myocardial infarction[91].

Finally, in infarct macrophages, early activation of Smad3 plays an important role in activation of a phagocytic phenotype and in an anti-inflammatory transition[70]. These effects of Smad3 on macrophages are important in the orchestration of the reparative response and in protection from adverse remodeling.

ROLE OF SMAD SIGNALING CASCADES IN CHRONIC HEART FAILURE

In chronic heart failure, activation of R-Smads has been implicated in the pathogenesis of hypertrophic and fibrotic cellular responses and in the regulation of cardiac function[92]. Left-ventricular pressure overload is the predominant pathophysiologic perturbation in patients with heart failure caused by hypertension or aortic stenosis. Prominent activation of Smad2/3 and Smad1 cascades has been reported in experimental models of pressure overload induced through transverse aortic constriction[93]. Studies using global loss-of-function approaches suggested that Smad3 mediates fibrosis and dysfunction in a model of angiotensin II infusion[94] and promotes fibrosis, while attenuating hypertrophy in a model of left-ventricular pressure overload[95]. Moreover, inhibition of ALK5 attenuated dysfunction and inhibited fibrosis in rodent models of left-ventricular pressure overload; these effects were attributed to the inhibition of Smad2/3 signaling[96,97,98]. Considering the wide range of Smad3 effects on all myocardial, immune, and vascular cells, the cellular basis for these actions remains poorly understood. Cell-specific loss-of-function studies are needed to understand the cell biological actions of R-Smads in the remodeling myocardium. Very limited information is available on the role of R-Smad signaling in heart failure cardiomyocytes. Although cardiomyocyte-specific TβRII signaling has been suggested to play a critical role in dysfunction and adverse remodeling following pressure overload[99], whether these actions are mediated through Smad-dependent mechanisms is not known.

Experiments in fibroblast- and myofibroblast-specific Smad3 KO mice have suggested a critical role for Smad3 signaling in fibroblast activation in failing and remodeling hearts. Although fibroblast Smad3 was involved in long-term fibrotic remodeling of the pressure-overloaded heart[100], early activation of Smad3 in myofibroblasts protected from systolic dysfunction by preserving the extracellular matrix through the downmodulation of collagenases. In the absence of fibroblast Smad3, increased protease activity generates extracellular matrix fragments and promotes collagen degradation, triggering inflammation and increasing cardiomyocyte injury (Figure 4.3)[63]. These observations suggest that activated myofibroblasts may play

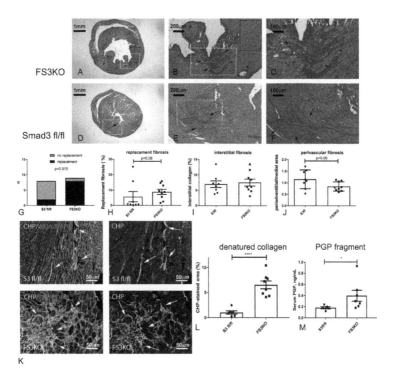

FIGURE 4.3 Fibroblast-specific Smad3 loss accentuates extracellular matrix degradation in the pressure-overloaded heart, resulting in collagen denaturation and the generation of matrix fragments. Sirius red staining labeled the collagen network in pressure-overloaded hearts. (A–F) In the transverse aortic constriction (TAC) model of left-ventricular pressure overload, fibrosis is typically interstitial and perivascular (arrows); there is minimal replacement fibrosis. In contrast to Smad3/fl/fl mice, animals lacking Smad3 in activated myofibroblasts (FS3KO) exhibited foci of replacement fibrosis (arrowheads) 7 days after TAC. (G) Quantitative analysis of replacement fibrosis areas showed that, after 7 days of TAC, 8 out of 9 FS3KO mice had >2.5% of the left ventricular myocardium replaced by scar ($p = 0.015$ vs. Smad3 fl/fl mice, $n = 8$–9/group). (H) The difference in the area of replacement fibrosis between pressure-overloaded FS3KO and Smad3 fl/fl mice did not reach statistical significance ($p = 0.09$). (I) Quantitative analysis of interstitial fibrosis was performed in areas with no evidence of replacement fibrosis (black rectangle, B) and showed no significant differences between Smad3 fl/fl and FS3KO animals. (J) FS3KO and Smad3 fl/fl mice did not have a statistically significant difference in the mean ratio of periadventitial collagen-stained area:medial area, an indicator of perivascular fibrosis ($p = 0.06$). (K–M) Fibroblast-specific Smad3 loss accentuated matrix degradation. In order to study the effects of fibroblast-specific Smad3 loss on collagen fragmentation and denaturation, we used two distinct methods: (1) fluorescent staining with collagen-hybridizing peptide (CHP), which binds only to unfolded, denatured collagen fibers (K, arrows), and (2) mass spectrometry to assess levels of the collagen-derived matrikine Pro-Gly-Pro (PGP). FS3KO mice had extensive collagen denaturation, as evidenced by a marked increase in the CHP-stained area in the pressure-overloaded cardiac interstitium after 7 days of TAC (K, arrows; M, ****$p < 0.0001$, $n = 7$–8/group). (M) Mass spectrometry of serum samples after 7 days of TAC showed that FS3KO mice had a twofold increase in the generation of PGP (*$p < 0.05$, $n = 5$/group).

Source: Reproduced with permission from Russo et al.[63].

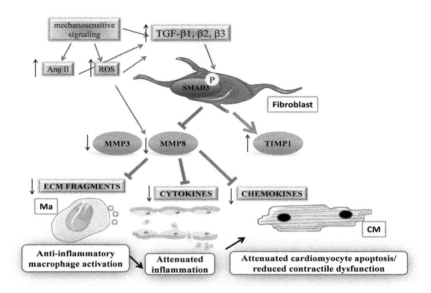

FIGURE 4.4   The protective effects of TGF-β/Smad3-activated fibroblasts in the pressure-overloaded myocardium. Mechanical stress following pressure overload stimulates angiotensin II (Ang II) and generates reactive oxygen species (ROS), activating proteases. TGF-β-mediated stimulation of fibroblasts promotes a matrix-preserving program, suppressing expression of the collagenases MMP3 and MMP8 and inducing TIMP1 synthesis. Reduced matrix degradation decreases the release of collagen-derived fragments and attenuates macrophage-driven inflammation, protecting cardiomyocytes from death and dysfunction. Moreover, restrained MMP activity may inhibit inflammation by decreasing the formation of bioactive cytokine and chemokine molecules.

Source: The cartoon was designed using Servier Medical Art (https:smart.servier.com) and was reproduced with permission from Russo et al.[63].

important reparative roles, even in the absence of myocardial infarction, by stabilizing the extracellular matrix network that surrounds the cardiomyocytes. Under conditions of stress, preservation of the endomysial and perimysial extracellular matrix is important to transduce prosurvival signals in cardiomyocytes, preventing cardiomyocyte death (Figure 4.4). Additional mechanisms involving matricellular proteins, secreted growth factors, and miRNA-containing exosomes may also contribute to the protective actions of fibroblasts in the pressure-overloaded hearts. Considering the remarkable heterogeneity of fibroblast populations[101,102,103], the protective actions of Smad3-activated fibroblasts in the early stages of cardiac remodeling may involve specific subsets of interstitial cells.

R-Smads in Diabetic Heart Disease

Diabetic patients have an increased incidence of heart failure, not exclusively related to accelerated atherosclerotic coronary disease but also caused by a distinct cardiomyopathic condition associated with fibrosis, hypertrophy, and diastolic dysfunction.

In animal models, diabetes is associated with TGF-β induction and R-Smad activation in many different tissues, including the heart[104,105,106]. R-Smad activation in diabetic tissues likely reflects the effects of hyperglycemia-mediated upregulation of TβRs[47]. Limited information is available on the role of Smad-dependent signaling in diabetic cardiomyopathy. Experiments using a global Smad3 haploinsufficiency model suggested that Smad3 mediates, at least in part, the increased collagen deposition noted in diabetic hearts by suppressing MMP activity. Smad3-dependent matrix deposition was involved in diastolic dysfunction but also preserved ventricular geometry, preventing chamber dilation[106]. Thus, TGF-β/R-Smad signaling may be involved in the pathogenesis of heart failure with preserved ejection fraction (HFpEF), which is typically associated with long-standing diabetes and obesity.

TGF-β/SMAD SIGNALING AS A THERAPEUTIC TARGET IN MYOCARDIAL DISEASE

Despite its critical role in a wide range of pathologic conditions, TGF-β remains a challenging therapeutic target[107,108,109]. Although pharmacologic inhibition of Smad2 and Smad3 signaling is feasible, the cell-specific effects of Smad cascades hamper the implementation of therapeutic interventions. In the infarcted heart, fibroblast and macrophage Smad3 activation appears to play important roles in repair, whereas cardiomyocyte Smad3 is protective[52,70]. We currently have very limited information regarding the role of Smad3 in the regulation of lymphocyte, dendritic cell, and vascular cell function following myocardial infarction. Moreover, we know very little regarding the potential role of endogenous Smad2 and Smad1 cascades in myocardial injury, repair, and remodeling.

Chronic heart failure, on the other hand exhibits remarkable pathophysiologic heterogeneity. In heart failure associated with hypertension, sustained or overactive Smad3 activation in interstitial cells is likely to be detrimental, promoting fibrosis and accentuating diastolic dysfunction. Thus, considering its profibrotic actions, inhibition of Smad3 in patients with HFpEF and prominent fibrotic changes may be a logical strategy. Unfortunately, experimental studies and the biology of R-Smads suggest caution regarding such approaches. In mouse models of left-ventricular pressure overload, early Smad3-dependent activation of myofibroblasts had protective matrix-preserving effects[63], raising concerns that overzealous Smad3 inhibition may result in the generation of matrix fragments with injurious properties. Thus, the implementation of strategies targeting Smad3 to inhibit fibrosis in patients with chronic heart failure requires pathophysiologic stratification and identification of patient sub-populations with excessive or unrestrained fibrogenic responses. Moreover, chronic therapy may carry significant risks, perturbing TGF-β-driven repair and abrogating important homeostatic signals that preserve aortic geometry.

CONCLUSIONS

Our current knowledge of the cell-specific actions of TGF-β/Smad signaling in vivo is not sufficient to design therapeutic interventions. Extensive experimental work is needed to study the role of Smad signaling cascades and their mechanisms of regulation in the cell types involved in myocardial disease. Moreover, we need to gain insight into the patterns of TGF-β/Smad activation in patients with myocardial diseases in order to identify subsets who may benefit from Smad targeting.

ACKNOWLEDGMENTS

Dr. Frangogiannis's laboratory is supported by National Institutes of Health (NIH) grants R01HL76246, R01HL85440, and R01HL149407 and by Department of Defense grants PR151029, PR151134, and PR181464. Dr. Humeres is supported by American Heart Association postdoctoral award 19POST34450144.

BIBLIOGRAPHY

1. Annes JP, Munger JS, Rifkin DB. Making sense of latent TGFbeta activation. J Cell Sci. 2003; 116:217–224.
2. Massague J. How cells read TGF-beta signals. Nat Rev Mol Cell Biol. 2000; 1:169–178.
3. Heldin CH, Moustakas A. Signaling Receptors for TGF-beta Family Members. Cold Spring Harb Perspect Biol. 2016; 8.
4. Heldin CH, Moustakas A. Signaling Receptors for TGF-β Family Members. Cold Spring Harb Perspect Biol. 2016; 8.
5. Feng XH, Derynck R. Specificity and versatility in tgf-beta signaling through Smads. Annu Rev Cell Dev Biol. 2005; 21:659–693.
6. Miyazono K, Maeda S, Imamura T. BMP receptor signaling: transcriptional targets, regulation of signals, and signaling cross-talk. Cytokine Growth Factor Rev. 2005; 16:251–263.
7. Rahimi RA, Leof EB. TGF-beta signaling: a tale of two responses. J Cell Biochem. 2007; 102:593–608.
8. Eickelberg O, Centrella M, Reiss M, Kashgarian M, Wells RG. Betaglycan inhibits TGF-beta signaling by preventing type I-type II receptor complex formation. Glycosaminoglycan modifications alter betaglycan function. J Biol Chem. 2002; 277:823–829.
9. Goumans MJ, Valdimarsdottir G, Itoh S, Rosendahl A, Sideras P, ten Dijke P. Balancing the activation state of the endothelium via two distinct TGF-beta type I receptors. Embo J. 2002; 21:1743–1753.
10. Zhang H, Du L, Zhong Y, Flanders KC, Roberts JD, Jr. Transforming growth factor-beta stimulates Smad1/5 signaling in pulmonary artery smooth muscle cells and fibroblasts of the newborn mouse through ALK1. Am J Physiol Lung Cell Mol Physiol. 2017; 313:L615-L627.
11. Nurgazieva D, Mickley A, Moganti K, Ming W, Ovsyi I, Popova A, Sachindra, Awad K, Wang N, Bieback K, Goerdt S, Kzhyshkowska J, Gratchev A. TGF-beta1, but not bone morphogenetic proteins, activates Smad1/5 pathway in primary human macrophages and induces expression of proatherogenic genes. J Immunol. 2015; 194:709–718.
12. Hata A, Chen YG. TGF-β signaling from receptors to Smads. Cold Spring Harb Perspect Biol. 2016; 8.
13. Wu G, Chen YG, Ozdamar B, Gyuricza CA, Chong PA, Wrana JL, Massague J, Shi Y. Structural basis of Smad2 recognition by the Smad anchor for receptor activation. Science. 2000; 287:92–97.
14. Xu L, Chen YG, Massagué J. The nuclear import function of Smad2 is masked by SARA and unmasked by TGFbeta-dependent phosphorylation. Nat Cell Biol. 2000; 2:559–562.

15. Xiao Z, Latek R, Lodish HF. An extended bipartite nuclear localization signal in Smad4 is required for its nuclear import and transcriptional activity. Oncogene. 2003; 22:1057–1069.

16. Curado F, Spuul P, Egana I, Rottiers P, Daubon T, Veillat V, Duhamel P, Leclercq A, Gontier E, Genot E. ALK5 and ALK1 play antagonistic roles in transforming growth factor beta-induced podosome formation in aortic endothelial cells. Mol Cell Biol. 2014; 34:4389–4403.

17. Finnson KW, Parker WL, ten Dijke P, Thorikay M, Philip A. ALK1 opposes ALK5/Smad3 signaling and expression of extracellular matrix components in human chondrocytes. J Bone Miner Res. 2008; 23:896–906.

18. Lebrin F, Goumans MJ, Jonker L, Carvalho RL, Valdimarsdottir G, Thorikay M, Mummery C, Arthur HM, ten Dijke P. Endoglin promotes endothelial cell proliferation and TGF-beta/ALK1 signal transduction. Embo J. 2004; 23:4018–4028.

19. Leask A, Abraham DJ, Finlay DR, Holmes A, Pennington D, Shi-Wen X, Chen Y, Venstrom K, Dou X, Ponticos M, Black C, Bernabeu C, Jackman JK, Findell PR, Connolly MK. Dysregulation of transforming growth factor beta signaling in scleroderma: overexpression of endoglin in cutaneous scleroderma fibroblasts. Arthritis Rheum. 2002; 46:1857–1865.

20. Rodriguez-Pena A, Eleno N, Duwell A, Arevalo M, Perez-Barriocanal F, Flores O, Docherty N, Bernabeu C, Letarte M, Lopez-Novoa JM. Endoglin upregulation during experimental renal interstitial fibrosis in mice. Hypertension. 2002; 40:713–720.

21. You HJ, Bruinsma MW, How T, Ostrander JH, Blobe GC. The type III TGF-beta receptor signals through both Smad3 and the p38 MAP kinase pathways to contribute to inhibition of cell proliferation. Carcinogenesis. 2007; 28:2491–2500.

22. Tazat K, Hector-Greene M, Blobe GC, Henis YI. TbetaRIII independently binds type I and type II TGF-beta receptors to inhibit TGF-beta signaling. Mol Biol Cell. 2015; 26:3535–3545.

23. Villalobos E, Criollo A, Schiattarella GG, Altamirano F, French KM, May HI, Jiang N, Nguyen NUN, Romero D, Roa JC, Garcia L, Diaz-Araya G, Morselli E, Ferdous A, Conway SJ, Sadek HA, Gillette TG, Lavandero S, Hill JA. Fibroblast primary cilia are required for cardiac fibrosis. Circulation. 2019; 139:2342–2357.

24. Huebener P, Abou-Khamis T, Zymek P, Bujak M, Ying X, Chatila K, Haudek S, Thakker G, Frangogiannis NG. CD44 Is Critically Involved in Infarct Healing by Regulating the Inflammatory and Fibrotic Response. J Immunol. 2008; 180:2625–2633.

25. Villar AV, Garcia R, Llano M, Cobo M, Merino D, Lantero A, Tramullas M, Hurle JM, Hurle MA, Nistal JF. BAMBI (BMP and activin membrane-bound inhibitor) protects the murine heart from pressure-overload biomechanical stress by restraining TGF-beta signaling. Biochim Biophys Acta. 2013; 1832:323–335.

26. Sekiya T, Oda T, Matsuura K, Akiyama T. Transcriptional regulation of the TGF-beta pseudoreceptor BAMBI by TGF-beta signaling. Biochem Biophys Res Commun. 2004; 320:680–684.

27. Yan X, Lin Z, Chen F, Zhao X, Chen H, Ning Y, Chen YG. Human BAMBI cooperates with Smad7 to inhibit transforming growth factor-beta signaling. J Biol Chem. 2009; 284:30097–30104.

28. Miyazawa K, Miyazono K. Regulation of TGF-β family signaling by inhibitory Smads. Cold Spring Harb Perspect Biol. 2017; 9.

29. Lin X, Duan X, Liang YY, Su Y, Wrighton KH, Long J, Hu M, Davis CM, Wang J, Brunicardi FC, Shi Y, Chen YG, Meng A, Feng XH. PPM1A functions as a Smad phosphatase to terminate TGFβ Signaling. Cell. 2016; 166:1597.

30. Luo K. Ski and SnoN: negative regulators of TGF-beta signaling. Curr Opin Genet Dev. 2004; 14:65–70.

31. Funaba M, Zimmerman CM, Mathews LS. Modulation of Smad2-mediated signaling by extracellular signal-regulated kinase. J Biol Chem. 2002; 277:41361–41368.
32. Liu S, Xu SW, Kennedy L, Pala D, Chen Y, Eastwood M, Carter DE, Black CM, Abraham DJ, Leask A. FAK is required for TGFbeta-induced JNK phosphorylation in fibroblasts: implications for acquisition of a matrix-remodeling phenotype. Mol Biol Cell. 2007; 18:2169–2178.
33. Shi-wen X, Parapuram SK, Pala D, Chen Y, Carter DE, Eastwood M, Denton CP, Abraham DJ, Leask A. Requirement of transforming growth factor beta-activated kinase 1 for transforming growth factor beta-induced alpha-smooth muscle actin expression and extracellular matrix contraction in fibroblasts. Arthritis Rheum. 2009; 60:234–241.
34. Hough C, Radu M, Dore JJ. Tgf-beta induced Erk phosphorylation of smad linker region regulates smad signaling. PLoS One. 2012; 7:e42513.
35. Leivonen SK, Hakkinen L, Liu D, Kahari VM. Smad3 and extracellular signal-regulated kinase 1/2 coordinately mediate transforming growth factor-beta-induced expression of connective tissue growth factor in human fibroblasts. J Invest Dermatol. 2005; 124:1162–1169.
36. Dolivo DM, Larson SA, Dominko T. Crosstalk between mitogen-activated protein kinase inhibitors and transforming growth factor-beta signaling results in variable activation of human dermal fibroblasts. Int J Mol Med. 2019; 43:325–335.
37. Luo K. Signaling cross talk between TGF-β/Smad and other signaling pathways. Cold Spring Harb Perspect Biol. 2017; 9.
38. Blyszczuk P, Muller-Edenborn B, Valenta T, Osto E, Stellato M, Behnke S, Glatz K, Basler K, Luscher TF, Distler O, Eriksson U, Kania G. Transforming growth factor-beta-dependent Wnt secretion controls myofibroblast formation and myocardial fibrosis progression in experimental autoimmune myocarditis. Eur Heart J. 2017; 38:1413–1425.
39. Aoyagi-Ikeda K, Maeno T, Matsui H, Ueno M, Hara K, Aoki Y, Aoki F, Shimizu T, Doi H, Kawai-Kowase K, Iso T, Suga T, Arai M, Kurabayashi M. Notch induces myofibroblast differentiation of alveolar epithelial cells via transforming growth factor-{beta}-Smad3 pathway. Am J Respir Cell Mol Biol. 2011; 45:136–144.
40. Pinto AR, Ilinykh A, Ivey MJ, Kuwabara JT, D'Antoni ML, Debuque R, Chandran A, Wang L, Arora K, Rosenthal NA, Tallquist MD. Revisiting cardiac cellular composition. Circ Res. 2016; 118:400–409.
41. Watkins SJ, Borthwick GM, Oakenfull R, Robson A, Arthur HM. Angiotensin II-induced cardiomyocyte hypertrophy in vitro is TAK1-dependent and Smad2/3-independent. Hypertens Res. 2012; 35:393–398.
42. Dai P, Nakagami T, Tanaka H, Hitomi T, Takamatsu T. Cx43 mediates TGF-beta signaling through competitive Smads binding to microtubules. Mol Biol Cell. 2007; 18:2264–2273.
43. Parker TG, Packer SE, Schneider MD. Peptide growth factors can provoke "fetal" contractile protein gene expression in rat cardiac myocytes. J Clin Invest. 1990; 85:507–514.
44. Long CS, Henrich CJ, Simpson PC. A growth factor for cardiac myocytes is produced by cardiac nonmyocytes. Cell Regul. 1991; 2:1081–1095.
45. Villarreal FJ, Lee AA, Dillmann WH, Giordano FJ. Adenovirus-mediated overexpression of human transforming growth factor-beta 1 in rat cardiac fibroblasts, myocytes and smooth muscle cells. J Mol Cell Cardiol. 1996; 28:735–742.
46. Ding J, Tang Q, Luo B, Zhang L, Lin L, Han L, Hao M, Li M, Yu L, Li M. Klotho inhibits angiotensin II-induced cardiac hypertrophy, fibrosis, and dysfunction in mice through suppression of transforming growth factor-beta1 signaling pathway. Eur J Pharmacol. 2019; 859:172549.
47. Wu L, Derynck R. Essential role of TGF-beta signaling in glucose-induced cell hypertrophy. Dev Cell. 2009; 17:35–48.

48. Sartori R, Milan G, Patron M, Mammucari C, Blaauw B, Abraham R, Sandri M. Smad2 and 3 transcription factors control muscle mass in adulthood. Am J Physiol Cell Physiol. 2009; 296:C1248–1257.

49. Xu J, Kimball TR, Lorenz JN, Brown DA, Bauskin AR, Klevitsky R, Hewett TE, Breit SN, Molkentin JD. GDF15/MIC-1 functions as a protective and antihypertrophic factor released from the myocardium in association with SMAD protein activation. Circ Res. 2006; 98:342–350.

50. Shimano M, Ouchi N, Nakamura K, Oshima Y, Higuchi A, Pimentel DR, Panse KD, Lara-Pezzi E, Lee SJ, Sam F, Walsh K. Cardiac myocyte-specific ablation of follistatin-like 3 attenuates stress-induced myocardial hypertrophy. J Biol Chem. 2011; 286:9840–9848.

51. Tsui H, Zi M, Wang S, Chowdhury SK, Prehar S, Liang Q, Cartwright EJ, Lei M, Liu W, Wang X. Smad3 couples Pak1 with the antihypertrophic pathway through the E3 ubiquitin ligase, Fbxo32. Hypertension. 2015; 66:1176–1183.

52. Kong P, Shinde AV, Su Y, Russo I, Chen B, Saxena A, Conway SJ, Graff JM, Frangogiannis NG. Opposing actions of fibroblast and cardiomyocyte Smad3 signaling in the infarcted myocardium. Circulation. 2018; 137:707–724.

53. Sekiguchi K, Tian Q, Ishiyama M, Burchfield J, Gao F, Mann DL, Barger PM. Inhibition of PPAR-alpha activity in mice with cardiac-restricted expression of tumor necrosis factor: potential role of TGF-beta/Smad3. Am J Physiol Heart Circ Physiol. 2007; 292:H1443–1451.

54. Chablais F, Jazwinska A. The regenerative capacity of the zebrafish heart is dependent on TGFbeta signaling. Development. 2012; 139:1921–1930.

55. Izumi M, Fujio Y, Kunisada K, Negoro S, Tone E, Funamoto M, Osugi T, Oshima Y, Nakaoka Y, Kishimoto T, Yamauchi-Takihara K, Hirota H. Bone morphogenetic protein-2 inhibits serum deprivation-induced apoptosis of neonatal cardiac myocytes through activation of the Smad1 pathway. J Biol Chem. 2001; 276:31133–31141.

56. Masaki M, Izumi M, Oshima Y, Nakaoka Y, Kuroda T, Kimura R, Sugiyama S, Terai K, Kitakaze M, Yamauchi-Takihara K, Kawase I, Hirota H. Smad1 protects cardiomyocytes from ischemia-reperfusion injury. Circulation. 2005; 111:2752–2759.

57. Sanders LN, Schoenhard JA, Saleh MA, Mukherjee A, Ryzhov S, McMaster WG, Jr., Nolan K, Gumina RJ, Thompson TB, Magnuson MA, Harrison DG, Hatzopoulos AK. BMP antagonist Gremlin 2 limits inflammation after myocardial infarction. Circ Res. 2016; 119:434–449.

58. Bujak M, Ren G, Kweon HJ, Dobaczewski M, Reddy A, Taffet G, Wang XF, Frangogiannis NG. Essential role of Smad3 in infarct healing and in the pathogenesis of cardiac remodeling. Circulation. 2007; 116:2127–2138.

59. Hao J, Ju H, Zhao S, Junaid A, Scammell-La Fleur T, Dixon IM. Elevation of expression of Smads 2, 3, and 4, decorin and TGF-beta in the chronic phase of myocardial infarct scar healing. J Mol Cell Cardiol. 1999; 31:667–678.

60. Huang S, Chen B, Su Y, Alex L, Humeres C, Shinde AV, Conway SJ, Frangogiannis NG. Distinct roles of myofibroblast-specific Smad2 and Smad3 signaling in repair and remodeling of the infarcted heart. J Mol Cell Cardiol. 2019; 132:84–97.

61. Frangogiannis NG. Transforming Growth Factor (TGF)-beta in tissue fibrosis. J Exp Med. 2020; 217:e20190103. https://doi.org/20190110.20191084/jem.20190103.

62. Dobaczewski M, Bujak M, Li N, Gonzalez-Quesada C, Mendoza LH, Wang XF, Frangogiannis NG. Smad3 signaling critically regulates fibroblast phenotype and function in healing myocardial infarction. Circ Res. 2010; 107:418–428.

63. Russo I, Cavalera M, Huang S, Su Y, Hanna A, Chen B, Shinde AV, Conway SJ, Graff J, Frangogiannis NG. Protective effects of activated myofibroblasts in the pressure-overloaded myocardium are mediated through smad-dependent activation of a matrix-preserving program. Circ Res. 2019; 124:1214–1227.

64. Chen H, Moreno-Moral A, Pesce F, Devapragash N, Mancini M, Heng EL, Rotival M, Srivastava PK, Harmston N, Shkura K, Rackham OJL, Yu WP, Sun XM, Tee NGZ, Tan ELS, Barton PJR, Felkin LE, Lara-Pezzi E, Angelini G, Beltrami C, Pravenec M, Schafer S, Bottolo L, Hubner N, Emanueli C, Cook SA, Petretto E. WWP2 regulates pathological cardiac fibrosis by modulating SMAD2 signaling. Nature communications. 2019; 10:3616.

65. Pannu J, Nakerakanti S, Smith E, ten Dijke P, Trojanowska M. Transforming growth factor-beta receptor type I-dependent fibrogenic gene program is mediated via activation of Smad1 and ERK1/2 pathways. J Biol Chem. 2007; 282:10405–10413.

66. Fan K, Ruan Q, Sensenbrenner L, Chen B. Transforming growth factor-beta 1 bifunctionally regulates murine macrophage proliferation. Blood. 1992; 79:1679–1685.

67. Wahl SM, Hunt DA, Wakefield LM, McCartney-Francis N, Wahl LM, Roberts AB, Sporn MB. Transforming growth factor type beta induces monocyte chemotaxis and growth factor production. Proc Natl Acad Sci U S A. 1987; 84:5788–5792.

68. Letterio JJ, Roberts AB. Regulation of immune responses by TGF-beta. Annu Rev Immunol. 1998; 16:137–161.

69. Kitamura M. Identification of an inhibitor targeting macrophage production of monocyte chemoattractant protein-1 as TGF-beta 1. J Immunol. 1997; 159:1404–1411.

70. Chen B, Huang S, Su Y, Wu YJ, Hanna A, Brickshawana A, Graff J, Frangogiannis NG. Macrophage Smad3 protects the infarcted heart, stimulating phagocytosis and regulating inflammation. Circ Res. 2019; 125:55–70.

71. Feinberg MW, Jain MK, Werner F, Sibinga NE, Wiesel P, Wang H, Topper JN, Perrella MA, Lee ME. Transforming growth factor-beta 1 inhibits cytokine-mediated induction of human metalloelastase in macrophages. J Biol Chem. 2000; 275:25766–25773.

72. Kehrl JH, Wakefield LM, Roberts AB, Jakowlew S, Alvarez-Mon M, Derynck R, Sporn MB, Fauci AS. Production of transforming growth factor beta by human T lymphocytes and its potential role in the regulation of T cell growth. J Exp Med. 1986; 163:1037–1050.

73. Lee G, Ellingsworth LR, Gillis S, Wall R, Kincade PW. Beta transforming growth factors are potential regulators of B lymphopoiesis. J Exp Med. 1987; 166:1290–1299.

74. Fantini MC, Becker C, Monteleone G, Pallone F, Galle PR, Neurath MF. Cutting edge: TGF-beta induces a regulatory phenotype in CD4+CD25- T cells through Foxp3 induction and down-regulation of Smad7. J Immunol. 2004; 172:5149–5153.

75. Dobaczewski M, Xia Y, Bujak M, Gonzalez-Quesada C, Frangogiannis NG. CCR5 signaling suppresses inflammation and reduces adverse remodeling of the infarcted heart, mediating recruitment of regulatory T cells. Am J Pathol. 2010; 176:2177–2187.

76. Saxena A, Dobaczewski M, Rai V, Haque Z, Chen W, Li N, Frangogiannis NG. Regulatory T cells are recruited in the infarcted mouse myocardium and may modulate fibroblast phenotype and function. Am J Physiol Heart Circ Physiol. 2014; 307:H1233–1242.

77. Weirather J, Hofmann UD, Beyersdorf N, Ramos GC, Vogel B, Frey A, Ertl G, Kerkau T, Frantz S. Foxp3+ CD4+ T cells improve healing after myocardial infarction by modulating monocyte/macrophage differentiation. Circ Res. 2014; 115:55–67.

78. Bansal SS, Ismahil MA, Goel M, Zhou G, Rokosh G, Hamid T, Prabhu SD. Dysfunctional and proinflammatory regulatory T-lymphocytes are essential for adverse cardiac remodeling in ischemic cardiomyopathy. Circulation. 2019; 139:206–221.

79. Hofmann U, Beyersdorf N, Weirather J, Podolskaya A, Bauersachs J, Ertl G, Kerkau T, Frantz S. Activation of CD4+ T lymphocytes improves wound healing and survival after experimental myocardial infarction in mice. Circulation. 2012; 125:1652–1663.

80. Nevers T, Salvador AM, Velazquez F, Ngwenyama N, Carrillo-Salinas FJ, Aronovitz M, Blanton RM, Alcaide P. Th1 effector T cells selectively orchestrate cardiac fibrosis in nonischemic heart failure. J Exp Med. 2017; 214:3311–3329.

81. Joetham A, Schedel M, Ning F, Wang M, Takeda K, Gelfand EW. Dichotomous role of TGF-beta controls inducible regulatory T-cell fate in allergic airway disease through Smad3 and TGF-beta-activated kinase 1. J Allergy Clin Immunol. 2020; 145:933–946 e934.

82. Pepper MS. Transforming growth factor-beta: vasculogenesis, angiogenesis, and vessel wall integrity. Cytokine Growth Factor Rev. 1997; 8:21–43.

83. Goumans MJ, Lebrin F, Valdimarsdottir G. Controlling the angiogenic switch: a balance between two distinct TGF-b receptor signaling pathways. Trends Cardiovasc Med. 2003; 13:301–307.

84. Lebrin F, Deckers M, Bertolino P, Ten Dijke P. TGF-beta receptor function in the endothelium. Cardiovasc Res. 2005; 65:599–608.

85. Pan CC, Kumar S, Shah N, Bloodworth JC, Hawinkels LJ, Mythreye K, Hoyt DG, Lee NY. Endoglin regulation of Smad2 function mediates Beclin1 expression and endothelial autophagy. J Biol Chem. 2015; 290:14884–14892.

86. Li J, Qu X, Yao J, Caruana G, Ricardo SD, Yamamoto Y, Yamamoto H, Bertram JF. Blockade of endothelial-mesenchymal transition by a Smad3 inhibitor delays the early development of streptozotocin-induced diabetic nephropathy. Diabetes. 2010; 59:2612–2624.

87. Medici D, Potenta S, Kalluri R. Transforming growth factor-beta2 promotes Snail-mediated endothelial-mesenchymal transition through convergence of Smad-dependent and Smad-independent signalling. Biochem J. 2011; 437:515–520.

88. Dunker N, Krieglstein K. Targeted mutations of transforming growth factor-beta genes reveal important roles in mouse development and adult homeostasis. Eur J Biochem. 2000; 267:6982–6988.

89. Huang S, Chen B, Humeres C, Alex L, Hanna A, Frangogiannis NG. The role of Smad2 and Smad3 in regulating homeostatic functions of fibroblasts in vitro and in adult mice. Biochim Biophys Acta Mol Cell Res. 2020; 1867:118703.

90. Bujak M, Kweon HJ, Chatila K, Li N, Taffet G, Frangogiannis NG. Aging-related defects are associated with adverse cardiac remodeling in a mouse model of reperfused myocardial infarction. J Am Coll Cardiol. 2008; 51:1384–1392.

91. Biernacka A, Frangogiannis NG. Aging and cardiac fibrosis. Aging Dis. 2011; 2:158–173.

92. Dobaczewski M, Chen W, Frangogiannis NG. Transforming growth factor (TGF)-beta signaling in cardiac remodeling. J Mol Cell Cardiol. 2011; 51:600–606.

93. Xia Y, Lee K, Li N, Corbett D, Mendoza L, Frangogiannis NG. Characterization of the inflammatory and fibrotic response in a mouse model of cardiac pressure overload. Histochem Cell Biol. 2009; 131:471–481.

94. Huang XR, Chung AC, Yang F, Yue W, Deng C, Lau CP, Tse HF, Lan HY. Smad3 mediates cardiac inflammation and fibrosis in angiotensin II-induced hypertensive cardiac remodeling. Hypertension. 2010; 55:1165–1171.

95. Divakaran V, Adrogue J, Ishiyama M, Entman ML, Haudek S, Sivasubramanian N, Mann DL. Adaptive and maladaptive effects of SMAD3 signaling in the adult heart after hemodynamic pressure overloading. Circ Heart Fail. 2009; 2:633–642.

96. Engebretsen KV, Skardal K, Bjornstad S, Marstein HS, Skrbic B, Sjaastad I, Christensen G, Bjornstad JL, Tonnessen T. Attenuated development of cardiac fibrosis in left ventricular pressure overload by SM16, an orally active inhibitor of ALK5. J Mol Cell Cardiol. 2014; 76:148–157.

97. Tan SM, Zhang Y, Connelly KA, Gilbert RE, Kelly DJ. Targeted inhibition of activin receptor-like kinase 5 signaling attenuates cardiac dysfunction following myocardial infarction. Am J Physiol Heart Circ Physiol. 2010; 298:H1415–1425.

98. Bjornstad JL, Skrbic B, Marstein HS, Hasic A, Sjaastad I, Louch WE, Florholmen G, Christensen G, Tonnessen T. Inhibition of SMAD2 phosphorylation preserves cardiac function during pressure overload. Cardiovasc Res. 2012; 93:100–110.

99. Koitabashi N, Danner T, Zaiman AL, Pinto YM, Rowell J, Mankowski J, Zhang D, Nakamura T, Takimoto E, Kass DA. Pivotal role of cardiomyocyte TGF-beta signaling in the murine pathological response to sustained pressure overload. J Clin Invest. 2011; 121:2301–2312.

100. Khalil H, Kanisicak O, Prasad V, Correll RN, Fu X, Schips T, Vagnozzi RJ, Liu R, Huynh T, Lee SJ, Karch J, Molkentin JD. Fibroblast-specific TGF-beta-Smad2/3 signaling underlies cardiac fibrosis. J Clin Invest. 2017; 127:3770–3783.

101. Farbehi N, Patrick R, Dorison A, Xaymardan M, Janbandhu V, Wystub-Lis K, Ho JW, Nordon RE, Harvey RP. Single-cell expression profiling reveals dynamic flux of cardiac stromal, vascular and immune cells in health and injury. Elife. 2019; 8.

102. McLellan MA, Skelly DA, Dona MSI, Squiers GT, Farrugia GE, Gaynor TL, Cohen CD, Pandey R, Diep H, Vinh A, Rosenthal NA, Pinto AR. High-resolution transcriptomic profiling of the heart during chronic stress reveals cellular drivers of cardiac fibrosis and hypertrophy. Circulation. 2020.

103. Humeres C, Frangogiannis NG. Fibroblasts in the infarcted, remodeling, and failing heart. JACC Basic Transl Sci. 2019; 4:449–467.

104. Talior-Volodarsky I, Connelly KA, Arora PD, Gullberg D, McCulloch CA. alpha11 integrin stimulates myofibroblast differentiation in diabetic cardiomyopathy. Cardiovasc Res. 2012; 96:265–275.

105. Gonzalez-Quesada C, Cavalera M, Biernacka A, Kong P, Lee DW, Saxena A, Frunza O, Dobaczewski M, Shinde A, Frangogiannis NG. Thrombospondin-1 induction in the diabetic myocardium stabilizes the cardiac matrix in addition to promoting vascular rarefaction through angiopoietin-2 upregulation. Circ Res. 2013; 113:1331–1344.

106. Biernacka A, Cavalera M, Wang J, Russo I, Shinde A, Kong P, Gonzalez-Quesada C, Rai V, Dobaczewski M, Lee DW, Wang XF, Frangogiannis NG. Smad3 signaling promotes fibrosis while preserving cardiac and aortic geometry in obese diabetic mice. Circ Heart Fail. 2015; 8:788–798.

107. Hanna A, Frangogiannis NG. The role of the TGF-beta superfamily in myocardial infarction. Front Cardiovasc Med. 2019; 6:140.

108. Frangogiannis NG. Targeting the transforming growth factor (TGF)-beta cascade in the remodeling heart: benefits and perils. J Mol Cell Cardiol. 2014; 76:169–171.

109. Huynh LK, Hipolito CJ, Ten Dijke P. A perspective on the development of TGF-beta inhibitors for cancer treatment. Biomolecules. 2019; 9.

5 Fibroblast and Immune Cell Cross Talk in Cardiac Repair

Stelios Psarras and Georgina Xanthou

CONTENTS

INTRODUCTION

Recent large-scale clinical studies have highlighted the contribution of inflammation to heart failure (HF) (1). Independent of the variable etiologies, the common ground remains the pronounced inability of the cardiomyocytes to proliferate and the failure of the cardiac tissue to regenerate, a fact dramatically translated in inefficient repair under conditions of injury or stress. Fibrosis, elicited by its effector cells the fibroblasts, plays a crucial role, sustaining adverse cardiac outcomes in the long term (2,3). However, fibrosis also contributes to cardiac repair in response to injury (4). To further complicate the cardiac milieu in the context of heart diseases, fibroblasts comprise multiple subpopulations and assume divergent functions, even antifibrotic, depending on the context and timing of the response. Notably, cells belonging to the innate and adaptive immune systems closely interact with fibroblasts (5) and, along with inflammation, can exhibit reparative and detrimental functions. Most of our current knowledge of fibroblast–immune cell interactions stems from studies of cardiac repair in animal models, wherein conditions of cardiac injury and stress are induced (following surgery or exposure to toxic agents) or generated through genetic

DOI: 10.1201/b22824-6

manipulation. Among the surgical models, myocardial infarction (MI) with or without reperfusion and thoracic aortic constriction (TAC) both recapitulate triggers that induce acute and chronic cardiac injury, leading to HF with reduced ejection faction (HFrEF) and HF with preserved ejection fraction (HFpEF), respectively, two different forms of HF characterized by distinct pathophysiologic features including diverse fibroblast phenotypes and functions (6). Experimental myocarditis models represent a setting wherein exposure to viruses and other infectious agents or forced deployment of autoantibodies against cardiac proteins recapitulates human inflammatory cardiomyopathy associated with cardiac dysfunction, which often leads to dilated cardiomyopathy and HF (7). Among the genetic models, the mouse deficient in desmin is a valuable tool wherein cardiomyocyte death due to mitochondrial defects leads to the development of a macrophage-driven inflammatory response (8) and features a combination of multiple cardiomyopathies, leading to HF (9,10). *Ex vivo* systems have also been used to study HF and associated fibrosis, while RNA-Seq analyses at the single-cell level are currently being employed to better understand human disease (11).

On the basis of reports from preclinical models and human studies, we discuss recent advances in the understanding of fibroblast and immune cell interactions in the context of heart diseases, explore fibroblast and immune cell phenotypic and functional plasticity and its effects on cardiac repair, and contemplate molecular pathways that can be exploited for the design of novel therapeutic approaches. Whereas parallel interactions involving cardiomyocytes, endothelial cells, and other cardiac cell populations are also pivotal in cardiac repair mechanisms (12), their description is beyond the scope of this chapter and the reader is referred to other sources (13–15).

PATHWAYS THROUGH WHICH CARDIAC FIBROBLASTS ALTER IMMUNE CELL PHENOTYPES

FIBROBLAST SUBPOPULATIONS

Although fibroblasts comprise less than one-sixth of the total number of cardiac cells (16), they orchestrate the fibrotic response and markedly contribute to pathologic remodeling (17). Fibroblast expansion following MI (18) forms part of a beneficial repair response under conditions of extended myocardial damage (4). In contrast, the proliferation of fibroblasts under pressure overload–mediated injury (18) promotes unfavorable fibrosis (19). In the TAC mouse model, and in HF patients, upregulation of small, proline-rich protein 2B (*Sprr2B*) expression regulates fibroblast proliferation (20). Elevation of SPRR2B, a component of the ubiquitin-specific peptidase 7/MDM2 proto-oncogene (USP7/MDM2) ubiquitination complex that mediates the degradation of p53, releases p53-mediated proliferation arrest on fibroblasts and induces cardiac pathology.

Cardiac fibroblasts are characterized by high plasticity under injury conditions: following MI, fibroblasts exhibit a pro-inflammatory gene expression profile associated with increased recruitment of immunocytes, whereas subsequently fibroblasts assume a beneficial pro-angiogenic phenotype that can later become anti-angiogenic via secretion of thrombospondin 1 (THBS1) (21). MI-triggered differentiation processes lead to the generation of matrifibrocytes, specialized fibroblast populations that express tenascin-C and induce scar rigidity to prevent ventricular wall rupture (22). Additional differentiation patterns of fibroblasts have been reported, including osteogenesis (23). In this context, cardiac fibroblasts express osteoblast markers and adopt an osteoblast-like fate, contributing to ectopic calcification of the cardiac tissue.

Alpha-smooth muscle actin-positive (α-SMA) myofibroblasts, emerging from resident fibroblasts, promote transforming growth factor-β-mediated (TGFβ) fibrosis (17,24). However, recent evidence suggests that they may not be exclusively responsible for the profibrotic responses in the heart. For example, in murine cardiac hypertrophy induced by profibrotic angiotensin II infusion, among six expression clusters representing fibroblast subpopulations, two were identified as being fibrogenic, with cartilage intermediate layer protein-1-positive (CILP) cells being the predominant ones mediating fibrosis (25). On the other hand, in MI models and biopsies, a subpopulation expressing collagen triple helix–containing 1 (*CTHRC1*) exhibits reparative functions (26). Moreover, fibroblast-specific protein-1-positive (FSP1) fibroblasts are distinct from α-SMA⁺ myofibroblasts and may represent a reparative population that exerts pro-angiogenic functions (27).

Fibroblast heterogeneity does not only arise post-injury. Early during the postnatal period, two distinct lineages were identified in the mouse that differentially affect cardiac homeostasis: (1) the highly proliferative periostin-positive (*Postn*+) lineage that transiently populates the heart and promotes neuronal development and cardiomyocyte maturation, and (2) the transcription factor-21-expressing (*Tcf21*) fibroblasts that specialize in extracellular matrix (ECM) regulation and promote immune cell cross talk (28). In the adult heart, overexpression of *Postn*, *Cthrc1*, cytoskeleton-associated protein 4 (*Ckap4*), and other gene products marks activated fibroblasts that contribute to cardiac repair and pathophysiology (26).

FIBROBLAST–IMMUNE CELL INTERACTIONS

Cardiac fibroblasts affect immune cell phenotype at multiple levels during injury and repair, but they can also switch to an inflammatory phenotype themselves (Figure 5.1). Indeed, fibroblasts cultured from HF biopsies readily upregulate pro-inflammatory cytokine expression upon exposure to bacterial lipopolysaccharides (29). Following an infarct, fibroblasts transiently secrete granulocyte-macrophage colony-stimulating factor (GM-CSF), which stimulates the local recruitment of monocytes and neutrophils while it also directs a myeloid-biased differentiation program in the bone marrow (BM) (30). These systemic and local changes induce cardiac inflammation and compromise tissue rigidity, promoting ventricular wall rupture (Figure 5.1). In experimental autoimmune myocarditis, interleukin-17A (IL-17A) secretion mediates pathogenesis by stimulating cardiac fibroblasts to secrete GM-CSF, which instructs local monocyte differentiation toward the pro-inflammatory subset (Ly6Cʰⁱ, expressing high levels of lymphocyte antigen 6/Ly6C) (31) (Figure 5.1). In co-culture studies, IL-17A inhibits the ability of cardiac fibroblasts to promote differentiation of monocytes to macrophages (32). Moreover, IL-17A trans-signaling stimulates the shedding of myeloid-epithelial-reproductive tyrosine kinase (MerTK) by macrophages,

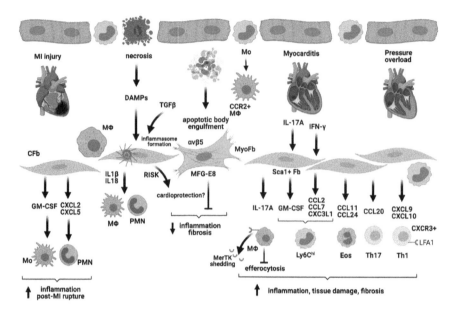

FIGURE 5.1 Fibroblasts modulate immune cell phenotype in cardiac repair. Left to right: In MI or I/R injury, activated cardiac fibroblasts (CFb) secrete GM-CSF and upregulate expression of CXCL2 and CXCL5 to recruit monocytes (Mo) and neutrophils (PMN), promoting myocardial inflammation and wall rupture. DAMPs released by necrotic cells or TGFβ1 activate inflammasomes in fibroblasts that release IL1β and IL18, recruiting neutrophils and macrophages (MΦ). NLRP3 inflammasome formation may also confer cardioprotection via the RISK pathway. Activated myofibroblasts (MyoFb) overexpressing MFG-E8 may dampen inflammation and fibrosis by engulfing apoptotic cells. In myocarditis, IL-17A from fibroblasts promotes MerTK shedding by macrophages, inhibiting efferocytosis and promoting inflammation. In myocarditis (and MI), IL-17A-dependent GM-CSF release by Sca1+ fibroblasts induces Ly6Chi monocyte recruitment. Pro-inflammatory IFN-γ activation induces expression of chemokines, preferentially recruiting Ly6C^{hi} monocytes. Fibroblasts produce eotaxins to recruit eosinophils (Eos) and secrete CCL20 to recruit Th17 cells. In pressure overload injury, fibroblasts secrete CXCL9 and CXCL10 to recruit detrimental CXCR3+ Th1 cells. Top: Intact cardiomyocytes, necrotic cells, and infiltrating monocytes undergoing differentiation to CCR2-expressing inflammatory macrophages. For details and further abbreviations see the main text.

Source: Figure created with BioRender.com.

reducing their ability to conduct efferocytosis (32). As efferocytosis enhances anti-inflammatory signaling following engulfment of apoptotic cells, IL-17A-mediated efferocytosis inhibition confers pro-inflammatory functions to macrophages, worsening myocarditis (Figure 5.1). A stem cell antigen-1-positive (*Sca1*) fibroblast population has been identified in the mouse that secretes GM-CSF in an IL-17A-dependent manner and induces pro-inflammatory Ly6C^{hi} monocyte recruitment (Figure 5.1). Importantly, IL-17A knockdown in Sca1$^+$ fibroblasts inhibited HF features not only in autoimmune myocarditis but also in MI (33), illuminating a central role for fibroblast-secreted IL-17A in cardiac damage.

Fibroblasts also secrete C-C motif chemokine ligand 20 (CCL20) to recruit detrimental IL-17A producing T helper cells (Th17) in murine myocarditis (34) (Figure 5.1). Moreover, cardiac fibroblasts, along with myeloid cells, secrete C-X-C motif chemokine ligands 9 (CXCL9) and 10 (CXCL10) to recruit Th1 cells. The latter express the chemokine receptor CXCR3 and induce adverse cardiac remodeling in pressure overload injury (35). The increased expression of lymphocyte function–associated-1 (LFA-1) integrin by CXCR3+ Th1 cells mediates their cardiotropic adhesion (35) (Figure 5.1).

Stimulation of cardiac fibroblasts in a pro-inflammatory milieu dictates the recruitment of immunocytes, promoting inflammation rather than repair. Indeed, the exposure of splenic monocytes to the secretomes of interferon-γ (IFN-γ)/TGFβ-stimulated fibroblasts reduced $Ly6C^{lo}/Ly6C^{hi}$ monocyte ratios compared to those achieved by fibroblasts stimulated with TGFβ alone (36). The IFN-γ/TGFβ regime increased the expression of the chemokines CCL2 and CCL7 and C-X3-C motif chemokine ligand 1 (CX3CL1) by cardiac fibroblasts, which preferentially elicit the recruitment of pro-inflammatory $Ly6C^{hi}$ over reparative $Ly6C^{lo}$ monocytes (36) (Figure 5.1).

However, activated fibroblasts may also drive anti-inflammatory functions that promote cardiac tissue repair. Similar to macrophages, cardiac myofibroblasts overexpress milk fat globule epidermal growth factor 8 (MFG-E8) and engulf apoptotic cells via αvβ5 integrin, thus reducing inflammatory cytokine production in MI (37) (Figure 5.1). Accordingly, MFG-E8 administration partially dampened inflammation and fibrosis, ameliorating cardiac function and survival (37).

There is evidence that neutrophil chemoattractants are overexpressed by cardiac fibroblasts in MI. Indeed, in mice lacking 11β-hydroxysteroid dehydrogenase type 1, CXCL2 and CXCL5 overexpression by cardiac fibroblasts was accompanied by increased neutrophilic inflammation (Figure 5.1), which was reversed by administration of corticosterone (38). Moreover, cardiac fibroblasts produce eotaxins (CCL11 and CCL24) and recruit eosinophils (Figure 5.1) in certain myocarditis conditions (39).

Fibroblasts can also assume an inflammatory phenotype during aging-associated cardiac fibrosis and dysfunction. Under this chronic stress condition, mesenchymal stem cell-derived (MSC) fibroblast-like cells in the murine heart show increased expression of interleukin-6 (IL-6). This results from activation of the farnesyltransferase-Ras-ERK pathway that elicits inflammation and interstitial fibrosis (40). Moreover, overexpression of CCL2 (also known as MCP1) stimulates leukocyte recruitment and promotes the generation of inflammatory fibroblast-like cells and aging-associated fibrosis via the same pathway (41).

Cardiac fibroblasts are also involved in inflammasome activation. This molecular platform is formed upon stimulation of intracellular pattern recognition receptors (PRRs), including NLR family pyrin containing 3 (NLRP3), by a diverse range of danger signals (DAMPs) released by necrotic or stressed cells and leads to interleukin-1β (IL-1β) and IL-18 secretion. Although inflammasome activation mainly takes place in macrophages, cardiac fibroblasts are readily activated even under exposure to TGFβ1 (42) and produce IL-1β and IL-18, mediating inflammatory cell infiltration in ischemia reperfusion (43) (Figure 5.1). Still, NLRP3-inflammasome activation by cardiac fibroblasts may confer cardioprotection via the reperfusion injury salvage kinase (RISK) pathway (Figure 5.1). Indeed, *Nlrp3*-deficient mice show increased infarct size despite similar levels of macrophage and neutrophil infiltration (44). BM-derived cells and cardiomyocytes also play crucial roles in inflammasome-mediated adverse remodeling (45,46), dictating complex interactions between cardiac cells. Given the central role of IL-1β- and IL-18-driven inflammation in HF outcome (1), further investigation is needed to clarify the precise role of inflammasome signaling in cardiac inflammation and repair.

The Involvement of the ECM

In accordance with the pronounced heterogeneity and plasticity observed in fibroblasts, ECM is also dynamically changing following cardiac injury. Collagens I and III are deposited to maintain cardiac tissue homeostasis, protecting from rupture post-MI but sustaining detrimental fibrosis in the long term. Other components, such as the proteoglycan agrin, support cardiac regeneration by promoting cardiomyocyte proliferation in the neonatal murine heart. Indeed, local agrin administration post-MI suppressed inflammation and fibrosis and improved cardiac function in preclinical models (47). Paradoxically, collagen V, a minor collagen species of the basement membrane upregulated upon MI injury, diminishes the infarct size by regulating fibroblast mechanosensing signaling in an integrin-dependent manner (48). The importance of ECM was clearly demonstrated in experiments in which decellularized ECM derived from regeneration-prone neonatal mouse hearts and injected into adult hearts alleviated cardiac dysfunction and scar expansion post-MI (49).

PATHWAYS THROUGH WHICH IMMUNE CELLS ALTER THE CARDIAC FIBROBLAST PHENOTYPE

Macrophage Subpopulations and Cardiac Repair

Macrophages critically contribute to cardiac homeostasis (50) by mediating electrical polarization of the cardiomyocytes in the conduction system and by promoting the maturation of the coronary vasculature. Macrophages via pro-angiogenic mediators contained in their secretomes also contribute to the regeneration of neonatal mammalian hearts, an ability maintained for an exceptionally short time frame post-partum and lost in the adult (51).

Macrophages display pronounced plasticity following cardiac injury (52), accompanied by altered gene expression and secretome composition that affect their functions. The ontogeny of cardiac macrophages includes primitive yolk sac-derived, fetal monocyte-derived, and adult monocyte-derived macrophages (53,54). Circulating or splenic monocytes populate the murine heart early on following injury and are broadly divided to pro-inflammatory Ly6C^{hi}, which appears first, followed by the reparative Ly6C^{lo} population (55). The latter subset can be generated from the former, and both can drive the differentiation of monocyte-derived macrophages *in situ*. Notably, whereas murine monocyte-derived macrophages express CCR2, the CCL2 receptor, cardiac-resident macrophages are CCR2 negative (56,57).

Depending on their origin and the disease context, cardiac macrophages mediate inflammation and tissue injury and sustain fibrosis, or they exert antifibrotic actions, protecting the heart from adverse remodeling. Indeed, monocyte-derived macrophages (CCR2$^+$) overcrowd the cardiac tissue, replacing the CCR2$^-$ resident ones early post-MI (57,58). CCR2$^+$ macrophages recruit monocytes to the injured heart and promote their differentiation to inflammatory macrophages (57). Furthermore, in the TAC model, CCR2$^+$ macrophages are mobilized early after pressure overload and promote LV remodeling and dysfunction, fibrosis, and CD4$^+$ and CD8$^+$ T cell expansion (59). In contrast, resident CCR2$^-$ macrophages are capable of self-renewal, expanding in a monocyte-independent manner. In fact, CCR2$^-$ resident macrophages inhibit the recruitment of circulating monocytes (57), and their depletion in MI results in cardiac systolic dysfunction, hypertrophy, and fibrosis (58). Thus, resident macrophages exert cardioprotective actions.

MACROPHAGE–FIBROBLAST INTERACTIONS

Recent expression analyses at the single-cell level revealed that several macrophage subpopulations emerge following cardiac injury (58,60). In a model of hypertension-mediated injury, an expanding MHC-II^{hi} population produces low levels of matrix metalloproteases (MMPs), protecting the ECM from extended reformation (Figure 5.2). More importantly, these macrophages produce the anti-inflammatory cytokine IL-10, which stimulates the production of osteopontin (OPN), a matricellular protein that promotes myofibroblast differentiation (61) (Figure 5.2). These events collectively induce collagen 1a2 and fibronectin-1 expression by cardiac fibroblasts, enhancing fibrosis and diastolic dysfunction (62). Similarly, our studies in the desmin-deficient mouse (des$^{-/-}$), a genetic model of HF wherein the necrotic death of cardiomyocytes leads to extended myocardial inflammation and fibrosis, revealed that overexpression of OPN by macrophages induces the expression of the profibrotic molecule galectin-3 and promotes cardiac fibrosis and dysfunction (8) (Figure 5.2). Macrophages in HFpEF biopsies produce TGFβ that transdifferentiates cardiac fibroblasts to myofibroblasts, increases collagen type I production, and decreases MMP-1 release to sustain fibrosis (63) (Figure 5.2).

Other subpopulations, such as the interferon-inducible cell (IFNIC) macrophages that emerge under the acute injury conditions of MI, sense DAMPs released by necrotic cardiomyocytes and activate type I IFN-stimulated gene expression that enhances inflammation, leading to myocardial wall rupture and death (60). However, pro-inflammatory macrophage activation is not always detrimental. In experimental myocarditis, interleukin-1 receptor-associated kinase-4 (IRAK-4), an adaptor acting downstream of MyD88 in pro-inflammatory gene expression pathways, inhibits the migration and function of pro-inflammatory CCR5-expressing monocytes, and this leads to disease exacerbation and extended cardiac damage (64). In fact, in IRAK-4-deficient mice, increased numbers of CCR5$^+$ monocyte-derived macrophages infiltrate the heart following coxsackievirus B3 infection, and macrophage-associated IFN-α and IFN-γ production eliminates the virus and attenuates disease severity. Moreover, in the TAC model, resident macrophages expand via Krüppel-like factor-4-dependent (KLF4) local proliferation, sustain angiogenesis, and protect

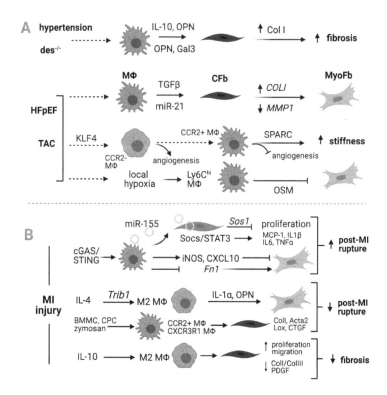

FIGURE 5.2 Macrophages affect cardiac fibroblasts and repair. (A) In hypertension-induced injury, macrophages (MΦ) produce IL-10 and OPN to promote collagen deposition in long-term fibrosis. In the des⁻ᐟ⁻ HF model, OPN and galectin-3 (Gal3) production promotes fibrosis. Macrophages also produce TGFβ1 in HFpEF and miR-21 in TAC injury. These mediators promote fibrosis by inducing fibroblast-to-myofibroblast (CFb-to-MyoFb) transdifferentiation and collagen expression or by reducing MMP expression. In TAC injury, CCR2⁻ macrophages expand via KLF4 to induce cardioprotective angiogenesis, while monocyte-derived CCR2⁺Ly6Cʰⁱ macrophages sequentially infiltrate the heart, exerting detrimental anti-angiogenic actions. Macrophage production of SPARC increases myocardial stiffness. OSM secreted by Ly6Cʰⁱ macrophages in hypoxic areas inhibits myofibroblast transdifferentiation. (B) In MI, macrophages release miR-155-containing exosomes, whose uptake inhibits fibroblast proliferation and induces inflammatory cytokine expression, promoting post-MI rupture. Macrophage activation by cGAS/STING induces expression of iNOS and CXCL10 and reduces expression of fibronectin-1, causing inhibited fibroblast-to-myofibroblast transdifferentiation and increased post-MI rupture. *Trib1*-dependent M2 activation of macrophages by IL-4 leads to IL-1α and OPN production, which induces myofibroblast transdifferentiation, protecting from rupture. Therapeutic injection of BM mononuclear cells (BMMC), cardiac progenitor cells (CPC), or zymosan mobilizes CCR2⁺ and CXCR3R1⁺ macrophages to induce profibrotic gene expression by cardiac fibroblasts, promoting early MI healing. IL-10-mediated M2 activation of macrophages promotes fibroblast proliferation and migration accompanied by a reduced collagen I/III ratio. M2 macrophage injection suppresses fibroblast activation via PDGF signaling, reducing fibrosis in the long term. For details and further abbreviations, see the main text.

Source: Figure created with BioRender.com.

cardiomyocytes against death, preserving cardiac function (65). Later on, monocyte-derived macrophages (CCR2$^+$Ly6C^{hi}CXC3CR1$^+$) infiltrate the heart and exert anti-angiogenic effects, compromising cardiac function. Other studies revealed that Ly6C^{hi} macrophages accumulate in hypoxic myocardial regions early after TAC and secrete oncostatin M, which impedes the transdifferentiation of fibroblasts to myofibroblasts and attenuates fibrosis (66) (Figure 5.2). A macrophage population expressing GATA-binding factor-6 (GATA6) of pericardial origin was recently identified as an additional subset exerting antifibrotic effects 1 month following MI (67). Overall, it becomes evident that the effects of macrophages and their subpopulations on cardiac repair are multifaceted and depend on the context, activation state, and time point examined.

Macrophage subpopulations at steady state and in failing myocardium do not conform with the so-called M1/M2 paradigm (68), particularly following MI injury (60). According to the M1/M2 paradigm, characteristic expression of surface and intracellular markers discriminates two major macrophage subtypes that assume either a pro-inflammatory (M1) "classical" or an anti-inflammatory/reparative (M2) alternative activation state, the latter being associated with the development of fibrosis. Despite reports highlighting the importance of M2 type, alternatively activated macrophages in cardiac repair (69), the paradigm is gradually replaced (70) by the notion that macrophage activation states represent a spectrum ranging between the M1 and M2 extremes. However, *ex vivo* activation protocols induce the M1 or M2 type of activation and their variations (M2a, M2b, M2c) and remain useful for the understanding of the biology of macrophages and their interactions with fibroblasts.

As mentioned previously, macrophages exert direct actions on fibroblasts affecting cardiac fibrosis and repair. In the murine MI model, exosomes secreted by macrophages contain miR-155 (71). Exosome uptake by fibroblasts restrains their proliferation by regulating the expression of son of sevenless-1 (*Sos1*), while it induces the expression of pro-inflammatory cytokines, such as IL-1β, IL-6, tumor necrosis factor-α (TNFα), and MCP-1/CCL2, through the inhibition of signaling by the suppressor of cytokine signaling 1 (Socs1)/signal transducer and activator of transcription 3 (STAT3) pathway. These events contribute to detrimental remodeling, promoting cardiac rupture in the post-MI heart, an effect abolished following miR-155 deficiency (71) (Figure 5.2). Another microRNA, miR-21, the most highly expressed microRNA in cardiac macrophages in healthy hearts, becomes further upregulated in HF. In fact, the cardiac dysfunction caused by pressure overload injury (TAC model) was partially rescued upon miR-21 knockdown in murine macrophages (72). Importantly, not only did miR-21 favor the M1 type of macrophage activation but its secretion was enhanced upon this pro-inflammatory activation and mediated the differentiation of cardiac fibroblasts to myofibroblasts (Figure 5.1), an event inhibited by locked nucleic acid (LNA)-anti-miR-21 inhibition (72).

Therapeutic infusion of IL-10 in MI induced an M2 alternative type of macrophage activation (73) and directly stimulated fibroblast proliferation and migration. Moreover, fibroblasts from IL-10-administered mice exhibited increased proliferation and a reduced collagen I/III ratio, associated with reduced fibrosis a week following MI (73) (Figure 5.2). Alternative macrophage activation regimes exhibit beneficial effects on fibroblasts and repair mechanisms in other settings as well.

Indeed, tribbles pseudokinase-deficient (*Tribl*) mice show reduced numbers of alternatively activated macrophage populations following MI, and this is accompanied by impaired collagen deposition, leading to catastrophic rupture (69). Whereas IL-4 administration induced alternatively activated macrophages in wt mice, protecting from post-MI rupture, it failed to do so in *Tribl*$^{-/-}$ mice. However, the protective effects of IL-4 were indirect, involving increased OPN and IL-1α secretion by alternatively activated macrophages that induced myofibroblast formation, reinforcing repair (69) (Figure 5.2).

The cardiac injury caused by MI also involves the cGAS/STING danger signal pathway. In this case, DNA released by necrotic myocardium is being sensed in macrophages by the cyclic GMP-AMP synthase (cGAS) PRR (60). This in turn leads to activation of the stimulator of interferon genes (STING) pathway and to elevated expression of interferon-stimulated genes, including those encoding inducible nitric oxide synthase (iNOS) and CXCL10 (74). Conversely, inhibition of the cGAS-STING axis protects from cardiac rupture (60) associated with a switch in macrophage phenotype from pro-inflammatory toward a reparative one. This switch is accompanied by the increased formation of myofibroblasts and dense collagen deposition in the infarct areas. The myofibroblast formation could be also facilitated by fibronectin, whose expression is elevated in reparative macrophages (74) (Figure 5.2). Interestingly, *ex vivo* generation of M2b alternatively activated macrophages and injection to the infarcted zones ameliorated MI repair by reducing platelet-derived growth factor–dependent (PDGF) activation of cardiac fibroblasts (75) (Figure 5.2).

Recent findings propose that macrophages can produce collagen, contributing to ECM formation during MI repair in a fibroblast-independent manner (76). Moreover, in the pressure overload model, macrophages were identified as the source of early expressed secreted protein and rich in cysteine (SPARC), which processes pro-collagen into insoluble fibrillar collagen and increases myocardial stiffness (77) (Figure 5.2). Intriguingly, macrophages have been shown to transdifferentiate into fibroblasts, or at least adopt a fibroblast-like phenotype, as shown both in murine MI and in prolonged cultures of human macrophages (78).

THE EFFECTS OF OTHER INNATE IMMUNE CELLS

During cardiac repair, neutrophils play a complex role that surpasses their phagocytic and inflammatory functions. During transient infiltration, neutrophils initially degranulate and induce protease-mediated tissue breakdown, while they gradually assume a reparative phenotype (79) and affect macrophage polarization, exerting protective effects against cardiac fibrosis and dysfunction (80). Neutrophils can also assume alternative polarization states. For example, whereas at day 1 post-MI the majority of neutrophils (termed N1) in the left-ventricular (LV) infarct show a pro-inflammatory phenotype, on days 5 and 7 another neutrophil population emerges (N2) that expresses anti-inflammatory markers (81). Notably, when co-cultured with cardiac fibroblasts, neutrophils alter their profibrotic response (increase fibronectin and TGFβ1 expression and reduce collagen type I expression) (82) (Figure 5.3). These findings provide opportunities for the design of novel therapeutic strategies, although direct *in vivo* evidence is still lacking.

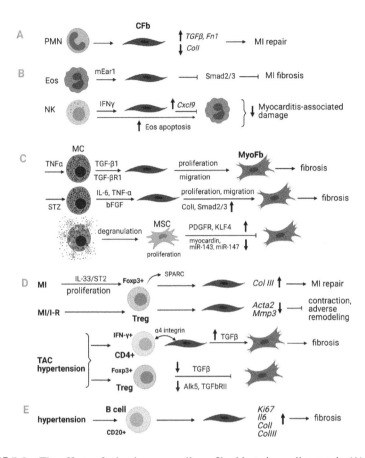

FIGURE 5.3 The effects of other immune cells on fibroblasts in cardiac repair. (A) Cardiac fibroblasts (CFb) co-cultured with neutrophils (PMN) show reduced collagen I (*ColI*) expression, while they increase fibronectin 1 (*Fn1*) and TGFβ1 expression to support MI repair. (B) In MI, eosinophils (Eos) secrete mEar1 to inhibit profibrotic Smad2/3 signaling by fibroblasts. In myocarditis, protective natural killer (NK) cells induce eosinophil apoptosis. IFN-γ produced by NK cells inhibits eosinophil migration by inducing CXCL9 expression in fibroblasts. (C) In TNFα-induced cardiomyopathy, mast cells (MC) overexpress TGFβ1 and TGFβR1 and induce proliferation, collagen expression, and myofibroblast (MyoFb) transdifferentiation of fibroblasts. In STZ-induced diabetic cardiomyopathy, mast cells produce IL-6, TNFα, and bFGF, inducing fibroblast proliferation, myofibroblast transdifferentiation, collagen expression, and Smad2/3 signaling. Mast cell degranulation stimulates MSC proliferation and inhibits myofibroblast transdifferentiation. (D) Treg cells expand by IL-33/ST2-dependent proliferation in MI injury, produce SPARC, and increase collagen III production by fibroblasts to support scar rigidity. Treg cells alter the expression and contractile activity of fibroblasts to reduce adverse remodeling. In pressure overload and hypertension injury, IFN-γ⁺ CD4⁺ T cells bind fibroblasts to activate TGFβ signaling and myofibroblast transdifferentiation, while Treg cells suppress TGFβ signaling and myofibroblast transdifferentiation. (E) In hypertension-induced HF, B cell secretomes induce profibrotic gene expression in fibroblasts, promoting fibrosis. For details and further abbreviations, see the main text.

Source: Figure created with BioRender.com.

Eosinophils accumulate in LV and appear to play a cardioprotective role in MI, as their depletion increases adverse remodeling and dysfunction (83). Although eosinophils act partially by facilitating the abundance of reparative macrophages (83) and protecting cardiomyocytes against apoptosis (84), they also secrete the cationic protein eosinophil-associated ribonuclease family member-1 (mEar1), which acts directly on cardiac fibroblasts, reducing TGFβ-mediated Smad family member-2 (Smad2)/Smad3 activation (84) (Figure 5.3). Eosinophils can exhibit detrimental functions in other cardiac disease settings, as is the case in experimental autoimmune myocarditis. In this context, natural killer cells (NK) accumulate in the heart and inhibit eosinophil influx by inducing apoptosis of the latter. Upon NK cell depletion, eosinophils infiltrate the murine hearts accompanied by increased myocardial fibrosis (85). Cardiac fibroblasts may interfere with this interaction as IFN-γ released by NK cells regulates their expression of CXCL9, a chemokine inhibiting eosinophil recruitment (Figure 5.3).

Mast cells can enhance fibrosis through direct actions on cardiac fibroblasts. In mice with cardiomyopathy due to the cardiac-specific overexpression of TNFα, adverse fibrosis is partially mediated by mast cells (86). More specifically, mast cells show increased expression of TGFβ1 and its receptor TGFβRI, and when co-cultured with fibroblasts originating from TNFα-overexpressing hearts, this enhanced their proliferation and profibrotic gene expression compared to normal fibroblasts (Figure 5.3). This pathologic mast cell–fibroblast cross talk was abrogated by an inhibitor of the type I TGFβ receptor (86). In diabetic cardiomyopathy induced by streptozotocin (STZ), increased myocardial fibrosis has been causally linked to the direct action of mast cell secretomes that contain TNFα and IL-6 on cardiac fibroblasts, which leads to Smad2/3 activation and collagens I and III and α-SMA (encoded by *Acta2*) upregulation (87) (Figure 5.3). Protective actions of mast cells post-MI have been reported involving basic fibroblast growth factor–mediated (bFGF) induction of cardiac fibroblast proliferation and TGFβ-mediated transdifferentiation into myofibroblasts (Figure 5.3); still, these effects are rather transient and vanish at later time points (88). On the other hand, mast cell granule contents suppress the differentiation of MSCs toward myofibroblasts, while increasing their proliferation. These effects are being mediated by the PDGF-receptor pathway and involve the downregulation of myocardin, miR-143, and miR-145 and the upregulation of KLF-4 expression (89) (Figure 5.3). The resulting accumulation of MSCs may enhance cardiac regeneration.

DENDRITIC CELLS

Dendritic cells (DCs), the specialized antigen-presenting cell population, are represented by multiple subsets in the heart and can exert cardioprotective actions or prime autoreactive T cells (90). Whereas CD103+ conventional type 1 DCs (cDC1) induce the differentiation of cardioprotective regulatory T cells (Tregs) at steady state, CD11b+ type 2 DCs (cDC2) become activated in MI and induce the priming of autoreactive CD4+ T cells that recognize cardiac α-myosin and produce IFN-γ and IL-17 (90). Depletion of cDCs reduces the infiltration of neutrophils and inflammatory macrophages and the associated IFN-γ and IL-1β production, ameliorating fibrosis and cardiac dysfunction following MI (91). Still, in virus-induced myocarditis, CD103⁺ cDCs protect the heart by inducing virus-specific CD8⁺ T cells that promote viral clearance and resolution of cardiac inflammation (92). In addition to cDCs, plasmatocytoid DC (pDC) levels are also increased following MI, yet their depletion does not affect cardiac fibrosis or function (91). Administration of *ex vivo*–generated, infarct-specific, tolerogenic DCs induces a systemic Treg activation and a macrophage switch toward the reparative phenotype, ameliorating post-MI remodeling (93). Whether the regulatory role of DCs in cardiac repair involves any direct interactions with fibroblasts remains to be elucidated.

ADAPTIVE IMMUNITY

T cells become activated and clonally expand in ischemic HF (94). CD4⁺ T cells play a detrimental role as their depletion attenuates post-MI adverse remodeling, while adoptive transfer of splenic CD4⁺ T cells or cardiac CD3⁺ T cells from donor mice with HF induces interstitial fibrosis and cardiac dysfunction in naive mice (95). Moreover, CD4⁻ γδ T cells accumulate and serve as a source of IL-17A, promoting cardiac fibrosis and dysfunction (96). In the TAC model, T cell depletion prevents HF development (97), and the detrimental action of CD4⁺ T cells involves their interaction with cardiac fibroblasts. In particular, IFN-γ-producing CD4⁺ T cells promote interstitial fibrosis by eliciting myofibroblast differentiation (98). The underlying mechanism includes the adhesion of activated T lymphocytes to cardiac fibroblasts via integrin subunit α4 and the subsequent activation of TGFβ signaling (Figure 5.3).

A well-known Treg cell subset, Foxp3⁺ Tregs, populates the heart following injury and exerts cardioprotective actions (99), altering inflammatory cell infiltration and activation status (100). However, under chronic inflammatory conditions, Tregs are reprogrammed and become dysfunctional, promoting adverse remodeling (101). In murine MI, cardioprotective Tregs expand in response to IL-33/suppression of tumorigenicity-2 (ST2) signaling and express increased amounts of SPARC, which supports the post-MI scar and prevents cardiac rupture (102). When co-cultured with cardiac fibroblasts, *Sparc*-overexpressing Tregs induce the expression of collagen type III by the fibroblasts (Figure 5.3), an effect suggesting that impaired ECM remodeling underlies the formation of immature scars in Treg-ablated mice (102). Moreover, Treg depletion results in increased apical remodeling following ischemia reperfusion that is partially attributed to a direct action on fibroblasts, as Tregs downregulate the expression of MMP3 and α-SMA in cardiac fibroblasts as well as the contractile activity of fibroblasts in collagen pads (Figure 5.3) (103). Whether these protective effects would vanish under a Treg phenotype switch during chronic cardiac injury is currently unknown. Nevertheless, in pressure-overload and hypertensive cardiac injury, adoptive transfer of Treg cells reduces the expression of TGFβ1 and its receptors TGFβRII and ALK5, leading to the inhibition of myofibroblast abundance and fibrosis (Figure 5.3) (104).

CD8⁺ T cells can induce cardiomyocyte apoptosis through granzyme-B release (105), leading to enhanced post-MI inflammation, adverse remodeling, and deterioration of cardiac function. Cross-priming functions of DCs are crucial for the activation of CD8⁺ T cell responses. Indeed, Clec9a-deficient mice, wherein DCs are unable to present antigen from necrotic cardiomyocytes in mediastinal lymph nodes (MLNs), are protected from CD8[+] T cell–mediated myocardial damage in the isoproterenol model of ischemic injury (106). However, induction of MI in transgenic mice deficient in CD8[+] T cells showed an accelerated inflammatory response and MMP activation, and despite better cardiac function and improved overall mouse survival, impaired scar formation was observed accompanying higher rates of myocardial rupture. These results suggest a more complex role of CD8[+] T cells in cardiac healing, including both beneficial and detrimental effects (107). Whether a direct interaction of CD8[+] T cells with cardiac fibroblasts is also involved is currently unknown. The same is true for invariant natural killer T cells (iNKT), which were shown to exert a protective, antifibrotic action post-MI (108).

B cells also become activated and accumulate in the heart following injury. In murine MI, maturation of B cells in MLN leads to autoantibody deposition in cardiac tissue, which is also evident in ischemic HF biopsies (109). Whereas autoantibody inhibition per se reduces inflammatory cell infiltration and fibrosis in murine MI (110), B cells modulate repair by additional, antibody-independent mechanisms. B cells recruit pro-inflammatory Ly6C[hi] monocytes through the production of CCL7 to induce myocardial damage and dysfunction (111). In myocarditis, an increased abundance of alternatively activated macrophages accompanied by reduced myocardial damage was observed in the absence of B cells, while B cell reconstitution enhanced disease severity (112). In the murine heart, there are three B cell subsets: a major CD19[+]CD11b[−] population and two CD19[+]CD11b[+] minor populations, called B1a and B1b. Following diphtheria toxin–mediated cardiomyocyte death or ischemia reperfusion, CD19[+]CD11b[−] B cells infiltrate the heart along with neutrophils and monocytes/macrophages. Treatment with the antifibrotic agent pirfenidone reduced the frequencies of B cells, but not those of the other immunocytes, while pirfenidone's protective action against adverse remodeling vanished upon B cell depletion, suggesting a rather complicated role of B cells in cardiac repair (113).

On the other hand, in a model of hypertension-induced HF, CD22 antibody–mediated B cell depletion attenuated the expression of IL-1β, TNFα, and IL-6, as well as cardiac adverse remodeling and dysfunction (114). Importantly, secretomes from B cells isolated from failing hearts and applied to cardiac fibroblasts upregulated the expression of genes involved in proliferation (*Ki67*), inflammation (*Il6*), and fibrosis (*Col1, Col3*) (Figure 5.3). The precise origins and the contribution of B cells to cardiac homeostasis are just starting to be elucidated, and further investigation of their interactions with fibroblasts is warranted to elucidate their role in cardiac repair.

TRANSLATIONAL PERSPECTIVES

The manipulation of the immune response is of paramount importance for cardiac output and HF fate (1). On the other hand, certain arms of the inflammatory response are definitively beneficial. When CD14[+]-activated macrophages were intramyocardially co-delivered along with CD90[+] MSCs in patients with HF of ischemic etiology, a

37% reduction in adverse cardiac events was achieved (115). Moreover, when murine hearts undergoing ischemia reperfusion were injected with fractionated BM mononuclear cells or c-Kit⁺ cardiac progenitor cells (CPCs), the mechanical properties of the infarcts were ameliorated and the extent of fibrosis was reduced (116). Notably, the same outcome was achieved by injecting zymosan, a cell-free agent activating the innate immune response. Mechanistically, the overall benefits could be attributed to the accumulation of two distinct populations of macrophages (CCR2⁺ and CXC3R1⁺) in murine hearts (116). When these populations were isolated and co-cultured with cardiac fibroblasts, CCR2⁺ macrophages induced the expression of collagen type I, αSMA, and the collagen cross-linking regulator lysyl oxidase (encoded by *Lox*) in stromal cells, while CXC3R1⁺ macrophages induced the expression of connective tissue growth factor (CTGF), a profibrotic molecule acting downstream of TGFβ1 (Figure 5.2).

Thus, the modulation of the immune response is capable of beneficially altering the activation status of fibroblasts, the pillars of cardiac fibrosis. Remarkably, established cardiac fibrosis can be modified, as myofibroblasts even from end-stage HF patients can partially reverse their pathogenic phenotype upon treatment with TGFβ1 inhibitors (117). More recent advances allow the *in vivo* targeting of pathogenic fibroblasts using T cells engineered to attack fibrotic fibroblasts with chimeric antigen receptor (CAR-T) technology (118). Given the scarcity of human cardiac samples, *ex vivo* systems using three-dimensional approaches (119), as well as cardiac biopsy material obtained during left-ventricular assist device (LVAD) implantation (120), may provide invaluable tools to study intercellular communication in the diseased heart and reveal novel therapeutic targets.

CONCLUSIONS

The interplay between cardiac fibroblasts and immune cells contributes to the regulation of cardiac repair following multiple types of insult (summarized in Table 5.1). Several lines of evidence suggest that these cell populations and the molecules or entities underlying their intercellular communication can be modified and/or targeted in favor of a more successful repair. However, the pronounced heterogeneity and plasticity of fibroblasts and immune cells, particularly macrophages, and their divergent effects during cardiac disease impose the need for a detailed characterization of their phenotypes and secretome. Such analyses should be conducted in a time-dependent manner following the cardiac insult, as emerging subpopulations of a particular cell type may exhibit opposing functions during the repair response. Animal models with defined injury time points are destined to provide important mechanistic insights. Still, conclusions from animal studies often are not fully translatable to human disease. Moreover, crucial details of the contribution of fibroblast–immune cell interplay in human cardiac repair remain elusive due to the scarcity of samples. Single-cell RNA seq and proteomic/metabolomic analyses, combined with *ex vivo* approaches using human clinical samples and clinically relevant cell culture systems, will facilitate a better understanding of the detrimental and beneficial arms of fibroblast–immune cell interplays, allowing the development of novel and more efficient therapeutic targets for heart diseases.

TABLE 5.1

Major Known Immunocyte Effects on Cardiac Fibroblasts Regulating Repair

Immunocyte Subset	Condition; Type of Injury; Time Point	Mediators and Pathways Involved	Effect on Fibroblasts	Effect on Cardiac Repair	Reference(s)
Resident macrophages	MI*; acute	Inhibition of monocyte recruitment		Inhibition of fibrosis and adverse remodeling	(57,58)
CCR2+ macrophages	MI; acute	Monocyte recruitment		Adverse remodeling	(57)
IFNIC macrophages	MI; acute	Type I IFN-stimulated gene expression		Wall rupture	(60)
Macrophages	MI; acute	miR-155	Proliferation; induced expression of IL-1β, IL-6, TNFα, MCP-1	Wall rupture	(71)
Proinflammatory macrophages	MI; acute	cGAS-STING; iNOS, CXCL10	Inhibition of MyoFb formation and collagen deposition	Wall rupture	(60,74)
CCR2+ macrophages	MI/therapeutic BMMC/CPC, zymosan; acute		Induced *ColI*, *Acta2*, *Lox* expression	Protection against wall rupture	(116)
CXC3R1+ macrophages	MI/therapeutic BMMC/CPC, zymosan; acute		Induced CTGF expression	Protection against wall rupture	(116)
M2 macrophages	MI; acute	IL4, *Trib1* OPN, IL-1α; Fn1	MyoFb formation; collagen production	Protection against wall rupture	(69)
	MI; acute	IL-10	Increased proliferation; reduced collagen I/III	Inhibition of fibrosis	(73)
	MI; chronic	PDGF	Inhibition of fibroblast activation	Improved repair	(75)
GATA6+ macrophages	MI; chronic			Inhibition of fibrosis	(67)

Immunocyte Subset	Condition; Type of Injury; Time Point	Mediators and Pathways Involved	Effect on Fibroblasts	Effect on Cardiac Repair	Reference(s)
Proinflammatory macrophages	Myocarditis; acute	IRAK4-mediated CCR5+ monocyte recruitment		IFN-mediated virus clearance; inhibition of fibrosis and adverse remodeling	(64)
Resident macrophages	TAC; early	KLF4-dependent proliferation; angiogenesis		Inhibition of fibrosis and adverse remodeling	(65)
Ly6C^{hi} macrophages	TAC; early	Oncostatin M	Inhibition of MyoFb formation	Inhibition of fibrosis	(66)
CCR2$^+$ macrophages	TAC; chronic	Inhibition of angiogenesis		Adverse remodeling	(65)
	TAC; chronic	T cell expansion		Fibrosis	(59)
M1 macrophages	TAC; chronic	miR-21	MyoFb formation	Fibrosis	(72)
MHC-II^{hi} macrophages	Hypertension, aging; chronic	IL-10, OPN	Induced *Col1a2, Fn1* expression	Fibrosis	(62)
Macrophages	desmin deficiency; chronic	OPN, Gal3		Fibrosis	(8)
Macrophages	HFpEF; chronic	TGFβ	induced ColI and MyoFb formation, reduced MMP1 release	Fibrosis	(63)
Neutrophils	MI; early	M1 macrophage polarization		Inflammation	(79–81)
	MI; late	M2 macrophage polarization		Inhibition of inflammation; induction of repair	(79–81)
	Co-culture		Increased *Tgfβ1, Fn1* and reduced *ColI* expression		(82)
Eosinophils	MI; late	mEar1	Smad2/3 inhibition	Inhibition of fibrosis	(84)
NK cells	Myocarditis; acute	IFN-γ	Induced *Cxcl9* expression	Inhibition of eosinophilia and myocarditis severity	(85)

(Continued)

TABLE 5.1
(Continued)

Immunocyte Subset	Condition; Type of Injury; Time Point	Mediators and Pathways Involved	Effect on Fibroblasts	Effect on Cardiac Repair	Reference(s)
Mast cells	MI; early	bFGF; TGFβ	Proliferation; MyoFb formation	Transient repair improvement	(88)
	MI	Myocardin; miR-143; miR145; KLF-4	Inhibition of MyoFb formation		(89)
	TNFα-induced cardiomyopathy; chronic	TGFβ1, TGFβRI	Proliferation; profibrotic gene expression	Fibrosis	(86)
	Diabetic cardiomyopathy; chronic	TNFα, IL6	Smad2/3 activation	Fibrosis	(87)
CD3+ T cells	MI; acute			Fibrosis; adverse remodeling	(95)
γδ T cells	MI; acute	IL-17A		Fibrosis	
CD4+ T cells	TAC; chronic	α4 integrin adhesion	TGFb activation; MyoFb formation	Fibrosis	(98)
Treg	MI; early	IL33/ST2; SPARC production	Induced *ColIII* expression	Inhibition of inflammation and wall rupture	(99,100,102)
	MI; early		MMP3 and α-SMA downregulation	Reduced Contractile activity; inhibition of adverse remodeling	(103)
	MI/IR; late			Adverse remodeling	(101)
	TAC, hypertension; chronic		TGFβ1, TGFβRII, ALK5 downregulation; MyoFb formation	Inhibition of fibrosis	(104)
B cells	Hypertension; chronic	IL-1β, TNFα, IL-6	Proliferation, induced *ColI, ColIII* expression	Inhibition of adverse remodeling	(114)

*MyoFb: myofibroblasts. For other abbreviations and details see main text.

BIBLIOGRAPHY

1. Everett BM, Cornel JH, Lainscak M, Anker SD, Abbate A, Thuren T, et al. Anti-inflammatory therapy with canakinumab for the prevention of hospitalization for heart failure. Circulation. 2019;139:1289–1299.
2. de Boer RA, De Keulenaer G, Bauersachs J, Brutsaert D, Cleland JG, Diez J, et al. Towards better definition, quantification and treatment of fibrosis in heart failure. Eur J Heart Fail 2019;21:272–285.
3. Xintarakou A, Tzeis S, Psarras S, Asvestas D, Vardas P. Atrial fibrosis as a dominant factor for the development of atrial fibrillation: facts and gaps. Europace. 2020;22:342–351.
4. Prabhu SD, Frangogiannis NG. The biological basis for cardiac repair after myocardial infarction. Circ Res. 2016;119:91–112.
5. Forte E, Furtado MB, Rosenthal N. The interstitium in cardiac repair: role of the immune—stromal cell interplay. Nat Rev Cardiol. 2018;15:601–616.
6. Oatmen KE, Cull E, Spinale FG. Heart failure as interstitial cancer: emergence of a malignant fibroblast phenotype. Nat Rev Cardiol. 2020;17:523–531.
7. Błyszczuk P. Myocarditis in humans and in experimental animal models. Front Cardiovasc Med. 2019;6:1–17.
8. Psarras S, Mavroidis M, Sanoudou D, Davos CH, Xanthou G, Varela AE, et al. Regulation of adverse remodelling by osteopontin in a genetic heart failure model. Eur Heart J. 2012;33:1954–1963.
9. Milner DJ, Taffet GE, Wang X, Pham T, Tamura T, Hartley C, et al. The absence of desmin leads to cardiomyocyte hypertrophy and cardiac dilation with compromised systolic function. J Mol Cell Cardiol. 1999;31:2063–2076.
10. Mavroidis M, Davos CH, Psarras S, Varela A, C Athanasiadis N, Katsimpoulas M, et al. Complement system modulation as a target for treatment of arrhythmogenic cardiomyopathy. Basic Res Cardiol. 2015;110:27.
11. Wang L, Yu P, Zhou B, Song J, Li Z, Zhang M, et al. Single-cell reconstruction of the adult human heart during heart failure and recovery reveals the cellular landscape underlying cardiac function. Nat Cell Biol. 2020;22:108–119.
12. Psarras S, Beis D, Nikouli S, Tsikitis M, Capetanaki Y. Three in a box: understanding cardiomyocyte, fibroblast, and innate immune cell interactions to orchestrate cardiac repair processes. Front Cardiovasc Med. 2019;6:32.
13. Tian Y, Morrisey EE. Importance of myocyte-nonmyocyte interactions in cardiac development and disease. Circ Res. 2012;110:1023–1034.
14. Talman V, Kivelä R. Cardiomyocyte—endothelial cell interactions in cardiac remodeling and regeneration. Front Cardiovasc Med. 2018;5:101.
15. Alex L, Frangogiannis NG. Pericytes in the infarcted heart. Vasc Biol. 2019;1:H23–31.
16. Pinto AR, Ilinykh A, Ivey MJ, Kuwabara JT, D'antoni ML, Debuque R, et al. Revisiting cardiac cellular composition. Circ Res. 2016;118:400–409.
17. Khalil H, Kanisicak O, Prasad V, Correll RN, Fu X, Schips T, et al. Fibroblast-specific TGF-β-Smad2/3 signaling underlies cardiac fibrosis. J Clin Invest. 2017;127:3770–3783.
18. Ivey MJ, Kuwabara JT, Pai JT, Moore RE, Sun Z, Tallquist MD. Resident fibroblast expansion during cardiac growth and remodeling. J Mol Cell Cardiol. 2018;114:161–174.
19. Teekakirikul P, Eminaga S, Toka O, Alcalai R, Wang L, Wakimoto H, et al. Cardiac fibrosis in mice with hypertrophic cardiomyopathy is mediated by non-myocyte proliferation and requires Tgf-β. J Clin Invest. 2010;120:3520–3529.
20. Burke RM, Lighthouse JK, Quijada P, Dirkx RA, Rosenberg A, Moravec CS, et al. Small proline-rich protein 2B drives stress-dependent p53 degradation and fibroblast proliferation in heart failure. Proc Natl Acad Sci. 2018;115:E3436–445.

21. Mouton AJ, Ma Y, Rivera Gonzalez OJ, Daseke MJ, Flynn ER, Freeman TC, et al. Fibroblast polarization over the myocardial infarction time continuum shifts roles from inflammation to angiogenesis. Basic Res Cardiol. 2019;114:6.

22. Fu X, Blaxall BC, Molkentin JD, Fu X, Khalil H, Kanisicak O, et al. Specialized fibroblast differentiated states underlie scar formation in the infarcted mouse heart. J Clin Invest. 2018;128:2127–2143.

23. Pillai ICL, Li S, Romay M, Lam L, Lu Y, Huang J, et al. Cardiac fibroblasts adopt osteogenic fates and can be targeted to attenuate pathological heart calcification. Cell Stem Cell. 2017;20:218–232.e5.

24. Kanisicak O, Khalil H, Ivey MJ, Karch J, Maliken BD, Correll RN, et al. Genetic lineage tracing defines myofibroblast origin and function in the injured heart. Nat Commun. 2016;7:1–14.

25. McLellan MA, Skelly DA, Dona MSI, Squiers GT, Farrugia GE, Gaynor TL, et al. High-resolution transcriptomic profiling of the heart during chronic stress reveals cellular drivers of cardiac fibrosis and hypertrophy. Circulation. 2020;142:1448–1463.

26. Ruiz-Villalba A, Romero JP, Hernandez SC, Vilas-Zornoza A, Fortelny N, Castro-Labrador L, et al. Single-cell RNA-seq analysis reveals a crucial role for collagen triple helix repeat containing 1 (CTHRC1) Cardiac fibroblasts after myocardial infarction. Circulation. 2020;1:1831–1847.

27. Saraswati S, Marrow SMW, Watch LA, Young PP. Identification of a pro-angiogenic functional role for FSP1-positive fibroblast subtype in wound healing. Nat Commun. 2019;10:3027.

28. Hortells L, Valiente-Alandi I, Thomas ZM, Agnew EJ, Schnell DJ, York AJ, et al. A specialized population of Periostin-expressing cardiac fibroblasts contributes to postnatal cardiomyocyte maturation and innervation. Proc Natl Acad Sci U S A. 2020;117:21469–21479.

29. Sandstedt J, Sandstedt M, Lundqvist A, Jansson M, Sopasakis VR, Jeppsson A, et al. Human cardiac fibroblasts isolated from patients with severe heart failure are immune-competent cells mediating an inflammatory response. Cytokine. 2019;113:319–325.

30. Anzai A, Choi JL, He S, Fenn AM, Nairz M, Rattik S, et al. The infarcted myocardium solicits GM-CSF for the detrimental oversupply of inflammatory leukocytes. J Exp Med. 2017;214:3293–3310.

31. Wu L, Ong S, Talor MV, Barin JG, Baldeviano GC, Kass DA, et al. Cardiac fibroblasts mediate IL-17A—driven inflammatory dilated cardiomyopathy. J Exp Med. 2014;211:1449–1464.

32. Hou X, Chen G, Bracamonte-Baran W, Choi HS, Diny NL, Sung J, et al. The cardiac microenvironment instructs divergent monocyte fates and functions in myocarditis. Cell Rep. 2019;28:172–189.e7.

33. Chen G, Bracamonte-Baran W, Diny NL, Hou X, Talor MV, Fu K, et al. Sca-1 + cardiac fibroblasts promote development of heart failure. Eur J Immunol. 2018;48:1522–1538.

34. Yu M, Hu J, Zhu MX, Zhao T, Liang W, Wen S, et al. Cardiac fibroblasts recruit Th17 cells infiltration into myocardium by secreting CcL20 in CVB3-induced acute viral myocarditis. Cell Physiol Biochem. 2013;32:1437–1450.

35. Ngwenyama N, Salvador AM, Velázquez F, Nevers T, Levy A, Aronovitz M, et al. CXCR3 regulates CD4+ T cell cardiotropism in pressure overload—induced cardiac dysfunction. JCI Insight. 2019;4:e125527.

36. Pappritz K, Savvatis K, Koschel A, Miteva K, Tschöpe C, Van Linthout S. Cardiac (myo) fibroblasts modulate the migration of monocyte subsets. Sci Rep. 2018;8:1–11.

37. Nakaya M, Watari K, Tajima M, Nakaya T, Matsuda S, Ohara H, et al. Cardiac myofibroblast engulfment of dead cells facilitates recovery after myocardial infarction. J Clin Invest. 2017;127:383–401.

38. Mylonas KJ, Turner NA, Bageghni SA, Kenyon CJ, White CI, McGregor K, et al. 11β-HSD1 suppresses cardiac fibroblast CXCL2, CXCL5 and neutrophil recruitment to the heart post MI. J Endocrinol. 2017;233:315–327.

39. Diny NL, Hou X, Barin JG, Chen G, Talor MV, Schaub J, et al. Macrophages and cardiac fibroblasts are the main producers of eotaxins and regulate eosinophil trafficking to the heart. Eur J Immunol. 2016;46:2749–2760.

40. Trial JA, Entman ML, Cieslik KA. Mesenchymal stem cell-derived inflammatory fibroblasts mediate interstitial fibrosis in the aging heart. J Mol Cell Cardiol. 2016;91:28–34.

41. Cieslik KA, Trial JA, Entman ML. Aicar treatment reduces interstitial fibrosis in aging mice: suppression of the inflammatory fibroblast. J Mol Cell Cardiol. 2017;111:81–85.

42. Boza P, Ayala P, Vivar R, Humeres C, Cáceres FT, Muñoz C, et al. Expression and function of toll-like receptor 4 and inflammasomes in cardiac fibroblasts and myofibroblasts: IL-1β synthesis, secretion, and degradation. Mol Immunol. 2016;74:96–105.

43. Kawaguchi M, Takahashi M, Hata T, Kashima Y, Usui F, Morimoto H, et al. Inflammasome activation of cardiac fibroblasts is essential for myocardial ischemia/reperfusion injury. Circulation. 2011;123:594–604.

44. Sandanger, Gao E, Ranheim T, Bliksøen M, Kaasbøll OJ, Alfsnes K, et al. NLRP3 inflammasome activation during myocardial ischemia reperfusion is cardioprotective. Biochem Biophys Res Commun. 2016;469:1012–1020.

45. Louwe MC, Olsen MB, Kaasbøll OJ, Yang K, Fosshaug LE, Alfsnes K, et al. Absence of NLRP3 inflammasome in hematopoietic cells reduces adverse remodeling after experimental myocardial infarction. JACC Basic to Transl Sci. 2020;5:1210–1224.

46. Suetomi T, Willeford A, Brand CS, Cho Y, Ross RS, Miyamoto S, et al. Inflammation and NLRP3 inflammasome activation initiated in response to pressure overload by Ca2+/calmodulin-dependent protein kinase II δ signaling in cardiomyocytes are essential for adverse cardiac remodeling. Circulation. 2018;138:2530–2544.

47. Baehr A, Umansky KB, Bassat E, Jurisch V, Klett K, Bozoglu T, et al. Agrin promotes coordinated therapeutic processes leading to improved cardiac repair in pigs. Circulation. 2020;142:868–881.

48. Yokota T, McCourt J, Ma F, Ren S, Li S, Kim TH, et al. Type V collagen in scar tissue regulates the size of scar after heart injury. Cell. 2020;1–18.

49. Wang Z, Long DW, Huang Y, Chen WCW, Kim K, Wang Y. Decellularized neonatal cardiac extracellular matrix prevents widespread ventricular remodeling in adult mammals after myocardial infarction. Acta Biomater. 2019;87:140–151.

50. Leuschner F, Nahrendorf M. Novel functions of macrophages in the heart: insights into electrical conduction, stress, and diastolic dysfunction. Eur Heart J. 2020;41:989–994.

51. Aurora AB, Porrello ER, Tan W, Mahmoud AI, Hill JA, Bassel-duby R, et al. Macrophages are required for neonatal heart regeneration. J Clin Invest. 2014;124:1382–1392.

52. Mouton AJ, DeLeon-Pennell KY, Rivera Gonzalez OJ, Flynn ER, Freeman TC, Saucerman JJ, et al. Mapping macrophage polarization over the myocardial infarction time continuum. Basic Res Cardiol. 2018;113:26.

53. Lavine KJ, Epelman S, Uchida K, Weber KJ, Nichols CG, Schilling JD, et al. Distinct macrophage lineages contribute to disparate patterns of cardiac recovery and remodeling in the neonatal and adult heart. Proc Natl Acad Sci. 2014;111:16029–16034.

54. Heidt T, Courties G, Dutta P, Sager HB, Sebas M, Iwamoto Y, et al. Differential contribution of monocytes to heart macrophages in steady-state and after myocardial infarction. Circ Res. 2014;115:284–295.

55. Nahrendorf M, Swirski FK, Aikawa E, Stangenberg L, Wurdinger T, Figueiredo J-L, et al. The healing myocardium sequentially mobilizes two monocyte subsets with divergent and complementary functions. J Exp Med. 2007;204:3037–3047.

56. Bajpai G, Schneider C, Wong N, Bredemeyer A, Hulsmans M, Nahrendorf M, et al. The human heart contains distinct macrophage subsets with divergent origins and functions. Nat Med [Internet]. 2018;24:1234–1245.

57. Bajpai G, Bredemeyer A, Li WW, Zaitsev K, Koenig AL, Lokshina II, et al. Tissue resident CCR2- and CCR2+ cardiac macrophages differentially orchestrate monocyte recruitment and fate specification following myocardial injury. Circ Res. 2019;124:263–278.

58. Dick SA, Macklin JA, Nejat S, Momen A, Clemente-Casares X, Althagafi MG, et al. Self-renewing resident cardiac macrophages limit adverse remodeling following myocardial infarction. Nat Immunol. 2019;20:29–39.

59. Patel B, Bansal SS, Ismahil MA, Hamid T, Rokosh G, Mack M, et al. CCR2+ monocyte-derived infiltrating macrophages are required for adverse cardiac remodeling during pressure overload. JACC Basic to Transl Sci. 2018;3:230–244.

60. King KR, Aguirre AD, Ye YX, Sun Y, Roh JD, Ng RP, et al. IRF3 and type i interferons fuel a fatal response to myocardial infarction. Nat Med [Internet]. 2017;23:1481–1487.

61. Lenga Y, Koh A, Perera AS, McCulloch CA, Sodek J, Zohar R. Osteopontin expression is required for myofibroblast differentiation. Circ Res. 2008;102:319–327.

62. Hulsmans M, Sager HB, Roh JD, Muñoz MV, Houstis NE, Iwamoto Y, et al. Cardiac macrophages promote diastolic dysfunction. J Exp Med. 2018;215:423–440.

63. Westermann D, Lindner D, Kasner M, Zietsch C, Savvatis K, Escher F, et al. Cardiac inflammation contributes to changes in the extracellular matrix in patients with heart failure and normal ejection fraction. Circ Hear Fail. 2011;4:44–52.

64. Valaperti A, Nishii M, Liu Y, Naito K, Chan M, Zhang L, et al. Innate immune interleukin-1 receptor-associated kinase 4 exacerbates viral myocarditis by reducing CCR5+CD11b+ monocyte migration and impairing interferon production. Circulation. 2013;128:1542–1554.

65. Liao X, Shen Y, Zhang R, Sugi K, Vasudevan NT, Alaiti MA, et al. Distinct roles of resident and nonresident macrophages in nonischemic cardiomyopathy. Proc Natl Acad Sci. 2018;115:E4661–4669.

66. Abe H, Takeda N, Isagawa T, Semba H, Nishimura S, Morioka MS, et al. Macrophage hypoxia signaling regulates cardiac fibrosis via Oncostatin M. Nat Commun. 2019;10:1–8.

67. Deniset JF, Belke D, Lee WY, Jorch SK, Deppermann C, Hassanabad AF, et al. Gata6+ pericardial cavity macrophages relocate to the injured heart and prevent cardiac fibrosis. Immunity [Internet]. 2019;51:131–140.e5.

68. Sager HB, Hulsmans M, Lavine KJ, Moreira MB, Heidt T, Courties G, et al. Proliferation and recruitment contribute to myocardial macrophage expansion in chronic heart failure. Circ Res. 2016;119:853–864.

69. Shiraishi M, Shintani Y, Shintani Y, Ishida H, Saba R, Yamaguchi A, et al. Alternatively activated macrophages determine repair of the infarcted adult murine heart. J Clin Invest. 2016;126:2151–2166.

70. Nahrendorf M, Swirski FK. Abandoning M1/M2 for a network model of macrophage function. Circ Res. 2016;119:414–417.

71. Wang C, Zhang C, Liu L, Xi A, Chen B, Li Y, et al. Macrophage-derived mir-155-containing exosomes suppress fibroblast proliferation and promote fibroblast inflammation during cardiac injury. Mol Ther. 2017;25:192–204.

72. Ramanujam D, Schön AP, Beck C, Vaccarello P, Felician G, Dueck A, et al. MiR-21-dependent macrophage-to-fibroblast signaling determines the cardiac response to pressure overload. Circulation. 2021;1513–1525.

73. Jung M, Ma Y, Iyer RP, DeLeon-Pennell KY, Yabluchanskiy A, Garrett MR, et al. IL-10 improves cardiac remodeling after myocardial infarction by stimulating M2 macrophage polarization and fibroblast activation. Basic Res Cardiol. 2017;112:33.

74. Cao DJ, Schiattarella GG, Villalobos E, Jiang N, May HI, Li T, et al. Cytosolic DNA sensing promotes macrophage transformation and governs myocardial ischemic injury. Circulation. 2018;137:2613–2634.

75. Yue Y, Huang S, Li H, Li W, Hou J, Luo L, et al. M2b macrophages protect against myocardial remodeling after ischemia/reperfusion injury by regulating kinase activation of platelet-derived growth factor receptor of cardiac fibroblast. Ann Transl Med. 2020;8:1409–1409.

76. Simões FC, Cahill TJ, Kenyon A, Gavriouchkina D, Vieira JM, Sun X, et al. Macrophages directly contribute collagen to scar formation during zebrafish heart regeneration and mouse heart repair. Nat Commun [Internet]. 2020;11:1–17.

77. McDonald LT, Zile MR, Zhang Y, Van Laer AO, Baicu CF, Stroud RE, et al. Increased macrophage-derived SPARC precedes collagen deposition in myocardial fibrosis. Am J Physiol Circ Physiol. 2018;315:H92–100.

78. Haider N, Boscá L, Zandbergen HR, Kovacic JC, Narula N, González-Ramos S, et al. Transition of macrophages to fibroblast-like cells in healing myocardial infarction. J Am Coll Cardiol. 2019;74:3124–3135.

79. Daseke MJ, Valerio FM, Kalusche WJ, Ma Y, DeLeon-Pennell KY, Lindsey ML. Neutrophil proteome shifts over the myocardial infarction time continuum. Basic Res Cardiol. 2019;114(5):1–13.

80. Horckmans M, Ring L, Duchene J, Santovito D, Schloss MJ, Drechsler M, et al. Neutrophils orchestrate post-myocardial infarction healing by polarizing macrophages towards a reparative phenotype. Eur Heart J. 2017;38:187–197.

81. Ma Y, Yabluchanskiy A, Iyer RP, Cannon PL, Flynn ER, Jung M, et al. Temporal neutrophil polarization following myocardial infarction. Cariovasc Res. 2016;110:51–61.

82. Curaj A, Schumacher D, Rusu M, Staudt M, Li X, Simsekyilmaz S, et al. Neutrophils modulate fibroblast function and promote healing and scar formation after murine myocardial infarction. Int J Mol Sci. 2020;21:3685.

83. Toor IS, Rückerl D, Mair I, Ainsworth R, Meloni M, Spiroski AM, et al. Eosinophil deficiency promotes aberrant repair and adverse remodeling following acute myocardial infarction. JACC Basic to Transl Sci. 2020;5:665–681.

84. Liu J, Yang C, Liu T, Deng Z, Fang W, Zhang X, et al. Eosinophils improve cardiac function after myocardial infarction. Nat Commun. 2020;11(1):6396.

85. Ong S, Ligons DL, Barin JG, Wu L, Talor MV, Diny N, et al. Natural killer cells limit cardiac inflammation and fibrosis by halting eosinophil infiltration. Am J Pathol. 2015;185:847–861.

86. Zhang W, Chancey AL, Tzeng HP, Zhou Z, Lavine KJ, Gao F, et al. The development of myocardial fibrosis in transgenic mice with targeted overexpression of tumor necrosis factor requires mast cell-fibroblast interactions. Circulation. 2011;124:2106–2116.

87. He A, Fang W, Zhao K, Wang Y, Li J, Yang C, et al. Mast cell-deficiency protects mice from streptozotocin-induced diabetic cardiomyopathy. Transl Res. 2019;208:1–14.

88. Shao Z, Nazari M, Guo L, Li SH, Sun J, Liu SM, et al. The cardiac repair benefits of inflammation do not persist: evidence from mast cell implantation. J Cell Mol Med. 2015;19:2751–2762.

89. Nazari M, Ni NC, Lüdke A, Li SH, Guo J, Weisel RD, et al. Mast cells promote proliferation and migration and inhibit differentiation of mesenchymal stem cells through PDGF. J Mol Cell Cardiol. 2016;94:32–42.

90. Van der Borght K, Scott CL, Nindl V, Bouché A, Martens L, Sichien D, et al. Myocardial infarction primes autoreactive T cells through activation of dendritic cells. Cell Rep. 2017;18:3005–3017.

91. Lee JS, Jeong SJ, Kim S, Chalifour L, Yun TJ, Miah MA, et al. Conventional dendritic cells impair recovery after myocardial infarction. J Immunol. 2018;20:1784–1798.

92. Clemente-Casares X, Hosseinzadeh S, Barbu I, Dick SA, Macklin JA, Wang Y, et al. A CD103+ conventional dendritic cell surveillance system prevents development of overt heart failure during subclinical viral myocarditis. Immunity. 2017;47:974–989.e8.

93. Choo E, Lee J, Park E, Park H, Jung N, Kim T, et al. Infarcted myocardium-primed dendritic cells improve remodeling and cardiac function after myocardial infarction by modulating the regulatory T cell and macrophage polarization. No title. Circulation. 2017;135:1444–1457.

94. Tang TT, Zhu YC, Dong NG, Zhang S, Cai J, Zhang LX, et al. Pathologic T-cell response in ischaemic failing hearts elucidated by T-cell receptor sequencing and phenotypic characterization. Eur Heart J. 2019;40:3924–3933.

95. Bansal SS, Ismahil MA, Goel M, Patel B, Hamid T, Rokosh G, et al. Activated T lymphocytes are essential drivers of pathological remodeling in ischemic heart failure. Circ Hear Fail. 2017;10:1–12.

96. Yan X, Shichita T, Katsumata Y, Matsuhashi T, Ito H, Ito K, et al. Deleterious effect of the IL-23/IL-17A axis and γδT cells on left ventricular remodeling after myocardial infarction. J Am Heart Assoc. 2012;1:1–22.

97. Nevers T, Salvador AM, Grodecki-Pena A, Knapp A, Velázquez F, Aronovitz M, et al. Left ventricular t-cell recruitment contributes to the pathogenesis of heart failure. Circ Hear Fail. 2015;8:776–787.

98. Nevers T, Salvador AM, Velazquez F, Ngwenyama N, Carrillo-Salinas FJ, Aronovitz M, et al. Th1 effector T cells selectively orchestrate cardiac fibrosis in nonischemic heart failure. J Exp Med. 2017;214:3311–3329.

99. Rieckmann M, Delgobo M, Gaal C, Büchner L, Steinau P, Reshef D, et al. Myocardial infarction triggers cardioprotective antigen-specific T helper cell responses. J Clin Invest. 2019;129:4922–4936.

100. Weirather J, Hoffmann U, Beyersdorf N, Ramos GC, Vogel B, Frey A, et al. Foxp3+ CD4+ T cells improve healing after myocardial infarction by modulating monocyte/macrophage differentiation. Circ Res. 2014;115:55–67.

101. Bansal SS, Ismahil MA, Goel M, Zhou G, Rokosh G, Hamid T, et al. Dysfunctional and proinflammatory regulatory T-lymphocytes are essential for adverse cardiac remodeling in ischemic cardiomyopathy. Circulation. 2019;139:206–221.

102. Xia N, Lu Y, Gu M, Li N, Liu M, Jiao J, et al. A unique population of regulatory T cells in heart potentiates cardiac protection from myocardial infarction. Circulation. 2020;142:1956–1973.

103. Saxena A, Dobaczewski M, Rai V, Haque Z, Chen W, Li N, et al. Regulatory T cells are recruited in the infarcted mouse myocardium and may modulate fibroblast phenotype and function. Am J Physiol—Hear Circ Physiol. 2014;307:H1233–1242.

104. Kanellakis P, Dinh T, Agrotis A, Bobik A. CD4+CD25+Foxp3+ regulatory T cells suppress cardiac fibrosis in the hypertensive heart. J Hypertens. 2011;29:1820–1828.

105. Santos-Zas I, Lemarié J, Zlatanova I, Cachanado M, Seghezzi J-C, Benamer H, et al. Cytotoxic CD8+ T cells promote granzyme B-dependent adverse post-ischemic cardiac remodeling. Nat Commun. 2021;12:1483.

106. Forte E, Perkins B, Sintou A, Kalkat HS, Papanikolaou A, Jenkins C, et al. Cross-priming dendritic cells exacerbate immunopathology after ischemic tissue damage in the heart. Circulation. 2020;143:821–836.

107. Ilatovskaya DV, Pitts C, Clayton J, Domondon M, Troncoso M, Pippin S, et al. CD8+ T-cells negatively regulate inflammation post-myocardial infarction. Am J Physiol—Hear Circ Physiol. 2019;317:H581–596.

108. Sobirin MA, Kinugawa S, Takahashi M, Fukushima A, Homma T, Ono T, et al. Activation of natural killer T cells ameliorates postinfarct cardiac remodeling and failure in mice. Circ Res. 2012;111:1037–1047.

109. Sintou A, Mansfield C, Iacob A, Chowdhury RA, Narodden S, Rothery SM, et al. Mediastinal lymphadenopathy, class-switched auto-antibodies and myocardial immune-complexes during heart failure in rodents and humans. Front Cell Dev Biol. 2020;8:1–12.

110. Haas MS, Alicot EM, Schuerpf F, Chiu I, Li J, Moore FD, et al. Blockade of self-reactive IgM significantly reduces injury in a murine model of acute myocardial infarction. Cardiovasc Res. 2010;87:618–627.

111. Zouggari Y, Ait-Oufella H, Bonnin P, Simon T, Sage AP, Guérin C, et al. B lymphocytes trigger monocyte mobilization and impair heart function after acute myocardial infarction. Nat Med. 2013;19:1273–1280.

112. Li Y, Huang Y, Wu W, Wei B, Qin L. B cells increase myocardial inflammation by suppressing M2 macrophage polarization in coxsackie virus B3-induced acute myocarditis. Inflammation. 2019;42:953–960.

113. Adamo L, Staloch LJ, Rocha-Resende C, Matkovich SJ, Jiang W, Bajpai G, et al. Modulation of subsets of cardiac B lymphocytes improves cardiac function after acute injury. JCI Insight. 2018;3:e120137.

114. Cordero-Reyes AM, Youker KA, Trevino AR, Celis R, Hamilton DJ, Flores-Arredondo JH, et al. Full expression of cardiomyopathy is partly dependent on B-cells: a pathway that involves cytokine activation, immunoglobulin deposition, and activation of apoptosis. J Am Heart Assoc. 2016;5:1–12.

115. Patel AN, Henry TD, Quyyumi AA, Schaer GL, Anderson RD, Toma C, et al. Ixmyelocel-T for patients with ischaemic heart failure: a prospective randomised double-blind trial. Lancet. 2016;387:2412–2421.

116. Vagnozzi RJ, Maillet M, Sargent MA, Khalil H, Johansen AKZ, Schwanekamp JA, et al. An acute immune response underlies the benefit of cardiac stem cell therapy. Nature. 2020;577:405–409.

117. Nagaraju CK, Robinson EL, Abdesselem M, Trenson S, Dries E, Gilbert G, et al. Myofibroblast phenotype and reversibility of fibrosis in patients with end-stage heart failure. J Am Coll Cardiol. 2019;73:2267–2282.

118. Aghajanian H, Kimura T, Rurik JG, Hancock AS, Leibowitz MS, Li L, et al. Targeting cardiac fibrosis with engineered T cells. Nature. 2019; 573:430–433.

119. Yu J, Seldin MM, Fu K, Li S, Lam L, Wang P, et al. Topological arrangement of cardiac fibroblasts regulates cellular plasticity novelty and significance. Circ Res. 2018;123:73–85.

120. Perbellini F, Thum T. Living myocardial slices: a novel multicellular model for cardiac translational research. Eur Heart J. 2019;49:2405–2408.

6 Inflammation, Stem Cell Therapy, and Cardiac Repair

Marcus J. Wagner, Jacob T. Menzer, and Sadia Mohsin

CONTENTS

CURRENT STATE AND MANAGEMENT OF CARDIOVASCULAR DISEASE

Cardiovascular disease (CVD) is the leading cause of death in the United States each year.[1] By the year 2035, the cost to treat and manage CVD in the United States is expected to reach $368 billion.[1] Coronary heart diseases (CHD) are manifested in the coronary arteries of the heart and account for ~43% of CVD-related diagnoses, making CHD the leading manifestation of CVD, with myocardial infarction (MI) being the most severe form of CHD.[1] A lack in treatment efficacy and timely ability to recognize and alleviate MI onset resulted in the death of 258.2 per 100,000 individuals in 2007.[1] Since the turn of the century, the development of new therapeutics such as ischemia reperfusion (IR) of the occluded coronary artery or coronary artery bypass graft (CABG) surgery has provided superior methods to

DOI: 10.1201/b22824-7

revascularize the tissue and reduce patient mortality during an adverse, ischemic myocardial event. Additionally, an increased emphasis on symptom onset recognition, early medical attention (cardiopulmonary resuscitation and defibrillation), and improved transport times to advanced medical care have reduced myocardial damage solicited during MIs, resulting in a 15% decrease in CVD-related deaths between 2007 to 2017.[1]

Unfortunately, the interventions employed during MI have only been effective in decreasing initial mortality, not the adverse cardiac remodeling or heart failure (HF) pathology that ensues following MI. Estimates for 2017 projected that approximately 5.7 million patients in the United States would be diagnosed with HF; however, 6.3 million patients, 500,000 more than the projected number, were actually diagnosed with HF in 2017.[1] The number of HF patients is expected to double by 2030.[1] Treatment options currently prescribed to patients only aid in the management of HF symptoms and are rather ineffective at preventing disease progression. The terminal therapeutic intervention for HF is heart transplantation, but the demand for heart transplants far outweighs the supply. Between the years 1987 and 2012, 40,253 patients were placed on the cardiac transplant list, but only 26,943 patients received cardiac transplantation.[1] The call for basic scientists to investigate and devise therapies that aim to replace, repair, or restore the myocardium damaged or lost during an ischemic attack is an immense necessity.

THE CURRENT STATE OF STEM CELL THERAPY

In the early 2000s, stem cells were introduced to the infarcted myocardium with the hope that stem cell progenitors would differentiate into new, functional tissue. However, mounting evidence collected over the last 20 years has identified the unwelcomed result that the adoptive transfer of progenitors into the infarcted heart do not result in the formation of *de novo*, functional myocardium; rather, the stem cells robustly influence processes that mediate angiogenesis, fibrotic tissue maturation, scar formation, and immune system response (Figure 6.1).[2,3] Below, we outline the different generations of cell-based therapies that have been implemented in the infarcted heart in both preclinical and clinical studies conducted over the last two decades. In addition, the key limitations, challenges, and unanswered questions that surround the efficacy of stem cell therapies in mediating cardiac repair and regeneration are discussed. Finally, we provide our insights on how stem cell therapy can be used to harness the inflammatory response of the infarcted heart to support cardiac wound healing post-MI.

At the turn of the twenty-first century, the first studies to incorporate the transfer of stem cells into the post-MI heart employed the use of progenitor cells isolated from skeletal muscle, skeletal myoblasts.[4] Adoptively transferred skeletal myoblasts into the MI heart failed to electrically integrate with the functional myocardium contributing to an increased incidence of ventricular fibrillation.[5] Consequently, skeletal myoblasts were determined to not be an advantageous cell type to orchestrate cardiac repair post-MI. Interest in other stem cell populations that could be harvested from hematopoietic origins (peripheral blood or bone

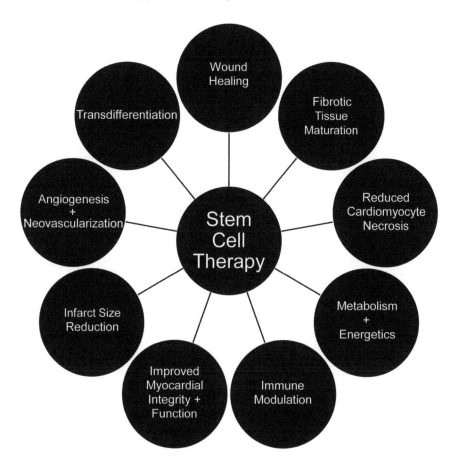

FIGURE 6.1 Stem cell therapies can solicit cardiac repair. Originally, stem cell therapies were implemented in the post-MI heart with the hope that the adoptively transferred stem cell populations would differentiate into functional myocardium to replace the myocardium damaged during an MI. Recent studies identify that stem cell populations undergo limited differentiation into functional myocardium, but rather modulate cardiac wound-healing processes, specifically angiogenesis, fibrotic tissue maturation, and immune cell trafficking.

marrow) were pursued, marking the birth of first generation cell-based therapies (Figure 6.2).

First-generation stem cell therapies are isolated from circulating blood pools and the bone marrow, which both contain heterogeneous populations of progenitors that are not standardized to specific cell identification marker expression.[6] The primary goal of first-generation cell-based therapies was to quickly isolate progenitors from patients experiencing an MI and reintroduce the isolated progenitors into the injured heart of the same patient, with the hope that an autoimmune response would not be mounted against the autologously transferred progenitors. Unfortunately, the reintroduction of heterogeneous progenitor populations into the MI heart only resulted in modest functional and wound-healing improvement.[6,7] Consequently, the race to

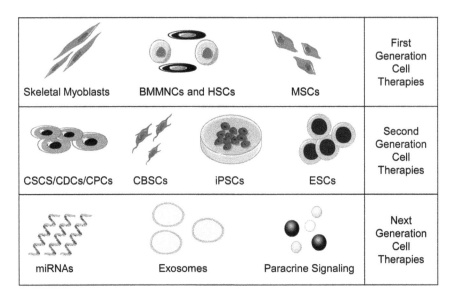

| | | | First Generation Cell Therapies |
| Skeletal Myoblasts | BMMNCs and HSCs | MSCs | |

FIGURE 6.2   Three generations of stem cell therapy. Over the last two decades, several generations of stem cell therapies have been implemented to modulate the repair of myocardium injured or lost during an MI. First-generation cell therapies incorporated the use of progenitors isolated from skeletal muscle or heterogeneous populations retained in the blood or bone marrow. Second-generation therapies implemented the use of progenitor cell populations isolated from other organ structures using stringent cell surface marker expression (CDCs and CBSCs), more primitive cell types (ESCs), or via chemically induced dedifferentiation of terminally differentiated cell types (iPSCs). Finally, next-generation cell-based therapies aim to harness the molecular signaling intermediates produced by stem cells to modulate cardiac repair.

isolate a more homogeneous stem cell therapy, selected on the basis of more stringent surface marker expression, was sought with the hope that the reintroduction of more unified populations would produce greater improvements in injury reduction and cardiac function post-MI. One of the main cell types investigated were mesenchymal stem cells (MSCs). These stem cells are isolated from bone marrow and purified via plastic adherence. Unfortunately, the incorporation of more purified, homogeneous stem cell populations, including MSCs, still only provided modest therapeutic improvement in cardiac function and injury reduction.[8] Therefore, stem cell biologists began searching for progenitor populations retained in other organ structures outside of the blood or bone marrow, marking the development of second-generation cell-based therapies (Figure 6.2).

Second-generation cell therapies encompass progenitors isolated from other organ structures that do not originate from the blood or bone marrow. Examples of second-generation cell-based therapies include progenitors isolated from cardiac tissue,[7] embryonic tissue,[9] cortical bone,[10,11] or those chemically derived from the dedifferentiation of primary cell types (iPSCs).[12] Given the multiplicity of cell types currently under investigation, an increase in understanding the fundamental biology of each progenitor population is essential before the efficacy of second-generation cell-based therapies can be adequately determined.[2] Further investigations that identify stem cell niches and their proliferative/differentiative capabilities, isolation and expansion practices, allogenic (donor) or autologous (self) sourcing, routes of administration, dosing level, homing and retention in the infarcted myocardium, and the standardization of surrogate end points to assess clinical efficacy must be addressed in future preclinical and clinical experimental designs to effectively unlock the maximum therapeutic potential of an ideal cell type retained in second-generation cell-based therapies.[13] Recently, an increased emphasis has been placed on the paracrine secretome produced by stem cells and the ability of the secretome to modulate cardiac wound healing.[2,14]

Next-generation cell-based therapies investigate the paracrine hypothesis, the belief that secretory factors produced by progenitors are the main source of the cardiogenic properties possessed by stem cell populations in the MI heart.[14,15] Investigations centered around the paracrine hypothesis have specifically inquired about the therapeutic applications of exosome production, miRNA secretion, and the cytokine and chemotactic signaling molecules produced by stem cell populations. Stem cells are diverse epicenters that produce numerous cytokine and chemotactic signaling molecules that can directly mediate the trafficking, localization, and function of immune cells.[16] The identification of how stem cell–mediated paracrine production can regulate the inflammatory cell infiltrate of the infarcted heart could have substantial therapeutic effects and provide a humbling anecdote of how next-generation cell-based therapies can be harnessed to regulate cardiac repair and function post-MI.[14] The initial implementation of stem cell therapy to modulate myocardial repair was fast tracked, and the basic, fundamental principles that regulate stem cell niche and function have been overlooked. Now, next-generation cell-based therapies are aiming to understand the fundamental biological properties of stem cell populations and how stem cells can be harnessed to enhance myocardial wound healing.

IMMUNE RESPONSE TO CARDIAC INJURY: FINDING THE GOLDILOCKS THERAPEUTIC

Ischemic injury to the myocardium results in the activation of a complex, interconnected, and essential inflammatory response that orchestrates necrotic cell clearance followed by the establishment of wound-healing processes, specifically: neovascularization, scar maturation, and cardiac tissue homeostasis.[17] The temporal regulation of the immune response to myocardial injury has proven to be essential for the shortening or suppression of the acute inflammatory stage or prolonged sustainment of the initial inflammatory response during chronic injury can greatly hinder cardiac repair.[17] Most therapies modulating cardiac repair following ischemic injury are designed to target the structural, functional, and molecular alterations that ensue during adverse cardiac remodeling and heart failure pathology. However, over the last decade, investigators have taken an interest in identifying therapeutic modalities that can be harnessed to modulate the inflammatory response mounted in the ischemic heart to improve endogenous cardiac repair.[14]

Initial, premature clinical observations coupled the inflammatory response to heart failure pathology; thus, the primitive thought was to administer pan-immunosuppressive agents to reduce the aggressive inflammatory response mounted following MI – permitting an improvement in patients' post-MI outcomes.[18] However, initial results collected from preliminary clinical trials reported minimal or lessened improvements in cardiac wound healing and function during the administration of broad immunosuppressive agents in the heart following ischemic injury. This emphasized that the sophisticated, interconnected, and multilayered immune responses mounted following cardiac injury cannot simply be modulated by pan-immunosuppression of all inflammatory cell types; rather, the punitive targeting of specific immune cell populations during cardiac injury is more advantageous.[18,19] The exact therapeutics that can target specific inflammatory cell responses in the ischemic heart are currently being investigated.

Intramyocardial injection of stem cell therapies permits the short-term engraftment of progenitor cell populations in the infarcted myocardium, allowing for an intimate relationship to form between the adoptively transferred progenitor cells and neighboring immune cells resident in the infarcted heart.[14] Stem cell therapy has proven to be a dynamic therapeutic that can provide the appropriate suppression of pro-inflammatory, pathogenic immune cell subsets while facilitating the expansion and preservation of anti-inflammatory, pro-reparative immune cell subsets that can orchestrate myocardial wound healing following MI (Figure 6.3).[20–24]

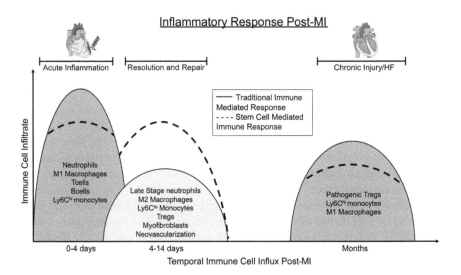

FIGURE 6.3 Stem cell therapies are a Goldilocks therapeutic. Cell-based therapies can effectively dampen pro-inflammatory cell types yet harness pro-reparative immune cell populations that enhance immune-mediated cardiac repair during acute and chronic stages of ischemic injury.

THE IMMUNOMODULATORY IMPLICATIONS OF STEM CELL THERAPY IN ISCHEMIC CARDIOMYOPATHIES

Stem cell therapies secrete paracrine profiles that can directly modify the recruitment, activation, phenotype, and function of neighboring immune cell populations occupying the injured heart, specifically: neutrophils, macrophages (MΦ), T cells, and B cells (Figure 6.4). The exact paracrine signaling molecules that are produced by stem cell progenitors and the mechanistic roles these factors serve in mediating immune cell dynamics and function are outlined in the following sections.

STEM CELLS AND NEUTROPHILS: THE INNATE IMMUNE RESPONSE

Neutrophils, within hours of ischemia onset, are one of the first populations to influx into the infarcted heart and release degradative enzymes that facilitate the clearance of necrotic myocardium.[25,26] Approximately 4 days following ischemic injury, late-stage neutrophils possessing pro-reparative signatures influx into the heart and

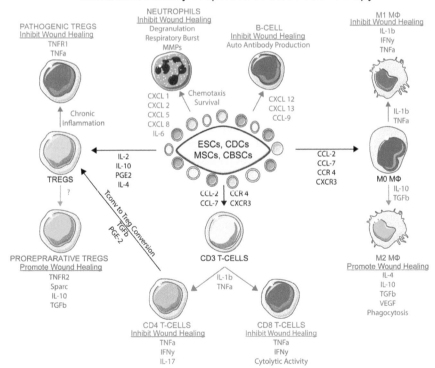

FIGURE 6.4 Stem cell secretome is a diverse epicenter of paracrine secretion. The paracrine secretome produced by cell-based therapies can directly interact with and modulate the function, recruitment, and phenotype of the inflammatory cell infiltrate that occupies the infarcted heart post-MI.

suppress the pro-inflammatory, degradative state previously established by the initial neutrophil infiltrate.[26] Late-stage neutrophils secrete scavenger receptors that clear the infarcted myocardium of pro-inflammatory, degradative signaling molecules, and enzymes that regulate necrotic cell clearance and tissue degradation.[17] This temporal shift in neutrophil phenotype facilitates a transition from a tissue degradative state to a reparative state that promotes scar formation, neovascularization, and tissue maturation.

Mesenchymal stem cells produce a paracrine secretome that can directly modulate the recruitment, retention, and viability of neutrophil populations. MSC secretome is enriched in chemotactic signaling molecules CXCL1, CXCL2, CXCL5, and CXCL8 – all of which elicit neutrophil recruitment.[27] Additionally, MSC-mediated production of IL-6 has been shown to directly affect neutrophil viability in co-culture systems.[28] Exposure of neutrophils to MSC cultures that are deficient in IL-6 compromises neutrophil viability.[29] Understanding how stem cells mediate the viability, recruitment, and phenotype of neutrophil populations in the infarcted heart can provide insight into how cell-based therapies can modulate the clearance of necrotic myocardium, cardiac rupture, and establishment of a pro-reparative state that promotes myocardial wound healing.

STEM CELLS AND MACROPHAGES: THE INNATE IMMUNE RESPONSE

Shortly after initial neutrophil influx, MΦs populate the infarcted myocardium.[2,30] Great heterogeneity exists among the MΦ subsets that occupy the infarcted heart, as each MΦ subset serves a specified role in mediating myocardial repair.[31] In general, M1 pro-inflammatory, classically activated MΦs possess a pro-inflammatory signature that is enriched in proteolytic enzymes that complement the harsh, pro-inflammatory microenvironment established by early neutrophil recruitment.[32,33] Approximately 4–7 days post-MI, anti-inflammatory, alternatively activated M2 MΦs prevail in the infarcted myocardium and possess anti-inflammatory signatures that support angiogenic processes that promote cardiac repair.[26,34,35]

Paracrine signaling molecules produced by MSCs can directly mediate M1, M2 MΦ polaraization.[36] The introduction of MSC secretome to MΦ cultures suppresses pro-inflammatory, M1 MΦ produced signaling molecules (TNFα, IL-1β, IL-6, IFNγ, and IL-2) and expands anti-inflammatory, pro-reparative, M2 MΦ produced signaling molecules (TGFβ and IL-10) which can either repress or promote myocardial wound healing respectively.[37] The MSC secretome is also enriched in PGE2, IL1rα, and TGFβ, all of which have been shown to induce M1 to M2 MΦ conversion.[36,38,39] Progenitor cells isolated from cardiac tissue, commonly referred to as cardiosphere-derived cells (CDCs), have also been shown to produce exosomes that can drive M1 to M2 MΦ polarization.[40,41] Additionally, MSC secretome is also enriched in chemotactic signaling molecules, CCL-3, CCL-7, and CCL-12, which support MΦ recruitment to the infarcted heart.[40,41] Another progenitor cell type isolated from the cortical bone (CBSCs) can also increase M2 MΦ residence in the infarcted myocardium 7 days following MI.[42]

The use of embryonic stem cells (ESCs) to regulate M1 to M2 MΦ dynamics is more ambiguous compared to the other stem cell types discussed earlier. Embryonic stem cells have not been shown to produce paracrine signaling factors that can directly induce MΦ polarization; however, due to the advanced primitive nature and greater differentiation capacities of ESCs, ESCs can easily differentiate into antigen-presenting cell lineages – a notorious property of MΦs. ESC administration into the infarcted heart expands antigen-presenting markers: MHCI and MHCII.[43] This expansion could be mediated by either: 1) increased recruitment of MΦ populations or other professional antigen-presenting cells to the infarcted heart following ESC administration or 2) the *de novo* formation of MHC-expressing cells from the adoptively transferred ESCs. Interestingly, another group identified that ESCs can diverge into a suppressor cell line that contains both M1 and M2 MΦ phenotype expression.[44] Exact lineage tracing of ESC therapies in the heart and the standardization of ESC heterogeneity must be assessed before cardiac immunologists can truly conclude the role that ESC cell therapy has in mediating MΦ response to ischemic injury. Fundamental studies have identified the potential for stem cells to regulate MΦ phenotype, function, and residence in the infarcted myocardium, which can permit the establishment of an anti-inflammatory, pro-reparative state that supports cardiac wound healing.

Stem Cells and T Cells: The Adaptive Immune Response

T-lymphocytes are retained in the adaptive immune response and do not populate the injured tissue immediately following injury onset; rather, they influx into the infarcted myocardium 4–7 days following injury onset.[45–47] T cell populations retain CD3+ expression and can be further divided into one of two subsets on the basis of either CD4+ (T-helper cell) or CD8+ (cytotoxic T cell) expression.[26] The literature surrounding the role T-lymphocytes serve in mediating cardiac repair post-MI shows great discrepancies.[26,48,49] Despite the simplistic characterization scheme proposed here; T cell populations are dynamic, and different transcription factor expression can drive T cell subset divergence with each subset exhibiting a specified phenotype and function in the context of myocardial repair.

Recently, much attention has been directed to the CD4+ T-helper cell subset that possesses FoxP3 transcription factor expression, commonly referred to as the T-regulatory (Treg) cell. The Treg is the main immunosuppressive T cell subset retained in the peripheral immune response and is responsible for suppressing other CD4+ T cell responses mounted against tissue damage or infection.[50,51] Recent reports have identified that Tregs can also possess extra-immunological processes by maintaining the homeostasis of the tissues they populate.[52] The idea that Tregs can mediate tissue homeostasis outside of immune regulation has resulted in the classification of new Treg subsets collectively referred to as tissue-specific Tregs or tissue Tregs (tsTregs) for short.[52]

The exact role that tsTregs serve in mediating tissue homeostasis is stringent on the tissue that the specific T-regulatory cell populates.[52] Each tsTreg population is functionally and phenotypically distinct from other tsTregs, as well as Treg counterparts that occupy traditional lymphoid stores. Tissue-specific Tregs have been identified in the visceral adipose tissue,[53,54] intestine,[55–59] skin,[60,61] skeletal muscle,[62,63] and most recently the heart (Figure 6.5).[64]

Heart-specific Tregs influx into the myocardium following ischemic injury and mirror the IL-33/ST2-dependent signaling axis of the skeletal muscle Treg.

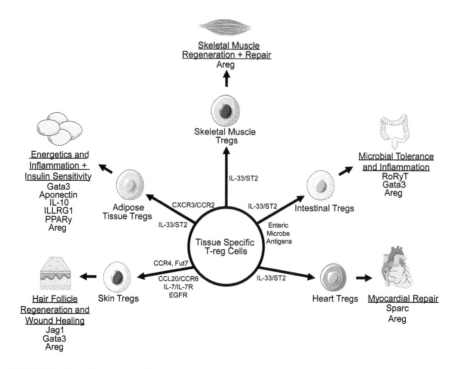

FIGURE 6.5 Tissue-specific Tregs are essential in mediating organ homeostasis. Each tsTreg is phenotypically and functionally distinct from other tsTregs as well as systemic Treg counterparts that occupy traditional lymphoid stores. TsTregs have been identified in the skeletal muscle, skin, adipose tissue, lamina propria, and heart. These populations are essential in mediating organ homeostasis during times of challenge or injury.

Additionally, heart-specific Tregs possess increased expression of secreted acidic cysteine-rich glycoprotein (SPARC), which is further identified as a critical element in mediating collagen deposition and infarct maturation.[64] Previous studies have identified that heart Tregs can diverge into a pathogenic, malfunctional phenotype that perpetuates adverse cardiac remodeling and compromised heart function when exposed to chronic ischemic injury.[65] Whether stem cell therapy administration can manage the inflammatory response mounted against chronic ischemia to preserve pro-reparative tsTreg phenotype and function has not yet been reported, but does provide a unique opportunity to corroborate studies that combine stem cell biology, tsTreg population dynamics, and cardiac wound-healing. However, for the rest of this section, we will focus our attention on the direct interactions that stem cell therapy has in modulating broad T cell and Treg dynamics in the MI heart.

MSCs possess co-inhibitory signaling molecules, FasL and TRAIL, on their cell surface. The binding of FasL and TRAIL to complementary receptors on neighboring T cell populations results in suppressed T cell activation and proliferation.[66,67] The MSC secretome is enriched in iNOS, IDO, TGFβ, and PGE-2, all of which have been shown to directly blunt T cell activation and proliferation in MSC, T cell co-cultured systems without requiring a physical interaction between the T cells and MSCs.[68,69] Additionally, MSC-produced TGFβ and PGE-2 can drive FoxP3+ Treg induction from pan, non-FoxP3+ T cells.[70] T-regulatory cells exposed to MSC secretome exhibit heightened immunosuppressive capacities as marked by increases in PD-1 receptor expression and IL-10 production.[71] Increased PD-1 receptor expression is also observed in Treg populations exposed to CDC-derived secretomes.[72] Additionally, ESCs have been shown to expand Treg compartments residing in the ischemic myocardium.[73,74] CBSC cell therapy can also expand CD4+ T cell content resident in the post-IR heart 7 days following injury onset, but whether CBSCs can directly facilitate Treg expansion has not been reported.[42] Further investigation into how stem cell therapy can modulate the plasticity and establishment of pro-reparative Treg cell types during cardiac wound healing or chronic injury exposure could unlock a strong therapeutic target, as more studies emphasize the importance of T cell population dynamics, phenotype plasticity, and function in the orchestration of myocardial wound healing and tissue homeostasis.

STEM CELLS AND B CELLS: THE ADAPTIVE IMMUNE RESPONSE

B-lymphocytes are also retained in the adaptive immune response; however, the exact temporal influx and role B cell populations have in response to cardiac ischemic injury are poorly understood.[75,76] Preliminary studies suggest that B cells serve a pathogenic role in the context of cardiac repair via their production of autoantibodies that target cardiac antigens released from or expressed by ischemic myocardium.[77,78] Autoantibody production against myocardial injury has been reported in several cardiac disease models, specifically: ischemic injury during IR/MI,[79,80] chronic heart failure,[81] Chagas disease,[82] and autoimmune myocarditis.[83] The exact role stem cell therapy plays in mediating B-lymphocyte phenotype and function in response to cardiac injury is a major gap in the field of cardiac immunology.

The MSC secretome can mediate B cell proliferation by causing G0/G1 cell cycle arrest and decreased expression in CD138, IgG, IgA, and IgM B cell maturation markers.[84,85] Additionally, as previously reviewed, stem cell therapies are influential in mediating MΦ recruitment, function, and phenotype. An essential role of MΦ populations is to serve as professional antigen-presenting cells, which in turn orchestrate B cell lineage commitment and function. Whether stem cell therapies can indirectly modulate B cell lineage commitment and function by regulating MΦ antigen presentation to B cells has not been assessed, but could provide unique regulatory insights into how B cell response following MI can be regulated.

STEM CELL IMMUNE MODULATION: A POSITIVE
FEEDBACK LOOP FOR STEM CELL EFFICACY

A large emphasis has been placed on the immunomodulatory capacities that stem cell therapy has on the remediation of inflammatory cell subsets in the MI heart in the context of cardiac repair rather than the immunomodulatory effects that stem cell therapy has on their own engraftment and functional capacity in the ischemic heart. Stem cell engraftment in the MI heart is a major challenge and the harsh, pro-inflammatory response mounted post-MI likely contributes to poor stem cell engraftment. Ideally, the early recruitment and expansion of anti-inflammatory, pro-reparative immune cells to repress degradative pro-inflammatory cell types would improve stem cell engraftment. Here, we briefly highlight how stem cells modulate the innate and adaptive immune response to support their engraftment and efficacy in the ischemic heart.

Neutrophils possess a pro-inflammatory signature that solicits the degradation and phagocytosis of necrotic myocardium. Consequently, neutrophil produced TNFα and IL-1β limit stem cell engraftment by causing TNFα- and IL-1β-mediated apoptosis of the adoptively transferred progenitors.[86] Studies that implemented the use of glucocorticoids prior to stem cell treatment identified enhanced stem cell engraftment, suggesting that the suppression of innate, pro-inflammatory cell types, like neutrophils, improve stem cell retention in the post-MI heart.[87] Macrophages have also been shown to modulate stem cell engraftment via the preservation of hemopoietic stem cell (HSC) transfers. The depletion of CD169+ MΦs compromises the long-term retention of HSC transfers, suggesting that CD169+ MΦs are essential for the maintenance of HSC engraftment.[88]

Studies that investigated the effects T cell populations have on neuronal stem cell function identified that that T cells secrete INFγ to inhibit neuronal stem cell proliferation.[89] During initial ischemic injury, pathogenic T cell types that express IFNγ have also been shown to influx into the myocardium and, in theory, could compromise the functional capacity of the adoptively transferred stem cells.[90] However, Treg produced adenosine has been shown to support HSC engraftment, suggesting Tregs are influential in promoting stem cell engraftment.[91] Literature surrounding the direct effects that B cells have in mediating stem cell engraftment is minimal. One study identified that B cell function is dependent on HSC transfer via IL-21-mediated signaling, but whether this affects HSC engraftment or efficacy is not clearly defined.[92]

Overall, the suppression of the inflammatory response during MI supports stem cell engraftment; however, numerous reports have highlighted that the broad immune suppression of the inflammatory response mounted following MI does not support cardiac wound healing. To date, how stem cells modulate inflammatory cell subsets to support myocardial wound healing is more developed, but how stem cells specifically alter immune cell responses to improve their function and engraftment post-MI is largely understudied. An increased emphasis is placed on how specific alterations in immune cell population dynamics can influence stem cell engraftment and efficacy in the ischemic heart.

FUTURE DIRECTIONS FOR STEM CELL THERAPY, IMMUNE MODULATION, AND CARDIAC REPAIR

Several immunomodulatory agents have been employed to modulate the post-MI inflammatory response with the hope that immune suppression would enhance myocardial repair.[19] Unfortunately, the use of pan-immunosuppressants did not improve myocardial wound healing and the development of therapeutics that can suppress pro-inflammatory cell types while sustaining pro-reparative immune cell types in the infarcted myocardium has yet to be identified. Stem cell therapies were originally designed with the intent that the adoptively transferred stem cell populations would differentiate into *de novo*, functional myocardium in the ischemic heart.[2,14] Unfortunately, the efficacy of this approach was low, but did identify that paracrine signaling factors produced by the adoptively transferred populations can enhance myocardial wound healing processes and improve cardiac function following MI.[16] Given the close proximity of transferred stem cell populations in the infarcted myocardium to the inflammatory cell infiltrate residing in the MI heart, it is reasonable to suggest that stem cell mediated paracrine signaling can directly modulate immune cell recruitment and function. Seminal studies have identified that stem cells can regulate the phenotype and function of neutrophils, MΦs, T lymphocytes, and B lymphocytes post-MI.[21–24,93] These effects can have a lasting impact on shaping the inflammatory microenvironment of the infarcted heart to better orchestrate myocardial repair. The identification of an ideal stem cell type and the direct effects this cell type has on immune cells following MI will have an immense impact on cardiac immune mediated myocardial repair.

ABBREVIATIONS

CVD, cardiovascular disease; CHD, coronary heart disease; MI, myocardial infarction; IR, ischemia reperfusion; CABG, coronary artery bypass graft surgery; MSCs, mesenchymal stem cells; HF, heart failure; iPSCs, inducible pluripotent stem cells; MΦ, macrophage; CDCs, cardiovascular-derived stem cells; CBSCs, cortical bone-derived stem cells; ESCs, embryonic stem cells; Treg, T-regulatory; tsTreg, tissue-specific Treg; Areg, amphiregulin; SPARC, secreted acidic cysteine-rich glycoprotein; HSC, hemopoietic stem cell.

BIBLIOGRAPHY

1. Virani SS, Alonso A, Aparicio HJ, Benjamin EJ, Bittencourt MS, Callaway CW, Carson AP, Chamberlain AM, Cheng S, Delling FN, Elkind MSV, Evenson KR, Ferguson JF, Gupta DK, Khan SS, Kissela BM, Knutson KL, Lee CD, Lewis TT, Liu J, Loop MS, Lutsey PL, Ma J, Mackey J, Martin SS, Matchar DB, Mussolino ME, Navaneethan SD, Perak AM, Roth GA, Samad Z, Satou GM, Schroeder EB, Shah SH, Shay CM, Stokes A, VanWagner LB, Wang N-Y, Tsao CW, null null. Heart disease and stroke statistics—2021 update. *Circulation*. 2021;143:e254–e743.
2. Mohsin S, Houser SR. Cortical bone derived stem cells for cardiac wound healing. *Korean Circulation J*. 2019;49:314–325.
3. Kraus L, Ma L, Yang Y, Nguyen F, Hoy RC, Okuno T, Khan M, Mohsin S. Cortical bone derived stem cells modulate cardiac fibroblast response via miR-18a in the heart after injury. *Front Cell Dev Biol*. 2020;8:494.
4. Menasché P, Hagège AA, Scorsin M, Pouzet B, Desnos M, Duboc D, Schwartz K, Vilquin J-T, Marolleau J-P. Myoblast transplantation for heart failure. *The Lancet*. 2001;357:279–280.
5. Menasché P, Alfieri O, Janssens S, McKenna W, Reichenspurner H, Trinquart L, Vilquin J-T, Marolleau J-P, Seymour B, Larghero J, Lake S, Chatellier G, Solomon S, Desnos M, Hagège AA. The myoblast autologous grafting in ischemic cardiomyopathy (MAGIC) trial: first randomized placebo-controlled study of myoblast transplantation. *Circulation*. 2008;117:1189–1200.

6. Perin EC, Dohmann HFR, Radovan B, Suzana AS, Sousa ALS, Mesquita CT, Rossi MID, Carvalho AC, Dutra HS, Dohmann HJF, Silva GV, Belém L, Vivacqua R, Rangel FOD, Esporcatte R, Geng YJ, Vaughn WK, Assad JAR, Mesquita ET, Willerson JT. Transendocardial, autologous bone marrow cell transplantation for severe, chronic ischemic heart failure. *Circulation*. 2003;107:2294–2302.

7. Quyyumi AA, Vasquez A, Kereiakes DJ, Klapholz M, Schaer GL, Abdel-Latif A, Frohwein S, Henry TD, Schatz RA, Dib N, Toma C, Davidson CJ, Barsness GW, Shavelle DM, Cohen M, Poole J, Moss T, Hyde P, Kanakaraj AM, Druker V, Chung A, Junge C, Preti RA, Smith RL, Mazzo DJ, Pecora A, Losordo DW. PreSERVE-AMI. *Circ Res*. 2017;120:324–331.

8. Mathiasen AB, Qayyum AA, Jørgensen E, Helqvist S, Fischer-Nielsen A, Kofoed KF, Haack-Sørensen M, Ekblond A, Kastrup J. Bone marrow-derived mesenchymal stromal cell treatment in patients with severe ischaemic heart failure: a randomized placebo-controlled trial (MSC-HF trial). *Eur Heart J*. 2015;36:1744–1753.

9. Segers VFM, Lee RT. Stem-cell therapy for cardiac disease. *Nature*. 2008;451:937–942.

10. Duran JM, Makarewich CA, Sharp TE, Starosta T, Zhu F, Hoffman NE, Chiba Y, Madesh M, Berretta RM, Kubo H, Houser SR. Bone-derived stem cells repair the heart after myocardial infarction through transdifferentiation and paracrine signaling mechanisms. *Circ Res*. 2013;113:539–552.

11. Sharp TE, Schena GJ, Hobby AR, Starosta T, Berretta RM, Wallner M, Borghetti G, Gross P, Yu D, Johnson J, Feldsott E, Trappanese DM, Toib A, Rabinowitz JE, George JC, Kubo H, Mohsin S, Houser SR. Cortical bone stem cell therapy preserves cardiac structure and function after myocardial infarction. *Circ Res*. 2017;121:1263–1278.

12. Zwi-Dantsis L, Gepstein L. Induced pluripotent stem cells for cardiac repair. *Cell Mol Life Sci*. 2012;69:3285–3299.

13. Tehzeeb J, Manzoor A, Ahmed MM. Is stem cell therapy an answer to heart failure: a literature search. *Cureus* [Internet]. [cited 2021 Mar 29];11. Available from: www.ncbi.nlm.nih.gov/pmc/articles/PMC6874291/

14. Wagner MJ, Khan M, Mohsin S. Healing the broken heart; the immunomodulatory effects of stem cell therapy. *Front Immunol* [Internet]. 2020 [cited 2020 Oct 23];11. Available from: www.frontiersin.org/articles/10.3389/fimmu.2020.00639/full

15. Kraus L, Mohsin S. Role of stem cell-derived microvesicles in cardiovascular disease. *J Cardiovasc Pharmacol*. 2020;76:650–657.

16. Sanganalmath SK, Bolli R. Cell therapy for heart failure: a comprehensive overview of experimental and clinical studies, current challenges, and future directions. *Circ Res*. 2013;113:810–834.

17. Prabhu Sumanth D, Frangogiannis Nikolaos G. The biological basis for cardiac repair after myocardial infarction. *Circ Res*. 2016;119:91–112.

18. Huang S, Frangogiannis NG. Anti-inflammatory therapies in myocardial infarction: failures, hopes and challenges. *Br J Pharmacol*. 2018;175:1377–1400.

19. Saxena A, Dobaczewski M, Rai V, Haque Z, Chen W, Li N, Frangogiannis NG. Regulatory T cells are recruited in the infarcted mouse myocardium and may modulate fibroblast phenotype and function. *Am J Physiol Heart Circ*. 2014;307:H1233–H1242.

20. Aurora AB, Olson EN. Immune modulation of stem cells and regeneration. *Cell Stem Cell*. 2014;15:14–25.

21. Blanc KL, Mougiakakos D. Multipotent mesenchymal stromal cells and the innate immune system. *Nat Rev Immunol*. 2012;12:383–396.

22. Cao W, Cao K, Cao J, Wang Y, Shi Y. Mesenchymal stem cells and adaptive immune responses. *Immunol Lett*. 2015;168:147–153.

23. Lin L, Du L. The role of secreted factors in stem cells-mediated immune regulation. *Cell Immunol*. 2018;326:24–32.

24. Volpe G, Bernstock JD, Peruzzotti-Jametti L, Pluchino S. Modulation of host immune responses following non-hematopoietic stem cell transplantation: translational implications in progressive multiple sclerosis. *J Neuroimmunol.* 2019;331:11–27.

25. Nikolaos GF, Anthony R. Regulation of the inflammatory response in cardiac repair. *Circ Res.* 2012;110:159–173.

26. Sattler S, Kennedy-Lydon T, editors. *The immunology of cardiovascular homeostasis and pathology* [Internet]. Springer International Publishing; 2017 [cited 2019 Dec 4]. Available from: www.springer.com/gp/book/9783319576114

27. Yu PF, Huang Y, Han YY, Lin LY, Sun WH, Rabson AB, Wang Y, Shi YF. TNFα-activated mesenchymal stromal cells promote breast cancer metastasis by recruiting CXCR2 + neutrophils. *Oncogene.* 2017;36:482–490.

28. Park YS, Lim G-W, Cho K-A, Woo S-Y, Shin M, Yoo E-S, Chan Ra J, Ryu K-H. Improved viability and activity of neutrophils differentiated from HL-60 cells by co-culture with adipose tissue-derived mesenchymal stem cells. *Biochem Biophys Res Commun.* 2012;423:19–25.

29. Raffaghello L, Bianchi G, Bertolotto M, Montecucco F, Busca A, Dallegri F, Ottonello L, Pistoia V. Human mesenchymal stem cells inhibit neutrophil apoptosis: a model for neutrophil preservation in the bone marrow niche. *STEM CELLS.* 2008;26:151–162.

30. Epelman S, Lavine KJ, Beaudin AE, Sojka DK, Carrero JA, Calderon B, Brija T, Gautier EL, Ivanov S, Satpathy AT, Schilling JD, Schwendener R, Sergin I, Razani B, Forsberg EC, Yokoyama WM, Unanue ER, Colonna M, Randolph GJ, Mann DL. Embryonic and adult-derived resident cardiac macrophages are maintained through distinct mechanisms at steady state and during inflammation. *Immunity.* 2014;40:91–104.

31. Mouton AJ, DeLeon-Pennell KY, Rivera Gonzalez OJ, Flynn ER, Freeman TC, Saucerman JJ, Garrett MR, Ma Y, Harmancey R, Lindsey ML. Mapping macrophage polarization over the myocardial infarction time continuum. *Basic Res Cardiol.* 2018;113:26.

32. Nahrendorf M, Pittet MJ, Swirski FK. Monocytes: protagonists of infarct inflammation and repair after myocardial infarction. *Circulation.* 2010;121:2437–2445.

33. Lavine KJ, Epelman S, Uchida K, Weber KJ, Nichols CG, Schilling JD, Ornitz DM, Randolph GJ, Mann DL. Distinct macrophage lineages contribute to disparate patterns of cardiac recovery and remodeling in the neonatal and adult heart. *PNAS USA.* 2014;111:16029–16034.

34. Shiraishi M, Shintani Y, Shintani Y, Ishida H, Saba R, Yamaguchi A, Adachi H, Yashiro K, Suzuki K. Alternatively activated macrophages determine repair of the infarcted adult murine heart. *J Clin Invest.* 2016;126:2151–2166.

35. Leblond A-L, Klinkert K, Martin K, Turner EC, Kumar AH, Browne T, Caplice NM. Systemic and cardiac depletion of m2 macrophage through CSF-1R signaling inhibition alters cardiac function post myocardial infarction. *PLoS ONE.* 2015;10:e0137515.

36. Vasandan AB, Jahnavi S, Shashank C, Prasad P, Kumar A, Prasanna SJ. Human mesenchymal stem cells program macrophage plasticity by altering their metabolic status via a PGE 2-dependent mechanism. *Sci Rep.* 2016;6:1–17.

37. Dayan V, Yannarelli G, Billia F, Filomeno P, Wang X-H, Davies JE, Keating A. Mesenchymal stromal cells mediate a switch to alternatively activated monocytes/macrophages after acute myocardial infarction. *Basic Res Cardiol.* 2011;106:1299–1310.

38. Maggini J, Mirkin G, Bognanni I, Holmberg J, Piazzón IM, Nepomnaschy I, Costa H, Cañones C, Raiden S, Vermeulen M, Geffner JR. Mouse bone marrow-derived mesenchymal stromal cells turn activated macrophages into a regulatory-like profile. *PLOS ONE.* 2010;5:e9252.

39. Luz-Crawford P, Djouad F, Toupet K, Bony C, Franquesa M, Hoogduijn MJ, Jorgensen C, Noël D. Mesenchymal stem cell-derived interleukin 1 receptor antagonist promotes macrophage polarization and inhibits b cell differentiation. *STEM CELLS.* 2016;34:483–492.

40. Barile L, Milano G, Vassalli G. Beneficial effects of exosomes secreted by cardiac-derived progenitor cells and other cell types in myocardial ischemia. *Stem Cell Investig* [Internet]. 2017 [cited 2019 Dec 4];4. Available from: http://sci.amegroups.com/article/view/17381

41. Ben-Mordechai T, Palevski D, Glucksam-Galnoy Y, Elron-Gross I, Margalit R, Leor J. Targeting macrophage subsets for infarct repair. *J Cardiovasc Pharmacol Ther.* 2015;20:36–51.

42. Hobby ARH, Sharp TE, Berretta RM, Borghetti G, Feldsott E, Mohsin S, Houser SR. Cortical bone-derived stem cell therapy reduces apoptosis after myocardial infarction. *Am J Physiol Heart Circ Physiol.* 2019;317:H820–H829.

43. Mosser DM, Edwards JP. Exploring the full spectrum of macrophage activation. *Nat Rev Immunol.* 2008;8:958–969.

44. Kudo H, Wada H, Sasaki H, Tsuji H, Otsuka R, Baghdadi M, Kojo S, Chikaraishi T, Seino K. Induction of macrophage-like immunosuppressive cells from mouse ES cells that contribute to prolong allogeneic graft survival. *PLoS ONE.* 2014;9:e111826.

45. Weirather J, Hofmann UDW, Beyersdorf N, Ramos GC, Vogel B, Frey A, Ertl G, Kerkau T, Frantz S. Foxp3+ CD4+ T cells improve healing after myocardial infarction by modulating monocyte/macrophage differentiation. *Circ Res.* 2014;115:55–67.

46. Seropian IM, Cerliani JP, Toldo S, Van Tassell BW, Ilarregui JM, González GE, Matoso M, Salloum FN, Melchior R, Gelpi RJ, Stupirski JC, Benatar A, Gómez KA, Morales C, Abbate A, Rabinovich GA. Galectin-1 controls cardiac inflammation and ventricular remodeling during acute myocardial infarction. *Am J Pathol.* 2013;182:29–40.

47. Homma T, Kinugawa S, Takahashi M, Sobirin MA, Saito A, Fukushima A, Suga T, Takada S, Kadoguchi T, Masaki Y, Furihata T, Taniguchi M, Nakayama T, Ishimori N, Iwabuchi K, Tsutsui H. Activation of invariant natural killer T cells by α-galactosylceramide ameliorates myocardial ischemia/reperfusion injury in mice. *J Mol Cell Cardiol.* 2013;62:179–188.

48. Yang Z, Day Y-J, Toufektsian M-C, Xu Y, Ramos SI, Marshall MA, French BA, Linden J. Myocardial infarct-sparing effect of adenosine A2A receptor activation is due to its action on CD4+ T lymphocytes. *Circulation.* 2006;114:2056–2064.

49. Lu L, Li G, Rao J, Pu L, Yu Y, Wang X, Zhang F. In vitro induced CD4+CD25+Foxp3+ Tregs attenuate hepatic ischemia—reperfusion injury. *Int Immunopharmacol.* 2009;9:549–552.

50. Bennett CL, Christie J, Ramsdell F, Brunkow ME, Ferguson PJ, Whitesell L, Kelly TE, Saulsbury FT, Chance PF, Ochs HD. The immune dysregulation, polyendocrinopathy, enteropathy, X-linked syndrome (IPEX) is caused by mutations of FOXP3. *Nat Genet.* 2001;27:20–21.

51. Liston A, Nutsch KM, Farr AG, Lund JM, Rasmussen JP, Koni PA, Rudensky AY. Differentiation of regulatory Foxp3+ T cells in the thymic cortex. *PNAS.* 2008;105:11903–11908.

52. Panduro M, Benoist C, Mathis D. Tissue tregs. *Annu Rev Immunol.* 2016;34:609–633.

53. Feuerer M, Herrero L, Cipolletta D, Naaz A, Wong J, Nayer A, Lee J, Goldfine A, Benoist C, Shoelson S, Mathis D. Fat Treg cells: a liaison between the immune and metabolic systems. *Nat Med.* 2009;15:930–939.

54. Cipolletta D, Cohen P, Spiegelman BM, Benoist C, Mathis D. Appearance and disappearance of the mRNA signature characteristic of Treg cells in visceral adipose tissue: age, diet, and PPARγ effects. *Proc Natl Acad Sci U S A.* 2015;112:482–487.

55. Geuking MB, Cahenzli J, Lawson MAE, Ng DCK, Slack E, Hapfelmeier S, McCoy KD, Macpherson AJ. Intestinal bacterial colonization induces mutualistic regulatory T cell responses. *Immunity.* 2011;34:794–806.

56. Atarashi K, Tanoue T, Shima T, Imaoka A, Kuwahara T, Momose Y, Cheng G, Yamasaki S, Saito T, Ohba Y, Taniguchi T, Takeda K, Hori S, Ivanov II, Umesaki Y, Itoh K, Honda K. Induction of colonic regulatory T cells by indigenous clostridium species. *Science*. 2011;331:337–341.

57. Sefik E, Geva-Zatorsky N, Oh S, Konnikova L, Zemmour D, McGuire AM, Burzyn D, Ortiz-Lopez A, Lobera M, Yang J, Ghosh S, Earl A, Snapper SB, Jupp R, Kasper D, Mathis D, Benoist C. MUCOSAL IMMUNOLOGY. Individual intestinal symbionts induce a distinct population of RORγ⁺ regulatory T cells. *Science*. 2015;349:993–997.

58. Lathrop SK, Bloom SM, Rao SM, Nutsch K, Lio C-W, Santacruz N, Peterson DA, Stappenbeck TS, Hsieh C-S. Peripheral education of the immune system by colonic commensal microbiota. *Nature*. 2011;478:250–254.

59. Cebula A, Seweryn M, Rempala GA, Pabla SS, McIndoe RA, Denning TL, Bry L, Kraj P, Kisielow P, Ignatowicz L. Thymus-derived regulatory T cells control tolerance to commensal microbiota. *Nature*. 2013;497:258–262.

60. Sather BD, Treuting P, Perdue N, Miazgowicz M, Fontenot JD, Rudensky AY, Campbell DJ. Altering the distribution of Foxp3(+) regulatory T cells results in tissue-specific inflammatory disease. *J Exp Med*. 2007;204:1335–1347.

61. Dudda JC, Perdue N, Bachtanian E, Campbell DJ. Foxp3+ regulatory T cells maintain immune homeostasis in the skin. *J Exp Med*. 2008;205:1559–1565.

62. Burzyn D, Kuswanto W, Kolodin D, Shadrach JL, Cerletti M, Jang Y, Sefik E, Tan TG, Wagers AJ, Benoist C, Mathis D. A special population of regulatory t cells potentiates muscle repair. *Cell*. 2013;155:1282–1295.

63. Kuswanto W, Burzyn D, Panduro M, Wang KK, Jang YC, Wagers AJ, Benoist C, Mathis D. Poor repair of skeletal muscle in aging mice reflects a defect in local, interleukin-33-dependent accumulation of regulatory T cells. *Immunity*. 2016;44:355–367.

64. Xia Ni, Lu Yuzhi, Gu Muyang, Li Nana, Liu Meilin, Jiao Jiao, Zhu Zhengfeng, Li Jingyong, Li Dan, Tang Tingting, Lv Bingjie, Nie Shaofang, Zhang Min, Liao Mengyang, Liao Yuhua, Yang Xiangping, Cheng Xiang. A unique population of regulatory t cells in heart potentiates cardiac protection from myocardial infarction. *Circulation*. 2020;142:1956–1973.

65. Shyam SB, Ameen IM, Mehak G, Guihua Z, Gregg R, Tariq H, Sumanth DP. Dysfunctional and proinflammatory regulatory t-lymphocytes are essential for adverse cardiac remodeling in ischemic cardiomyopathy. *Circulation*. 2019;139:206–221.

66. Akiyama K, Chen C, Wang D, Xu X, Qu C, Yamaza T, Cai T, Chen W, Sun L, Shi S. Mesenchymal-stem-cell-induced immunoregulation involves FAS-ligand-/FAS-mediated T cell apoptosis. *Cell Stem Cell*. 2012;10:544–555.

67. Lee RH, Yoon N, Reneau JC, Prockop DJ. Preactivation of human MSCs with TNF-α enhances tumor-suppressive activity. *Cell Stem Cell*. 2012;11:825–835.

68. Ren G, Zhang L, Zhao X, Xu G, Zhang Y, Roberts AI, Zhao RC, Shi Y. Mesenchymal stem cell-mediated immunosuppression occurs via concerted action of chemokines and nitric oxide. *Cell Stem Cell*. 2008;2:141–150.

69. Xu G, Zhang Y, Zhang L, Ren G, Shi Y. Bone marrow stromal cells induce apoptosis of lymphoma cells in the presence of IFNγ and TNF by producing nitric oxide. *Biochem Biophys Res Commun*. 2008;375:666–670.

70. English K, Wood KJ. Mesenchymal stromal cells in transplantation rejection and tolerance. *Cold Spring Harb Perspect Med*. 2013;3:a015560.

71. Yan Z, Zhuansun Y, Chen R, Li J, Ran P. Immunomodulation of mesenchymal stromal cells on regulatory T cells and its possible mechanism. *Exp Cell Res*. 2014;324:65–74.

72. Lauden L, Boukouaci W, Borlado LR, López IP, Sepúlveda P, Tamouza R, Charron D, Al-Daccak R. Allogenicity of human cardiac stem/progenitor cells orchestrated by programmed death ligand 1novelty and significance. *Circ Res*. 2013;112:451–464.

73. Wada H, Kojo S, Kusama C, Okamoto N, Sato Y, Ishizuka B, Seino K. Successful differentiation to T cells, but unsuccessful B-cell generation, from B-cell-derived induced pluripotent stem cells. *Int Immunol.* 2011;23:65–74.

74. Kofidis T, deBruin JL, Tanaka M, Zwierzchoniewska M, Weissman I, Fedoseyeva E, Haverich A, Robbins RC. They are not stealthy in the heart: embryonic stem cells trigger cell infiltration, humoral and T-lymphocyte-based host immune response. *Eur J Cardiothorac Surg.* 2005;28:461–466.

75. Yan X, Anzai A, Katsumata Y, Matsuhashi T, Ito K, Endo J, Yamamoto T, Takeshima A, Shinmura K, Shen W, Fukuda K, Sano M. Temporal dynamics of cardiac immune cell accumulation following acute myocardial infarction. *J Mol Cell Cardiol.* 2013;62:24–35.

76. Lin L, Du L. The role of secreted factors in stem cells-mediated immune regulation. *Cell Immunol.* 2018;326:24–32.

77. De Scheerder I, Vandekerckhove J, Robbrecht J, Algoed L, De Buyzere M, De Langhe J, De Schrijver G, Clement D. Post-cardiac injury syndrome and an increased humoral immune response against the major contractile proteins (actin and myosin). *Am J Cardiol.* 1985;56:631–633.

78. O'Donohoe TJ, Schrale RG, Ketheesan N. The role of anti-myosin antibodies in perpetuating cardiac damage following myocardial infarction. *Int J Cardiol.* 2016;209:226–233.

79. Busche MN, Pavlov V, Takahashi K, Stahl GL. Myocardial ischemia and reperfusion injury is dependent on both IgM and mannose-binding lectin. *Am J Physiol Heart Circ Physiol.* 2009;297:H1853–H1859.

80. Haas MS, Alicot EM, Schuerpf F, Chiu I, Li J, Moore FD, Carroll MC. Blockade of self-reactive IgM significantly reduces injury in a murine model of acute myocardial infarction. *Cardiovasc Res.* 2010;87:618–627.

81. Ziya K, Christoph L, Hugo AK, Anthony R. Autoantibodies in heart failure and cardiac dysfunction. *Circ Res.* 2012;110:145–158.

82. Medei EH, Nascimento JHM, Pedrosa RC, de Carvalho ACC. Role of autoantibodies in the physiopathology of chagas' disease. *Arq Bras Cardiol.* 2008;91:257–286.

83. Rose NR. Myocarditis: infection versus autoimmunity. *J Clin Immunol.* 2009;29:730–737.

84. Che N, Li X, Zhou S, Liu R, Shi D, Lu L, Sun L. Umbilical cord mesenchymal stem cells suppress B-cell proliferation and differentiation. *Cell Immunol.* 2012;274:46–53.

85. Corcione A, Benvenuto F, Ferretti E, Giunti D, Cappiello V, Cazzanti F, Risso M, Gualandi F, Mancardi GL, Pistoia V, Uccelli A. Human mesenchymal stem cells modulate B-cell functions. *Blood.* 2006;107:367–372.

86. Li X, Tamama K, Xie X, Guan J. Improving cell engraftment in cardiac stem cell therapy. *Stem Cells Int.* 2015;2016:e7168797.

87. Guo B, Huang X, Broxmeyer HE. Enhancing human cord blood hematopoietic stem cell engraftment by targeting nuclear hormone receptors. *Curr Opin Hematol.* 2018;25:245–252.

88. Kaur S, Raggatt LJ, Millard SM, Wu AC, Batoon L, Jacobsen RN, Winkler IG, MacDonald KP, Perkins AC, Hume DA, Levesque J-P, Pettit AR. Self-repopulating recipient bone marrow resident macrophages promote long-term hematopoietic stem cell engraftment. *Blood.* 2018;132:735–749.

89. Dulken BW, Buckley MT, Navarro Negredo P, Saligrama N, Cayrol R, Leeman DS, George BM, Boutet SC, Hebestreit K, Pluvinage JV, Wyss-Coray T, Weissman IL, Vogel H, Davis MM, Brunet A. Single-cell analysis reveals T cell infiltration in old neurogenic niches. *Nature.* 2019;571:205–210.

90. Bansal SS, Ismahil MA, Goel M, Patel B, Hamid T, Rokosh G, Prabhu SD. Activated T lymphocytes are essential drivers of pathological remodeling in ischemic heart failure. *Circ Heart Fail.* 2017;10:e003688.

91. Hirata Y, Furuhashi K, Ishii H, Li HW, Pinho S, Ding L, Robson SC, Frenette PS, Fujisaki J. CD150high bone marrow tregs maintain hematopoietic stem cell quiescence and immune privilege via adenosine. *Cell Stem Cell*. 2018;22:445–453.e5.

92. Miggelbrink AM, Logan BR, Buckley RH, Parrott RE, Dvorak CC, Kapoor N, Abdel-Azim H, Prockop SE, Shyr D, Decaluwe H, Hanson IC, Gillio A, Dávila Saldaña BJ, Eibel H, Hopkins G, Walter JE, Whangbo JS, Kohn DB, Puck JM, Cowan MJ, Griffith LM, Haddad E, O'Reilly RJ, Notarangelo LD, Pai S-Y. B-cell differentiation and IL-21 response in IL2RG/JAK3 SCID patients after hematopoietic stem cell transplantation. *Blood*. 2018;131:2967–2977.

93. Drago D, Basso V, Gaude E, Volpe G, Peruzzotti-Jametti L, Bachi A, Musco G, Andolfo A, Frezza C, Mondino A, Pluchino S. Metabolic determinants of the immune modulatory function of neural stem cells. *J Neuroinflammation*. 2016;13:232.

7 Cardiovascular Complications of Immune Checkpoint Inhibitors

Sultan Tousif, Anand Prakash Singh,
Prachi Umbarkar, and Hind Lal

CONTENTS

INTRODUCTION

The immune system is the host defense machinery that fights against pathogens and keeps our body healthy. The immune system comprises a variety of cells categorized as innate and adaptive immune cells. Natural or nonspecific defense mechanisms facilitated with immune cells like monocytes, macrophages, dendritic cells (DCs), natural killer cells (NK), neutrophils, mast cells, and innate lymphoid cells (ILCs) fall under the innate immune system. Adaptive immunity develops throughout our life upon response to different pathogens or foreign substances and is primarily mediated via the B cells and T cells. Whereas T cells orchestrate the cell-mediated immune response, B cells are responsible for the humoral immune response. Adaptive immune responses are needed when innate immunity is not sufficient to

DOI: 10.1201/b22824-8

129

combat pathogens or foreign substances. Acquired immune cells can only mobilize when innate immune cells assist them. T cells (CD4 and CD8) become activated once antigen-presenting cells (e.g., DCs, macrophages, and B cells) present antigens to the T cell receptor (TCR). Antigen-presenting cells (APCs) must present antigens to TCR through major histocompatibility complexes I and II (MHC-I and MHC-II), and they also require co-stimulatory signals to support them.

The co-stimulatory signal, which regulates the recognition of antigens by the TCR, can also be termed as an immune checkpoint. Immune checkpoints can be either co-stimulatory or co-inhibitory. CD27, CD37, CD40, GITR (CD278), and OX40 (CD134) are co-stimulatory immune checkpoints that fall under the tumor necrosis factor (TNF) superfamily, whereas CD28 and ICOS stimulatory signals belong to the B7-CD28 superfamily. Programmed death-1 (PD-1), cytotoxic T-lymphocyte-associated protein-4 (CTLA-4), lymphocyte activation gene-3 (LAG-3), adenosine A2A receptor (A2AR), indoleamine 2,3-dioxygenase (IDO), nicotinamide adenine dinucleotide phosphate (NADPH) oxidase isoform 2 (NOX-2), and V-domain Ig suppressor of T cell activation (VISTA) are considered as co-inhibitory immune checkpoints. On exposure to pathogens, adaptive immune cells are activated by antigen presentation and the signals induced by co-stimulatory immune checkpoints to protect the healthy tissues from damage [1]. The inhibitory immune checkpoint competes with the co-stimulatory molecule to diminish host immunity during pathogenic attacks, cancer, or other deadly diseases that hijack the host immune system [2]. This concerted action of co-stimulatory and inhibitory signals ensures that the immune system does not keep firing once the offending pathogen or disease stimulus has been neutralized. Pathogens and cancer cells have devised smart ways to exploit such inhibitory immune checkpoints to evade host immune response [3, 4]. Therefore, immune checkpoint therapy relies on reactivation of immune function by using either an agonist of the co-stimulatory signal or an antagonist of inhibitory immune checkpoint molecules [5].

The last decade has seen a resurgence in novel immunotherapies against cancer and other deadly diseases [6, 7]. Among the new immunotherapies, PD-1 (CD279) and CTLA-4 (CD152) are the two immune checkpoint molecules that are studied most actively. Their corresponding antibodies inhibit the activities of these receptors to boost anticancer immunity [6, 7]. Several additional immune checkpoint inhibitors (ICI) that show promising results for anticancer therapy are under active development and on the way to the market [5]. However, enhanced activities of T cells with the use of ICIs can promote systemic autoimmune complications [8–10]. The autoimmune adverse effects of PD-1 and CTLA-4 inhibition are well documented; these include ocular inflammation, pneumonitis, hyperthyroidism, vitiligo, hepatitis, etc. [8–10]. In this regard, adverse effects related to cardiac events and fatal myocarditis have received only limited recognition. Emerging evidence has shown that ICI-mediated myocarditis occurs with an expansion of a specific clone of T (antigen-specific T cells) cells within the myocardium [11–13]. Interestingly, the antigen-specific T cells are identical in the tumor and the skeletal muscle of ICI-treated patients, strongly suggesting that these T cells are targeted by the antigens common to the tumor, skeletal muscle, and cardiac tissues [12]. Recent data from clinical studies have established that patients treated with ICIs have elevated levels of cardiac troponin, a well-established marker of cardiotoxicity [14]. The clinical strategies to manage

ICI-induced myocarditis include a high dose of steroids or other immunosuppressive agents and plasmapheresis. These strategies have been employed only in limited cases. Having said that, intense research is ongoing worldwide to further validate the comparative outcome of these agents. Importantly, the underlying mechanism behind ICI-associated cardiotoxicity is not well defined and, therefore, warrants further investigation. An improved understanding of the fundamental mechanism of ICI-induced myocarditis will be critical to develop innovative tools for their clinical management for favorable outcomes.

BASIC PRINCIPLES OF IMMUNE CHECKPOINT BLOCKADE IN CANCER: THE CONCEPT OF IMMUNE SURVEILLANCE

Cancer is currently one of the deadliest diseases in the world. The tumor microenvironment (TME) (represented by tumor cells, infiltrating innate and adaptive immune cells, fibroblasts, signaling molecules, and the extracellular matrix) plays a dynamic role in regulating immune responses during cancer progression [15, 16]. Tumor-infiltrating immune cells are known to both inhibit and promote tumor growth [15, 16]. A wide range of immunosuppressive cells can populate TME. Examples of immunosuppressive cells in TME include tumor-associated macrophages (TAM) or M2, myeloid-derived suppressor cells (MDSCs), regulatory T cells (Tregs), and regulatory B cells (Bregs). Infiltrating effector T cells (cytotoxic CD8 and helper CD4) in TME respond to tumor antigens presented by MHC (MHC-I and MHC-II) on the surface of diseased cells in the presence of immune checkpoints (co-stimulatory and co-inhibitory). Helper CD4 T cells assist cytotoxic CD8 T cells by the production of IL-2, IL-12, and interferon-gamma (IFN-γ). These activities promote the effector function of CD8 T cells through the production of TNF-mediated apoptosis-inducing ligands (TRAILs), reactive oxygen species (ROS), and perforin [17]. Tumor cells express co-inhibitory immune checkpoint ligands such as the programmed death-ligand 1 (PD-L1) and CD80 on their surface. These ligands, in turn, can bind with co-inhibitory immune checkpoint receptors PD-1 and CTLA-4 expressed on CD8 T cells [18]. The interactions between co-inhibitory ligands and receptors inhibit the function of effector CD8+ T cells and, thereby, allow tumor cells to evade immune surveillance [19, 20].

Here, we discuss the current state of knowledge on regulatory mechanisms governing the co-inhibitory immune checkpoints CTLA-4 and PD-1 (Figures 7.1 and 7.2). As discussed previously, CTLA-4 is a co-inhibitory immune checkpoint receptor expressed over T cells, which is upregulated with the induction of signal 1 (antigen presentation or antigen-MHC engagement with TCR) [21–24]. T cells are activated and become effector T cells once they achieve signal 2 [i.e., the interaction of co-stimulatory immune checkpoint molecule CD28 with ligands CD80 (B7-1) and CD86 (B7-2) of superfamily B7] (Figure 7.1) [21–25]. CTLA-4 has a higher affinity and avidity (200 times more than CD28) for B7 superfamily ligands and, therefore, inhibits TCR signaling by competing with the co-stimulatory molecule (Figure 7.1) [21–25]. The difference in binding strength between CTLA-4 and CD28 allows CTLA-4 to limit downstream signaling of CD28 (PI3K and AKT pathways) by attenuating the interaction of CD28 and B7 ligands (Figure 7.1) [22, 26]. This cell-intrinsic function through CTLA-4 results in the impairment of TCR signaling

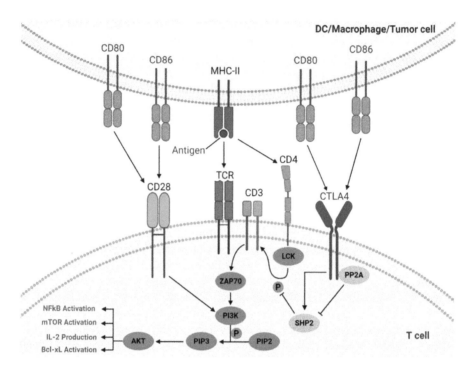

FIGURE 7.1   Known molecular mechanism of the CD28/CTLA-4 pathway showing activation/attenuation of T cells induced by downstream signaling upon antigen recognition and interaction of CD28/CTLA-4 and their ligands. Ligand CD80 (B7-1) or CD86 (B7-2) expressed over professional APCs or tumor cells interacts with CTLA-4 and recruits SHP2 and PP2A in the cytoplasm of T cells. Recruitment of SHP2 navigates attenuation of TCR signaling by dephosphorylation of the CD3ζ chain. PP2A recruitment results inhibit T cell activation through the dephosphorylation of AKT. Abbreviations: LCK, lymphocyte-specific protein tyrosine kinase; SHP2, Src homology region 2 domain-containing phosphatase-2; PI3K, phosphoinositide 3-kinase; PIP3 phosphatidylinositol (3,4,5)-trisphosphate; ZAP70, zeta-chain-associated protein kinase 70; AKT, protein kinase B; Bcl-xl, B cell lymphoma xl.

amplitude and, thus, inhibits T cell activity [22, 26]. Several reports have indicated that CTLA-4 can also modulate T cell activity through other cell-extrinsic regulatory mechanisms. A majority of cell-extrinsic suppressive functions of CTLA-4 are mediated by Treg [22, 27]. Recent evidence has shown that specific inhibition of CTLA-4 on Tregs promotes T cell activity and results in autoimmunity [28]. On the other hand, Treg expansion also inhibits autoimmunity, suggesting that Treg-CTLA-4 maintains T cell–mediated tolerance [29, 30]. CTLA-4 on Tregs inhibits effector T cell activation through a cell-extrinsic manner by limiting the availability of CD80 and CD86 ligands for CD28-mediated co-stimulation [31, 32]. However, in reference to cancer immunity, the contribution of cell-extrinsic properties of CTLA-4 to T cell tolerance remains to be explored entirely.

Programmed cell death protein 1 (PD-1, CD279) is a negative regulator of the CD28 immune checkpoint receptor superfamily. It is predominantly expressed by exhausted

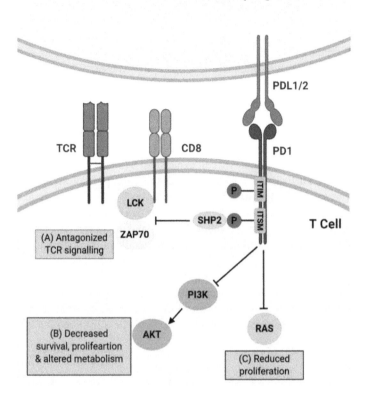

FIGURE 7.2 Known molecular mechanism of the PD-1 signaling pathway. PD-1 ligands PD-L1 or PD-L2 expressed over professional APCs or tumor cells interact with PD-1 of T cells and recruit SHP2 to ITSM domain, resulting in the attenuation of TCR signaling by dephosphorylation of LCK and ZAP70. PD-1 and its ligand interaction also causes inhibition of PI3K/AKT and the RAS/MAPK/Erk pathway, leading to impaired metabolism in T cells. Abbreviations: LCK, lymphocyte-specific protein tyrosine kinase; SHP2, Src homology region 2 domain-containing phosphatase-2; PI3K, phosphoinositide 3-kinase; ZAP70, zeta-chain-associated protein kinase 70; AKT, protein kinase B; ITIM, immunoreceptor tyrosine-based inhibition motif; ITSM, immunoreceptor tyrosine-based switch motif; MAPK, mitogen-activated protein kinases; Erk, extracellular signal–regulated kinase.

or activated T cells, B cells, macrophages, and mesenchymal stem cells (MSCs). PD-1 interacts with its ligands, programmed death-ligands 1 and 2 (PD-L1 and PD-L2), expressed on APCs and nonlymphoid tissues (tumor cells, cardiomyocytes, fibroblasts, and other cells) [33–36]. During tumor progression and various infections, PD-1 interaction with its ligand PD-L1 inhibits T cell activation and leads to their exhaustion [36–38]. Pro-inflammatory cytokine IFN-γ is known to induce PD-L1 and, to a lesser degree, PD-L2 expression [19, 37]. PD-L1 expressed on tumor cells engages with PD-1 of T cells in TME and inhibits apoptosis of cancer cells and effector T cell activation, allowing cancer cells to escape from the immune response [39, 40]. PD-1 interaction with PD-L1 and PD-L2 triggers a negative co-stimulatory signal, which results in the recruitment of tyrosine phosphatase SHP2 and subsequent inactivation of T cells. This event occurs via attenuation of TCR signaling through dephosphorylation of proximal signaling elements (Figure 7.2) [41]. This molecular mechanism highlights a fundamental difference in the PD-1 and CTLA-4 regulatory mechanisms. PD-1 directly regulates TCR signaling to attenuate T cell activity, whereas CTLA-4 inhibits T cell activity by attenuating CD28 downstream signaling. Furthermore, PD-1 also targets CD28 to inhibit T cell activity [42]. PD-1 primarily targets CD28 dephosphorylation via SHP2 rather than affecting TCR signaling (Figure 7.2) [43]. Thus, PD-1 operates with molecular mechanisms similar to those of CTLA-4, at least in part, for attenuating signal 2 (CD28-mediated co-stimulation). PD-1 signaling is also critical to metabolomics. Specifically, PD-1 promotes T cell exhaustion by inducing metabolic restrictions (Figure 7.2) [44]. Furthermore, PD-1 signaling can impair glycolysis and induce other modes of energy derivation, such as fatty acid oxidation (FAO) and lipid catabolism [45]. PD-L1 on macrophages engages with PD-1 to evict T cells from TME, suggesting that PD-1 signaling can regulate T cell trafficking and migration [46]. However, future studies are required to determine other intricate details of non-classical mechanisms that contribute to the efficacy of T cell–mediated immunotherapies.

Cancer treatment via immunotherapy is one of the most promising strategies to achieve prolonged-to-lasting disease remission. Currently, the Food and Drug Administration (FDA) has approved several ICIs against a broad spectrum of hematological malignancies and solid cancers (Table 7.1). These immunotherapies are very

TABLE 7.1
FDA-Approved Immune Checkpoint Inhibitors for Cancer and Common Adverse Effects

ICI (Drug)	Target	Approval Year	Cancer Type	Common Adverse Events
Ipilimumab	CTLA-4	2011	Melanoma (fourth stage and metastatic melanoma)	Enterocolitis, hepatitis, dermatitis, endocrinopathy, neuropathy
Nivolumab	PD-1	2014	Melanoma, NSCLC, renal cell carcinoma, urothelial carcinoma	Encephalitis, colitis, hepatitis, nephritis, endocrinopathy
Pembrolizumab	PD-1	2014	Melanoma, NSCLC, urothelial carcinoma gastric and cervical cancer	Pneumonitis, colitis, hepatitis, nephritis, encephalitis, endocrinopathy
Atezolizumab	PD-L1	2016	NSCLC, urothelial carcinoma	Pneumonitis, colitis hepatitis, endocrinopathy
Avelumab	PD-L1	2017	Markel cell carcinoma, urothelial carcinoma	Pneumonitis, colitis, hepatitis, endocrinopathy, nephritis, arthritis
Durvalumab	PD-L1	2017	Urothelial carcinoma	Pneumonitis, colitis, endocrinopathy, dermatitis
Cemiplimab	PD-1	2018	Cutaneous squamous cell carcinoma	Pneumonitis, hepatitis colitis, nephritis

effective; some patients even show complete responses (8.9–33.0%) [47, 48]. Most of the FDA-approved immune checkpoint blockade are the antibodies against CTLA-4 (ipilimumab; the first ICI approved by the FDA in 2011), PD-1 (nivolumab and pembrolizumab), and PD-L1 (atezolizumab, durvalumab, and avelumab) (Table 7.1). ICI-mediated immunotherapy suppresses co-inhibitory signals that inhibit the activation of T cells. This allows tumor antigen–specific activation of T cells and mounts a robust antitumor response against the cancer cells [49–51]. Both molecular and clinical studies have revealed that tumor cells devise ingenious mechanisms to evade immune surveillance achieved by a single ICI. To overcome this challenge, a combination of ICIs has been suggested as a viable strategy to improve clinical outcomes [52]. Indeed, significant improvements in antitumor immune response and enhanced patient survival profiles have been recorded in patients that have received combination therapy (anti-CTLA4 and anti-PD-1) [53].

Immune checkpoint blockades employing antibodies against TIM-3, VISTA, BTLA-B, and LAG-3 are under investigation and have shown promising results in preclinical studies [54]. TIM-3 includes IC inhibitory molecules predominantly expressed on CD4+ helper T cells and CD8+ T cells. TIM-3 binds with its ligand galectin-9 expressed on tumor cells and inhibits T cell proliferation [55]. Its blockade promotes hyperproliferation of T cells and results in improved antitumor immunity [56]. VISTA is primarily expressed on tumor cells and shares homology with PD-L1. Its blockade facilitates the infiltration and activation of T cells in TME and subsequently leads to better antitumor immunity [57]. T cell lymphocyte attenuator (BTLA) is a co-inhibitory molecule expressed on T cells that engage with the B7 superfamily of ligands on APCs and the TNF superfamily. Blocking of BTLA-B leads to better antitumor immune response through enhancement of CD8+ T cell function [58]. Lymphocyte-activation gene 3 (LAG-3), mostly expressed on B cells but to a lesser extent on T cells, induces inhibitory signals in T cells upon MHC-II interaction. Combination treatment employing LAG-3 blockade and anti-PD-1 (nivolumab) has shown promising results in patients with advanced melanoma and those who had no response with anti-PD-1 monotherapy [54]. The therapeutic potential of several other IC targets is currently being investigated in preclinical models and clinical studies. A deeper understanding of the underlying biology of immune checkpoint molecules will aid in the rational development of new inhibitors.

CARDIOVASCULAR DISEASE (CVD) ADVERSE EFFECTS WITH ICIS

The occurrence of cardiovascular adverse events or cardiotoxicity following conventional anticancer treatment and radiotherapy is well established [59]. As ICI-mediated immunotherapy emerged, ICI-associated toxicities influencing various aspects of cardiac function (e.g., cardiomyopathy, congestive heart failure, hypertension, rhythm disturbance, and myocarditis) are also being reported [59, 60]. Immune checkpoints on the PD-1 and CTLA-4 axis follow a natural negative feedback mechanism to inhibit appropriate immune responses, thereby protecting against excessive autoimmune reactions. During tumor progression, cancer cells hijack these pathways to evade immune surveillance and promote their proliferation. Treatment with ICIs releases this brake to stimulate strong antitumor immunity. However, as expected, it also alters immunologic tolerance and promotes inflammatory and autoimmune responses (or autoreactivity). Collectively, these side effects are referred as immune-related adverse events (IRAEs) [61]. Due to this concern, autoimmune patients are usually excluded from ICI clinical trials. The ICI-mediated IRAEs are a systemic response that occurs with a variable frequency, depending on the type and location of the cancer, the type of ICI, and the patient's immune responses. These pleiotropic factors make it very challenging to predict which patients will develop these adverse effects. The underlying mechanism of ICI-associated cardiotoxicity is currently a subject of intense investigation. Most patients (~94%) displaying ICI-induced cardiac adverse effects showed elevated levels of troponins [53, 62]. Furthermore, recent clinical data have shown that an elevated troponin level is a more consistent surveillance metric than the decline in ejection fraction (EF). Indeed, up to 50% of ICI-associated cardiac adverse event cases do not display any ejection fraction decline. This observation encourages clinicians and scientists to investigate the potential of cardiac troponin as a monitoring tool for the prompt diagnosis of myocarditis in ICI recipients. However, further research is warranted to confirm this hypothesis and to estimate the optimal timing and frequency of troponin measurements. With the growing popularity of ICI-mediated immunotherapy and the increasing frequency of adverse cases, significant collaboration among cardiologists, immunologists, statisticians, and oncologists is required for developing improved management approaches against ICI-mediated cardiotoxicities.

Preclinical Studies: The Lesson Learned from PD-1 and CTLA-4 Knockout Animals

Preclinical validation of novel therapeutic targets in animal models is imperative for bench-to-bedside translation. The vast research in the field of autoimmunity has established that it is especially true for this field. Most of the previous studies on myocarditis have been performed using mouse models in which autoimmunity is induced either by immunization with a cocktail combining cardiac myosin (CM) and appropriate adjuvants or by injection of cardiotropic viruses [63–65]. Therefore, a mouse model of spontaneous myocarditis is warranted to capture the natural mechanisms underlying human myocarditis. More recently, mouse models deficient in some critical genes, such as PD-1, CTLA-4, and TGF-β, have been identified as spontaneous myocarditis models [66–68]. However, T cells in these animals are activated nonspecifically and develop antigen-independent inflammation. PD-1 or CTLA-4 deficiency leads to elevated T cell activation and diminished peripheral tolerance [69]. Indeed, mice deficient for CTLA-4, PD-1, or its ligand PD-L1 demonstrate an enhanced activity of T cells that leads to severe autoimmune phenotypes, including myocarditis and dilated cardiomyopathy (DCM) [66–68].

Once T cells have been activated and achieved the desired therapeutic outcome, disengagement of PD-1 co-receptor and the therapeutic agents is equally important to reduce autoimmune complications. The evidence for this comes from the PD-1-deficient mouse (PD-1$^{-/-}$), which displays a wide range of autoimmune reactions [70, 71]. In addition, it also develops autoimmune cardiomyopathy similar to human dilated cardiomyopathy (DCM) [70]. Mechanistically, PD-L1 expressed on cardiomyocytes engages with the PD-1 receptor and downregulates T cell function, thereby protecting the host from myocarditis [12, 19, 70, 72]. Studies in rat models have also suggested the strong association between PD-1 and autoimmune myocarditis, as evidenced by the significant upregulation of PD-1 and PD-L1 upon myocardial injury [73]. Importantly, PD-1 deletion not only leads to autoimmunity but also induces functional impairment in antigen-specific T cells during chronic viral, fungal, and tuberculosis infections [74–78]. A growing body of literature has established that PD-1 global KO mice exhibit increased inflammation, elevated serum markers of myocardial damage, and enhanced infiltration of inflammatory immune cells in the heart [79]. Furthermore, the presence of PD-1 significantly limits T cell responses in the heart [79]. The significance of PD-1 in the heart was further confirmed by the fatal inflammatory myocarditis phenotype in an engineered mouse model of myocarditis (MRL-Pdcd-1$^{-/-}$) [80]. Additionally, the adoptive transfer of genetically engineered CD8$^+$PD-1$^-$ T cells into a murine model of autoimmune myocarditis exacerbated myocardial inflammation [79]. Recently, autoantibodies directed against troponin 1 have been recognized in PD-1$^{-/-}$ mice and are believed to be the primary mediator of myocarditis [81]. This is evident through the observation that the administration of monoclonal antibodies against troponin 1 in wild type (WT) mice triggers myocarditis [81]. Additionally, the presence of antibodies against cardiac myosin is identified in PD-L1-deficient mice, supporting the concept of autoantibody-induced myocarditis [82]. Considering all of these preclinical studies performed on mice and rats, the PD-1–PD-L1 axis seems critical to the study of autoimmune myocarditis. Indeed, all of the genetically modified PD-1 and PD-L1 models reported to date are global manipulation and, therefore, complicated by systemic effects. The creation and characterization of cardiac-specific PD-1/PD-L1 mouse models are needed to further understand the role of the PD-1–PD-L1 axis in cardiac pathophysiology.

CTLA-4, a member of the CD28 family, is an indispensable co-inhibitory immune checkpoint that displays T cell downregulation properties. It is most frequently expressed on activated conventional T cells and Foxp3+ Tregs [26, 83, 84]. CTLA-4 has been associated with a variety of autoimmune disorders, including diabetes mellitus, rheumatoid arthritis, autoimmune endocrinopathies, and heart diseases [85–90]. CTLA-4 is crucial for immune homeostasis and well-known to regulate immune activation and self-tolerance through various autonomous and nonautonomous mechanisms. The autonomous pathway involves the interaction of CTLA-4 with its ligands CD80 or CD86 on APC. This interaction induces inhibitory signals within T cells and brings about their apoptosis. Additionally, CTLA-4-expressing Tregs are sufficient for restricting T cell activity and keeping them calm and inactive. The nonautonomous mechanism of CTLA-4 is regulated partly by the modulation of ligands CD80 and CD86 in APC and partly by the release of immunosuppressive metabolites like L-kynurenine [32, 91, 92]. Furthermore, recent studies have documented the critical role of CTLA-4 in the regulation of all stages of collagen-induced arthritis (CIA) without affecting T and B cell responses, suggesting a T cell–independent mechanism of CTLA-4-mediated regulation [93]. Taken together, the CTLA-4 function is complicated and possibly operated by multiple mechanisms to promote different levels of tolerance in a wide range of cell populations. Therefore, more CTLA-4-specific *in vivo* studies are warranted to elucidate its multiple roles and underlying mechanisms.

Several autoimmune diseases, including cardiotoxicities, have been broadly reported in CTLA-4-deficient mice [85–89]. Germ line deficiency of CTLA-4 in a murine model leads to the spontaneous development of a lethal lymphoproliferative autoimmune disorder characterized by multiorgan leukocyte infiltration. This manifests in severe myocarditis and pancreatitis, which lead to early fatality within 3–4 weeks [67, 68]. In an *in vitro* setting, CTLA-4-deficient T cells exhibit an activated phenotype (CD69low, CD62Llow, CD44high) and proliferate spontaneously [94, 95]. Consistently, CTLA-4-deficient animals exhibit accumulation of the activated T cells due to an uncontrolled expansion of peripheral T cells [94, 96]. As discussed previously, CTLA-4 deficiency on Tregs is sufficient to induce lymphoproliferation that can consequently lead to the death of these mice at around 8 weeks of age. This suggests a key role of CTLA-4 in mediating the immunosuppressive functions of Tregs [93, 96]. Tamoxifen-induced conditional deletion of CTLA-4 in adult mice rapidly promotes subvert immune activation, autoantibody production, and multiorgan leukocyte infiltration. Consistently, mice born with CTLA-4 deficiency develop spontaneous myocarditis and succumb to death with pancreatitis [67, 68]. Taken together, these studies suggest that CTLA-4 abolition in adult mice leads to autoimmune disease due to the disruption of central and peripheral tolerance mechanisms as well as by the CTLA-4-regulated immunosuppressive functions of Tregs. Of note, although inducible deletion of CTLA-4 in adulthood unleashes T cells and impairs Tregs' homeostasis, it does not result in multiorgan lymphocytic infiltration-mediated lethal autoimmune consequences observed in congenic CTLA-4 knockouts [29, 93]. Thus, the conditional deletion of CTLA-4 from the adult mouse promises to be a better approach for investigating CTLA-4-mediated autoimmune disorders. Collectively, studies with CTLA-4 KO animals (both global embryonic KO and inducible conditional CTLA-4 KOs) played a key role in illustrating the complex mechanism of CTLA-4 biology in tempering immune responses against various tumors and self-tissues (autoimmune response). The studies also show that a higher precision in controlling the CD28/CTLA-4 axis is required for improving the therapeutic exploitation of this pathway.

ICI-MEDIATED ADVERSE CARDIOVASCULAR EFFECT: REPORTS FROM RANDOMIZED CONTROLLED TRIALS

Clinical studies have revealed several cases of heart failure in cancer patients treated with ICIs [12, 61, 97–100]. The underestimated cardiac side effects translate into several life-threatening complications, including heart failure, hemodynamic instability, and myocardial infarction [12, 61, 97–100].

Previous case studies and meta-analysis from randomized clinical trials with ICIs have documented higher incidences of gastrointestinal, endocrine, and cutaneous complications but reported relatively few cases of cardiotoxicity [61, 101, 102]. Six cases of cardiotoxicity and late onset of pericarditis were reported in melanoma patients treated with ipilimumab [103, 104]. This study further revealed fatality in two out of a total of six cases, despite intensive treatment [103]. Moreover, one case of myocarditis was recognized after combined therapy of CTLA-4 blockade with ipilimumab and PD-1 inhibitor nivolumab [105]. Spontaneous cardiac arrest was identified in a patient with melanoma who was enrolled in a clinical trial involving the ICI ipilimumab [106]. In another study, one patient with non-small-cell lung cancer (NSCLC) who was treated with Pembrolizumab succumbed to fatal myocardial infarction [107]. In a multicenter, phase II, randomized clinical trial, 26 patients in advanced stages of Markel cell carcinoma were treated with anti-PD-1 Pembrolizumab. In this study, just after the first dose of PD-1 blockade, a case of myocarditis was identified. Additionally, 77% of patients demonstrated other adverse events [108]. These cases were reported to be fatal even after intensive treatment. Importantly, these patients were initially diagnosed to have only hypertension and no history of previous cardiac risk factors. Histological analysis demonstrated the infiltration of macrophages, CD4+, and CD8+ T cells in the myocardium. As expected, these patients showed an increased expression of PD-L1 on injured cardiomyocytes and CD8+ T cells. This recapitulates preclinical findings with mouse models wherein significant upregulation of PD-L1 expression was observed on injured cardiomyocytes in a T cell–mediated myocarditis mouse model [12]. The infiltration of CD4+ and CD8+ T cells in the myocardium promotes the overexpression of IFN-γ, TNF-α, and CD8+-mediated granzyme B. These soluble mediators are critical to further cardiac damage. These events collectively lead to myocarditis [109]. Recently, two cases of myositis and fulminant myocarditis were described in patients treated with a combination therapy of ipilimumab and nivolumab, blockers of PD-1 and CTLA-4, respectively [12]. It is important to note that some predisposing factors might affect the incidence of ICI-associated cardiotoxicity and mortality. In a case series, Mahmood et al. (62) identified more frequent myocarditis with preexisting cardiovascular risk factors [62]. In contrast, Moslehi et al. [110] recently reported that 75% of all cases developed ICI-associated myocarditis without any predisposing factors [110]. However, in some patients, myocarditis occurs early, just after 12–15 days of initiation of ipilimumab (anti-CTLA-4) and nivolumab (anti-PD-1) both [12, 62, 111]. Of note, 20–30% of patients with preexisting autoimmune disorders experienced exacerbated complications after treatment with ipilimumab and nivolumab [112, 113]. In general, patients with autoimmune complications are recommended to be excluded from ICI therapy. Taken together, findings from these studies highlight the potential importance of preexisting risk factors in ICI-mediated myocarditis and CV events. The increased prevalence of cardiac abnormalities following ICI therapy highlights the need for gaining a deeper mechanistic understanding of cardio-oncology. This will be essential for the minimization of cardiac toxicities and the effective development of therapeutic interventions. The frequencies of the reported cardiac events increased in the postapproval phases following the widespread use of ICIs. Thus, oncologists and cardiologists must carefully consider the risk versus the therapeutic outcome of ICI-based immunotherapy in assessing the best option for improving survival and minimizing cardiotoxic-mediated morbidities in patients.

Case Reports of ICI-Mediated Cardiotoxicity

There is conflicting evidence concerning the occurrence of cardiac-related adverse events in ICI-treated patients. For example, myocarditis was not observed in a meta-analysis of 448 patients treated with a combination therapy of nivolumab and ipilimumab [114]. In contrast, a comparatively large study with 20,594 patients reported 18 (0.09%) myocarditis cases in recipients of PD-1 blockade nivolumab or in combined therapy with nivolumab and CTLA-4 inhibitor ipilimumab [12]. Having said that, the cardiotoxicities associated with ICIs are underreported [60, 62]. Table 7.2 depicts the cardiac events in ICI-treated patients [103, 115–131]. A case series of ICI recipients has reported 99 patients with cardiotoxic events [132]. There were 34% (19 recipients) who reported as female of these 56 patients. The most common malignancy observed in this case report was melanoma at 41% (41 out of 99–100 patients). NSCLC and multiple myeloma were observed in 26% (26 cases) and 9% (9 cases) of patients, respectively. The distribution of ICI in this subset of patients was as follows: (1) PD-1 blockade [nivolumab, 30% ($n = 30$); pembrolizumab, 25% ($n = 25$)]; (2) CTLA-4 inhibitor (ipilimumab, 24%; tremelimumab, 2%); (3) PD-L1 blockade (atezolizumab, 3%; avelumab, 1%; durvalumab, 2%); and (4) combination therapy with anti-PD-1 and anti-CTLA-4 antibodies (nivolumab and ipilimumab, 12%). Forty-five percent (~45 cases) were reported with myocarditis, while 20% showed other forms of cardiotoxicity. About 27% of patients presented with congestive heart failure, including cardiomyopathy, without proven myocarditis. Conduction complications were reported in 12% of patients. The other 15% showed pericardial disease.

CheckMate 067 was a milestone study examining the combinational effects of nivolumab plus ipilimumab as first-line immunotherapy for advanced melanoma [133, 134]. Results from the phase 3 CheckMate 067 showed a significant improvement in overall survival of the patients with advanced melanoma who received combinational therapy vs. nivolumab or ipilimumab alone [135]. Most of the adverse

---

TABLE 7.2
Published Case Reports of Cardiotoxicity Related to Immune Checkpoint Inhibitors

ICI (Drug)	Reported Cardiotoxicity	Documented Symptoms	References
Ipilimumab	Myocarditis, fulminant myocarditis, atrial fibrillation (AF), heart failure (HF)	Dyspnea, anasarca, lower extremity edema, chest pain, cough	104, 112–114
Nivolumab	Myocarditis, AF, HF, fulminant myocarditis	Chest pain, Severe asthenia, dyspnea, palpitations	115–121
Pembrolizumab	Myocarditis, cardiac arrhythmia, pericarditis, vasculitis, bradycardia, cardiac arrest	Dyspnea, chest pain, sweats, fever, fatigue, myalgia	104, 119, 122–125
Atezolizumab	Myocarditis	Dyspnea, fatigue	126
Avelumab	Hypertension, cardiac arrest	Fatigue, constipation	127
Durvalumab	Myocarditis, HF	Dyspnea	128

events were skin related. There were a total of four reported deaths; one of them was with cardiomyopathy in the nivolumab plus ipilimumab group [136].

In a French case series, 30 cases of ICI-mediated cardiotoxic events were identified within 2 years [137]. These adverse effects include cardiomyopathy and conduction abnormalities, and they occurred 65 days after starting ICIs [137]. Another study of 964 ICI recipients documented a 1.14% prevalence of myocarditis after 34 days of treatment [62]. As per the WHO global database (VigiBase) of drug-related adverse events, 75% of the total number of drug-associated cardiotoxicities in 2017 were due to ICI-mediated myocarditis, vasculitis, pericardial disease, and supraventricular arrhythmias [138]. However, a comparative study of randomized controlled trials analyzing PD-1/PD-L1 or CTLA-4 blockade vs. control failed to report cardiotoxic events. On the other hand, a growing body of evidence suggests that cancerous cells themselves mediate an immune response against cardiomyocytes [12, 139]. Therefore, it is conceivable that the occurrence of cardiotoxic events reported in ICI recipients is underreported. Quality control in detection methods would be useful in revising estimates of cardiotoxic events and resolving discrepancies in expected and observed numbers of cardiotoxicities.

Retrospective and Surveillance Studies

ICI therapy has revolutionized cancer management, with favorable outcomes for many advanced-stage malignancies; hence, the number of ICI recipients has rapidly increased. However, the augmented use of ICIs has led to an increased prevalence of IRAEs. Retrospective studies have suggested that ICI-mediated IRAEs typically occur in the early phase or within 12 weeks of starting therapy and are rarely observed after 1 year of treatment [140]. IRAEs range from asymptomatic laboratory findings to life-threatening fulminant heart failure [141]. These ICI-associated IRAEs are designated as low, high, or lethal grade as per terminology criteria of adverse events [142]. The nature of complications of IRAEs differs between PD-1 blockade and CTLA-4 blockade. Previous data suggest that high-grade adverse events became three times more intense with combined therapy compared to anti-PD-1 monotherapy [134]. Retrospective studies of ICI therapy showed that CTLA-4 inhibitors are comparatively more toxic than anti-PD-1 or anti-PD-L1 inhibitors [141, 143]. In the same line of thought, 90% of anti-CTLA-4 recipients reported low-grade IRAEs in comparison to 70% of the patients receiving anti-PD-1 or anti-PD-L1 [141, 143]. About 10–15% of ICI recipients demonstrated high-grade or major IRAEs, and lethal-grade adverse events (0–3.2%) were observed in very few cases [141, 143]. Recently, data collected from a WHO-based pharmacovigilance program covering clinical trials on cancer patients receiving anti-PD-1/PD-L1 and anti-CTLA-4 therapy showed that 52 out of 613 ICI-mediated lethal adverse events were cardiac-related IRAEs [140]. Myocarditis had the highest mortality rate (39.7%). A retrospective, multicenter study with 3,545 patients who were treated with ICIs revealed a 0.6% fatality rate with cardiac adverse events [140]. We present a brief overview of ICI-mediated adverse events in Table 7.3 [12, 53, 98, 100, 103, 104, 106, 117, 144–151]. Cardiovascular complications detected in the patients treated with ICIs are relatively rare but have the highest fatality rate [138]. As

TABLE 7.3
Summary of Common Cardiovascular Adverse Events Associated with ICIs

ICI (Drug)	Study Population	Cardiovascular Adverse Events	References
Ipilimumab	676 patients with metastatic melanoma	0.2% recipients developed myocarditis, 0.3% cardiac arrest, Takotsubo syndrome, pericarditis, and asymptomatic LVD documented as case reports	101, 105, 107, 114, 138
Nivolumab	120 patients with melanoma when ipilimumab did not work	0.06% myocarditis, myocardial fibrosis, lymphocytic myocarditis, heart block, and pericarditis reported as case reports	12, 99, 139–142
Pembrolizumab	834 patients with melanoma	3.8% myocarditis, cardiac arrest, 0.6% hypertension, 0.4% stable angina	104, 143
Atezolizumab	310 patients with urothelial carcinoma	Heart failure, cardiac arrest, pericarditis	144, 145
Avelumab	1,738 patients with Merkel cell carcinoma	<1% immune myocarditis	53
Durvalumab	182 patients with urothelial carcinoma	<1% immune myocarditis	53

discussed previously, the widespread use of ICI therapy has led to increased reporting of the frequency of ICI-associated myocarditis in various case series and reports [138, 140]. According to Bristol Myers Squibb's corporate safety database, 0.09% of ICI-mediated myocarditis was recorded in 2016 [12, 152]. However, as reported in a multicenter case registry recently, the incidence increased to 1.14% [62]. ICI-induced myocarditis is the lethal form of IRAEs, with a fatality rate of 27–46% [110, 137]. ICI-induced myocarditis develops in an early phase of treatment and eventually turns to lethal disease, with severely depressed left-ventricular function that requires urgent intensive care [62, 153]. Although myocarditis is the primary adverse effect associated with ICIs, growing evidence collected from clinical trials indicates other potential ICI-associated cardiovascular complications. These include myocardial infarction, inflamed atherosclerotic plaques, Takotsubo syndrome, and pericardial diseases [152]. A retrospective study reported that 14% of ICI-treated patients showed a Takotsubo syndrome–like phenotype [137]. Pericardial disease, also known as pericarditis, is a well-documented adverse event of ICI therapy [154]. The WHO global database (VigiBase) suggests that pericardial disease accounts for 13.6% of all cardiac adverse drug reactions. A retrospective study of patients treated with ICIs reported that pericarditis phenotypes were seen in 7% of cases [137]. Furthermore, this study reported that 21% of the fatalities could be accounted for by pericarditis or perimyocarditis events [138]. Histopathological analysis of heart sections from three patients with ICI-associated pericarditis demonstrated leukocytic infiltration and fibrinous exudates [155]. More detailed retrospective studies and surveillance of ICI recipients are needed to elucidate the underlying mechanisms behind ICI-mediated cardiotoxic events that might facilitate improved outcomes in cancer patients.

DIAGNOSIS OF ICI-INDUCED CARDIOVASCULAR TOXICITIES

Due to its inconsistent nature, the diagnosis of ICI-mediated cardiotoxicity is challenging. Detailed patient history and physical examination are required to exclude other immune manifestations, such as viral and autoimmune cardiac disease, infectious myocarditis, and myocardial infarction. An accurate or comprehensive diagnostic method is needed to identify a specific treatment to improve symptoms. Early diagnosis of ICI-related myocarditis entails regular laboratory tests, electrocardiograms (ECGs), and transthoracic echocardiograms (TTEs). Laboratory tests typically monitor cardiac troponin I (cTnI), troponin T (cTnT), creatine phosphokinase (CPK), creatine kinase (CK), creatine kinase-myocardial band (CK-MB), brain natriuretic peptide (BNP), and N-terminal pro-brain natriuretic peptide (NT-proBNP). Cardiac troponins are considered to be the most sensitive marker to diagnose ICI-associated myocarditis [62, 153]. Several reports have previously demonstrated that 94% of the cases of myocarditis have elevated levels of troponins [62, 153]. Also, 89% of patients with ICI-mediated cardiac adverse events showed an elevated concentration of cTnI with abnormal ECG [62]. Many previous studies suggest that a higher level of serum cTnI can serve as a critical indicator for cardiac injury and is a preferred marker for ICI-associated cardiotoxicities [62, 153]. BNP and proBNP predict clinical outcomes in all stages of heart failure. Acute HF decompensation patients have high BNP values (BNP ≥ 1,730 pg/mL) and were reported to have 2.23-fold greater mortality compared to patients with the lowest BNP values (<430 pg/mL) [156, 157]. Therefore, NT-proBNP level is strongly associated with short- and long-term clinical outcomes [156, 157]. As per Mahmood et al., 66% of patients with ICI-associated myocarditis had elevated BNP and pro-BNP concentrations [62]. Clinical data highlighted that BNP is a critical adjunct to HF markers in patients hospitalized in the emergency department with cardiac complications, and if initial troponin-1 is nondiagnostic [158]. Multiple studies have also indicated that BNP or NT-proBNP is elevated in most patients and suggest its applicability as a sensitive marker for ICI-mediated adverse events [62, 159]. However, contrasting reports indicated that BNP is elevated not only in patients with acute cardiac injury and noninflammatory left-ventricular dysfunction but also in most cancer patients who have cardiac problems [160]. Therefore, BNP might not be a suitable marker due to its nonspecificity for the diagnosis of ICI-associated cardiotoxicities. Enhanced creatine kinase (CK) was also observed in ICI-induced myocarditis [121, 122, 161]. Several studies have detected mild to massive CK elevations in the serum of patients diagnosed with ICI-mediated myositis or myasthenia gravis [162–164]. Thus, an elevated level of CK also might not be considered as a preferred marker due to a lack of specificity. ECG is a popular method that is easy to perform and is considered a first-line diagnostic tool for identifying ICI-mediated myocarditis in suspected patients [165]. Previous observations indicated that 40–89% of patients with ICI-mediated cardiac adverse events had an abnormal ECG; however, the impairments noted on ECG were nonspecific [62, 137]. TTE is another useful tool for monitoring left-ventricular ejection fraction (LVEF) impairments, pericardial effusions, and wall motion abnormalities. However, typical TTE results in patients cannot completely rule out the possibility of ICI-related myocarditis [166, 167].

Cardiac magnetic resonance imaging (CMRI) is considered the gold standard tool to diagnose myocarditis accurately [168–171]. However, this technique also has some limitations. For instance, CMR imaging might not be feasible in patients who need respiratory or circulatory support. Furthermore, concerns over its sensitivity are another limitation with CMRI. For instance, a negative report on CMRI cannot completely rule out the possibility of ICI-mediated myocarditis [111, 137, 139].

An endomyocardial biopsy (EMB) is another highly preferred technique to diagnose myocarditis. EMB allows the detection of various features of interstitial inflammation, including interstitial fibrosis and lymphocyte infiltration [172–175]. Thus, EMB facilitates examination of the infiltration of T cells (CD4+, CD8+) and macrophage into the myocardium [12, 139]. Indeed, hyperactivated T cell–mediated cardiac tissue damage is critical to ICI- induced myocarditis. Of note, sometimes inflammatory infiltration can be inaccessible, which results in a false-negative diagnosis [173]. Therefore, an EMB is often suggested to justify unexplained progressive heart failure [172].

As discussed previously, ICI-associated cardiotoxicity has been observed by a wide range of clinical manifestations. The nature of the clinical manifestation primarily depends on the extent of cardiac involvement, and therefore early diagnosis of cardiotoxic events is challenging. Hence, it is of paramount importance to develop sensitive monitoring guidelines for the early diagnosis of ICI-associated cardiotoxicity.

MANAGEMENT OF ICI-ASSOCIATED MYOCARDITIS

ICI-associated cardiotoxic events are rare, but fatal in a majority of cases. Therefore, the timing of diagnosis and management is critical. However, the management of ICI-associated cardiotoxic events is particularly challenging. To date, there are no established guidelines for the management of ICI-mediated cardiotoxic events. A few case series have reported that ICI therapy also causes conduction-related disease and noninflammatory LV dysfunction [176, 177]. Additionally, electrical irregularities related to ICI-mediated cardiotoxicities may include lethal ventricular arrhythmias, atrial fibrillation, and supraventricular tachycardia. However, these complications have rarely been reported during ICI therapy [138, 178, 179]. This is primarily due to limited data on its diagnosis and relatively rare occurrence. Therefore, close monitoring of cardiotoxicity in ICI-treated patients is highly recommended. The management strategy for ICI-associated cardiotoxic effects depends on the severity of the cardiotoxic manifestation. Therefore, the first step in the management of ICI-mediated toxicities is to recognize and estimate the severity and grade of cardiac-related complications. As discussed earlier, several diagnostic tools have been employed to establish the extent of damage caused by cardiotoxic events. Examples of such monitoring tools include regular cardiac biomarkers (troponin, creatine kinase), inflammatory biomarkers (ESR, CRP, and WBC counts), BNP, ECG, chest X-ray, and echocardiogram. Of note, clinical studies have reported a normal left-ventricular ejection fraction (LVEF) for half of the patients with myocarditis [62]. Therefore, cardiac MRI with a sequence of inflammatory biomarkers and gadolinium enhancement is recommended [180]. As alluded to in the diagnosis section, cardiac MRI is not feasible for patients who require the support of ventilator or have an intravenous pacemaker. In this situation, a CT scan is advised to detect myocardial inflammation. In some uncertain cases of ICI-mediated cardiotoxicity, an endomyocardial biopsy is recommended to confirm the final diagnosis [172–174]. The ICI recipients who show laboratory abnormalities (cardiac biomarkers and ECG) without any significant adverse symptoms fall in the category of grade 1 cardiotoxicity. Patients with mild symptoms and abnormal lab results are classified as having grade 2 cardiotoxicity. Patients with mild symptoms displaying moderate-to-abnormal cardiac lab results are classified as having grade 3 cardiotoxicity, and those with moderate-to-severe decompensation symptoms and life-threatening symptoms fall in grade 4. Most clinicians suggest holding off ICI therapy after the detection of a cardiac complication of grade 3 or 4. However, considering the high mortality rate of ICI-mediated cardiotoxicity, the American Society of Clinical Oncology (ASCO) guidelines suggest holding off on ICI therapy even after a diagnosis of grade 1 cardiotoxicity [142]. Decisions regarding discontinuing and restarting ICI therapy require collaboration among the primary treatment team, oncologist, cardiologist, and safety management team to ensure that the intervention leads to a fruitful outcome and is associated with minimal or preferably no cardiotoxicity. In contrast to ASCO guidelines, the National Comprehensive Cancer Network (NCCN) recommends permanent discontinuation of ICI treatment only if patients have grades 3 and 4 toxicity [181].

Immunosuppressive therapy is one of the vital approaches to dealing with ICI-associated myocarditis. This therapy is focused on targeting hyperactivated T cells. Corticosteroids have been proposed as first-line immunosuppressive therapy for reversing ICI-related left-ventricular dysfunction [182]. Therefore, a high dose of steroids has been suggested to treat severe cases of ICI-induced myocarditis. Many institutions, however, discourage the use of a high dose of steroids for the treatment of ICI-mediated myocarditis due to a minor risk of rare mortality [62, 183]. But reasonably, a high dose of steroids is often followed to treat the third and fourth grades of life-threatening complications [181]. In parallel with immunosuppressive therapy, standard cardiac care such as β-blocker and angiotensin receptor blockers for the treatment of LV dysfunction, diuretics for fluid overload, and mineralocorticoids/ aldosterone receptor inhibitor for decreased LVEF is also suggested to treat ICI-mediated cardiotoxicities [184, 185]. ICI recipients diagnosed with troponin elevation with conduction abnormalities are advised to transfer to a coronary care unit directly [186]. In summary, ICI-mediated myocarditis should be managed depending on the severity of clinical symptoms at the time of diagnosis. More robust clinical trials focusing on the effects of ICI-mediated cardiovascular disease are required to improve the therapeutic management of this complication.

CONCLUSION AND FUTURE PERSPECTIVES

ICI therapy is being used to treat a variety of cancer types. Therefore, the number of patients receiving ICI therapy is continuously growing. The use of ICIs, either alone or in combination with other therapeutic agents, carries a significant risk of adverse cardiac reactions, such as myocarditis, cardiomyopathy, acute coronary syndrome, pericarditis, and other cardiotoxicities. Among these, myocarditis is the most common and is highly fatal. Although the risk of ICI-mediated cardiac adverse events is low, it can have dangerous to disastrous consequences once it develops. Usually, ICI-mediated cardiotoxicity is recorded in the early stage of therapy, with pathological outcomes ranging from asymptomatic cardiac biomarker elevations to fatal cardiac arrest. Clinical features of ICI-mediated cardiotoxicity are evaluated with regular laboratory tests (cTnI, cTnT, BNP, NT-proBNP, CK) and the use of extensive imaging technology (ECG, TTE, CMR). EMB is only recommended for the final confirmatory diagnosis. Serum troponin level is one of the most promising and sensitive markers for the early diagnosis of ICI-associated myocardial damage. ECG and EMB are widely used as standard diagnostic tests to monitor ICI-related cardiac complications. Thus, ICI-mediated cardiac syndromes have gained increased recognition with widespread improvements in diagnostic technologies. A detailed assessment of cardiac risk factors must be completed before initiating ICI therapy, especially for patients with preexisting cardiac complications. Following a confirmed diagnosis of ICI-associated cardiotoxicity, patients can be effectively treated with a high dose of steroids or with agents of standard cardiac care.

The absence of knowledge of the specific pathophysiological mechanisms underlying the development and progression of ICI-associated adverse events necessitates future research. This is required to gain a deeper understating of the pathophysiological mechanisms and the predisposing risk factors underlying the development of ICI-induced cardiac syndrome. As discussed earlier, a comprehensive surveillance protocol must be developed to detect ICI-induced cardiac complications at their earliest to facilitate a prompt treatment plan. It is also essential to spread awareness among clinicians about ICI-related cardiotoxicity. Therefore, fruitful collaboration and extensive discussion among oncologists, immunologists, cardiologists, and toxicity management teams are needed to improve the clinical outcomes of ICI therapy. Most of the current data about ICI-associated cardiotoxicity are deduced from small cohort studies and case reports. Hence, it is crucial to fill these knowledge gaps with well-designed, prospective, multi-cohort studies. The results of these studies will be critical for developing new therapies with minimal or no ICI-mediated cardiotoxicities.

ACKNOWLEDGMENTS

This work is supported by research grants to HL from the NHLBI (R01HL133290, R01HL119234). PU is supported by an American Heart Association (AHA) Postdoctoral Fellowship (19POST34460025).

BIBLIOGRAPHY

1. Gaudino, S.J. and P. Kumar, *Cross-talk between antigen presenting cells and T cells impacts intestinal homeostasis, bacterial infections, and tumorigenesis.* Front Immunol, 2019. **10**: p. 360.
2. Davis, R.J., R.L. Ferris, and N.C. Schmitt, *Costimulatory and coinhibitory immune checkpoint receptors in head and neck cancer: unleashing immune responses through therapeutic combinations.* Cancers Head Neck, 2016. **1**: p. 12.

3. Patel, S.A. and A.J. Minn, *Combination cancer therapy with immune checkpoint block-ade: mechanisms and strategies.* Immunity, 2018. **48**(3): p. 417–433.

4. Wong, J., et al., *Potential therapies for infectious diseases based on targeting immune evasion mechanisms that pathogens have in common with cancer cells.* Front Cell Infect Microbiol, 2019. **9**: p. 25.

5. Marin-Acevedo, J.A., et al., *Next generation of immune checkpoint therapy in cancer: new developments and challenges.* J Hematol Oncol, 2018. **11**(1): p. 39.

6. Dimberu, P.M. and R.M. Leonhardt, *Cancer immunotherapy takes a multi-faceted approach to kick the immune system into gear.* Yale J Biol Med, 2011. **84**(4): p. 371–380.

7. Yan, L. and H.X. Chen, *Cancer immunotherapy.* Chin J Cancer, 2014. **33**(9): p. 413–415.

8. Weinmann, S.C. and D.S. Pisetsky, *Mechanisms of immune-related adverse events dur-ing the treatment of cancer with immune checkpoint inhibitors.* Rheumatology (Oxford), 2019. **58**(Suppl 7): p. vii59–vii67.

9. Postow, M.A., R. Sidlow, and M.D. Hellmann, *Immune-related adverse events associ-ated with immune checkpoint blockade.* N Engl J Med, 2018. **378**(2): p. 158–168.

10. Trinh, S., et al., *Management of immune-related adverse events associated with immune checkpoint inhibitor therapy: a minireview of current clinical guidelines.* Asia Pac J Oncol Nurs, 2019. **6**(2): p. 154–160.

11. Brustle, K. and B. Heidecker, *Checkpoint inhibitor induced cardiotoxicity: manag-ing the drawbacks of our newest agents against cancer.* Oncotarget, 2017. **8**(63): p. 106165–106166.

12. Johnson, D.B., et al., *Fulminant myocarditis with combination immune checkpoint blockade.* N Engl J Med, 2016. **375**(18): p. 1749–1755.

13. Varricchi, G., et al., *Cardiotoxicity of immune checkpoint inhibitors.* ESMO Open, 2017. **2**(4): p. e000247.

14. Chahine, J., et al., *Myocardial and pericardial toxicity associated with immune check-point inhibitors in cancer patients.* JACC: Case Reports, 2020. **2**: p. 191–199.

15. Hanahan, D. and L.M. Coussens, *Accessories to the crime: functions of cells recruited to the tumor microenvironment.* Cancer Cell, 2012. **21**(3): p. 309–322.

16. Spill, F., et al., *Impact of the physical microenvironment on tumor progression and metastasis.* Curr Opin Biotechnol, 2016. **40**: p. 41–48.

17. Maimela, N.R., S. Liu, and Y. Zhang, *Fates of CD8+ T cells in tumor microenvironment.* Comput Struct Biotechnol J, 2019. **17**: p. 1–13.

18. Alsaab, H.O., et al., *PD-1 and PD-L1 checkpoint signaling inhibition for cancer immu-notherapy: mechanism, combinations, and clinical outcome.* Front Pharmacol, 2017. **8**: p. 561.

19. Freeman, G.J., et al., *Engagement of the PD-1 immunoinhibitory receptor by a novel B7 family member leads to negative regulation of lymphocyte activation.* J Exp Med, 2000. **192**(7): p. 1027–1034.

20. Topalian, S.L., C.G. Drake, and D.M. Pardoll, *Targeting the PD-1/B7-H1(PD-L1) path-way to activate anti-tumor immunity.* Curr Opin Immunol, 2012. **24**(2): p. 207–212.

21. Fallarino, F., P.E. Fields, and T.F. Gajewski, *B7–1 engagement of cytotoxic T lymphocyte antigen 4 inhibits T cell activation in the absence of CD28.* J Exp Med, 1998. **188**(1): p. 205–210.

22. Linsley, P.S., et al., *Intracellular trafficking of CTLA-4 and focal localization towards sites of TCR engagement.* Immunity, 1996. **4**(6): p. 535–543.

23. Masteller, E.L., et al., *Structural analysis of CTLA-4 function in vivo.* J Immunol, 2000. **164**(10): p. 5319–5327.

24. Schneider, H., et al., *Reversal of the TCR stop signal by CTLA-4.* Science, 2006. **313**(5795): p. 1972–1975.

25. Buchbinder, E.I. and A. Desai, *CTLA-4 and PD-1 pathways: similarities, differences, and implications of their inhibition*. Am J Clin Oncol, 2016. **39**(1): p. 98–106.

26. Rudd, C.E., A. Taylor, and H. Schneider, *CD28 and CTLA-4 coreceptor expression and signal transduction*. Immunol Rev, 2009. **229**(1): p. 12–26.

27. Wang, C.J., et al., *Cutting edge: cell-extrinsic immune regulation by CTLA-4 expressed on conventional T cells*. J Immunol, 2012. **189**(3): p. 1118–1122.

28. Walker, L.S., *Treg and CTLA-4: two intertwining pathways to immune tolerance*. J Autoimmun, 2013. **45**: p. 49–57.

29. Wing, K., et al., *CTLA-4 control over Foxp3+ regulatory T cell function*. Science, 2008. **322**(5899): p. 271–275.

30. Jain, N., et al., *Dual function of CTLA-4 in regulatory T cells and conventional T cells to prevent multiorgan autoimmunity*. Proc Natl Acad Sci U S A, 2010. **107**(4): p. 1524–1528.

31. Corse, E. and J.P. Allison, *Cutting edge: CTLA-4 on effector T cells inhibits in trans*. J Immunol, 2012. **189**(3): p. 1123–1127.

32. Qureshi, O.S., et al., *Trans-endocytosis of CD80 and CD86: a molecular basis for the cell-extrinsic function of CTLA-4*. Science, 2011. **332**(6029): p. 600–603.

33. Keir, M.E., et al., *PD-1 and its ligands in tolerance and immunity*. Annu Rev Immunol, 2008. **26**: p. 677–704.

34. Keir, M.E., L.M. Francisco, and A.H. Sharpe, *PD-1 and its ligands in T-cell immunity*. Curr Opin Immunol, 2007. **19**(3): p. 309–314.

35. Keir, M.E., et al., *Programmed death-1 (PD-1):PD-ligand 1 interactions inhibit TCR-mediated positive selection of thymocytes*. J Immunol, 2005. **175**(11): p. 7372–7379.

36. Keir, M.E. and A.H. Sharpe, *The B7/CD28 costimulatory family in autoimmunity*. Immunol Rev, 2005. **204**: p. 128–143.

37. Latchman, Y., et al., *PD-L2 is a second ligand for PD-1 and inhibits T cell activation*. Nat Immunol, 2001. **2**(3): p. 261–268.

38. Latchman, Y.E., et al., *PD-L1-deficient mice show that PD-L1 on T cells, antigen-presenting cells, and host tissues negatively regulates T cells*. Proc Natl Acad Sci U S A, 2004. **101**(29): p. 10691–10696.

39. Pardoll, D.M., *The blockade of immune checkpoints in cancer immunotherapy*. Nat Rev Cancer, 2012. **12**(4): p. 252–264.

40. Zou, W. and L. Chen, *Inhibitory B7-family molecules in the tumour microenvironment*. Nat Rev Immunol, 2008. **8**(6): p. 467–477.

41. Yokosuka, T., et al., *Programmed cell death 1 forms negative costimulatory microclusters that directly inhibit T cell receptor signaling by recruiting phosphatase SHP2*. J Exp Med, 2012. **209**(6): p. 1201–1217.

42. Hui, E., et al., *T cell costimulatory receptor CD28 is a primary target for PD-1-mediated inhibition*. Science, 2017. **355**(6332): p. 1428–1433.

43. Rota, G., et al., *Shp-2 is dispensable for establishing T cell exhaustion and for PD-1 signaling in vivo*. Cell Rep, 2018. **23**(1): p. 39–49.

44. Bengsch, B., et al., *Bioenergetic insufficiencies due to metabolic alterations regulated by the inhibitory receptor PD-1 are an early driver of CD8(+) T cell exhaustion*. Immunity, 2016. **45**(2): p. 358–373.

45. Patsoukis, N., et al., *PD-1 alters T-cell metabolic reprogramming by inhibiting glycolysis and promoting lipolysis and fatty acid oxidation*. Nat Commun, 2015. **6**: p. 6692.

46. Kortlever, R.M., et al., *Myc cooperates with Ras by programming inflammation and immune suppression*. Cell, 2017. **171**(6): p. 1301–1315 e14.

47. Haslam, A. and V. Prasad, *Estimation of the percentage of US patients with cancer who are eligible for and respond to checkpoint inhibitor immunotherapy drugs*. JAMA Netw Open, 2019. **2**(5): p. e192535.

48. Emens, L.A., et al., *Cancer immunotherapy: opportunities and challenges in the rapidly evolving clinical landscape.* Eur J Cancer, 2017. **81**: p. 116–129.
49. Pitt, J.M., et al., *Resistance mechanisms to immune-checkpoint blockade in cancer: Tumor-intrinsic and -extrinsic factors.* Immunity, 2016. **44**(6): p. 1255–1269.
50. Hurst, J.H., *Cancer immunotherapy innovator James Allison receives the 2015 Lasker~DeBakey Clinical Medical Research Award.* J Clin Invest, 2015. **125**(10): p. 3732–3736.
51. Ribas, A. and J.D. Wolchok, *Cancer immunotherapy using checkpoint blockade.* Science, 2018. **359**(6382): p. 1350–1355.
52. Postow, M.A., et al., *Nivolumab and ipilimumab versus ipilimumab in untreated melanoma.* N Engl J Med, 2015. **372**(21): p. 2006–2017.
53. Zarifa, A., et al., *Cardiotoxicity of FDA-approved immune checkpoint inhibitors: a rare but serious adverse event.* Journal of Immunotherapy and Precision Oncology, 2018.
54. Ascierto, P.A., et al., *Initial efficacy of anti-lymphocyte activation gene-3 (anti—LAG-3; BMS-986016) in combination with nivolumab (nivo) in pts with melanoma (MEL) previously treated with anti—PD-1/PD-L1 therapy.* Journal of Clinical Oncology, 2017. **35**(15_suppl): p. 9520–9520.
55. Elahi, S., et al., *Galectin-9 binding to Tim-3 renders activated human CD4+ T cells less susceptible to HIV-1 infection.* Blood, 2012. **119**(18): p. 4192–4204.
56. Ngiow, S.F., et al., *Anti-TIM3 antibody promotes T cell IFN-gamma-mediated antitumor immunity and suppresses established tumors.* Cancer Res, 2011. **71**(10): p. 3540–3551.
57. Le Mercier, I., et al., *VISTA regulates the development of protective antitumor immunity.* Cancer Res, 2014. **74**(7): p. 1933–1944.
58. Fourcade, J., et al., *CD8(+) T cells specific for tumor antigens can be rendered dysfunctional by the tumor microenvironment through upregulation of the inhibitory receptors BTLA and PD-1.* Cancer Res, 2012. **72**(4): p. 887–896.
59. Kang, Y.J., *Molecular and cellular mechanisms of cardiotoxicity.* Environ Health Perspect, 2001. **109** (Suppl 1): p. 27–34.
60. Moslehi, J.J., *Cardiovascular toxic effects of targeted cancer therapies.* N Engl J Med, 2016. **375**(15): p. 1457–1467.
61. Hofmann, L., et al., *Cutaneous, gastrointestinal, hepatic, endocrine, and renal side-effects of anti-PD-1 therapy.* Eur J Cancer, 2016. **60**: p. 190–209.
62. Mahmood, S.S., et al., *Myocarditis in patients treated with immune checkpoint inhibitors.* J Am Coll Cardiol, 2018. **71**(16): p. 1755–1764.
63. Neu, N., et al., *Coxsackievirus induced myocarditis in mice: cardiac myosin autoantibodies do not cross-react with the virus.* Clin Exp Immunol, 1987. **69**(3): p. 566–574.
64. Neu, N., et al., *Cardiac myosin induces myocarditis in genetically predisposed mice.* J Immunol, 1987. **139**(11): p. 3630–3636.
65. Pummerer, C.L., et al., *Identification of cardiac myosin peptides capable of inducing autoimmune myocarditis in BALB/c mice.* J Clin Invest, 1996. **97**(9): p. 2057–2062.
66. Shull, M.M., et al., *Targeted disruption of the mouse transforming growth factor-beta 1 gene results in multifocal inflammatory disease.* Nature, 1992. **359**(6397): p. 693–699.
67. Tivol, E.A., et al., *Loss of CTLA-4 leads to massive lymphoproliferation and fatal multiorgan tissue destruction, revealing a critical negative regulatory role of CTLA-4.* Immunity, 1995. **3**(5): p. 541–547.
68. Waterhouse, P., et al., *Lymphoproliferative disorders with early lethality in mice deficient in Ctla-4.* Science, 1995. **270**(5238): p. 985–988.
69. Keir, M.E., et al., *Tissue expression of PD-L1 mediates peripheral T cell tolerance.* J Exp Med, 2006. **203**(4): p. 883–895.

70. Nishimura, H., et al., *Development of lupus-like autoimmune diseases by disruption of the PD-1 gene encoding an ITIM motif-carrying immunoreceptor.* Immunity, 1999. **11**(2): p. 141–151.

71. Wang, J., et al., *Establishment of NOD-Pdcd1-/- mice as an efficient animal model of type I diabetes.* Proc Natl Acad Sci U S A, 2005. **102**(33): p. 11823–11828.

72. Dong, H., et al., *B7-H1, a third member of the B7 family, co-stimulates T-cell proliferation and interleukin-10 secretion.* Nat Med, 1999. **5**(12): p. 1365–1369.

73. Baban, B., et al., *Upregulation of programmed death-1 and its ligand in cardiac injury models: interaction with GADD153.* PLoS One, 2015. **10**(4): p. e0124059.

74. Brown, K.E., et al., *Role of PD-1 in regulating acute infections.* Curr Opin Immunol, 2010. **22**(3): p. 397–401.

75. Finnefrock, A.C., et al., *PD-1 blockade in rhesus macaques: impact on chronic infection and prophylactic vaccination.* J Immunol, 2009. **182**(2): p. 980–987.

76. Trautmann, L., et al., *Upregulation of PD-1 expression on HIV-specific CD8+ T cells leads to reversible immune dysfunction.* Nat Med, 2006. **12**(10): p. 1198–1202.

77. Velu, V., et al., *Enhancing SIV-specific immunity in vivo by PD-1 blockade.* Nature, 2009. **458**(7235): p. 206–210.

78. Tousif, S., et al., *T cells from Programmed Death-1 deficient mice respond poorly to Mycobacterium tuberculosis infection.* PLoS One, 2011. **6**(5): p. e19864.

79. Tarrio, M.L., et al., *PD-1 protects against inflammation and myocyte damage in T cell-mediated myocarditis.* J Immunol, 2012. **188**(10): p. 4876–4884.

80. Wang, J., et al., *PD-1 deficiency results in the development of fatal myocarditis in MRL mice.* Int Immunol, 2010. **22**(6): p. 443–452.

81. Okazaki, T., et al., *Autoantibodies against cardiac troponin I are responsible for dilated cardiomyopathy in PD-1-deficient mice.* Nat Med, 2003. **9**(12): p. 1477–1483.

82. Lucas, J.A., et al., *Programmed death ligand 1 regulates a critical checkpoint for autoimmune myocarditis and pneumonitis in MRL mice.* J Immunol, 2008. **181**(4): p. 2513–2521.

83. Takahashi, T., et al., *Immunologic self-tolerance maintained by CD25(+)CD4(+) regulatory T cells constitutively expressing cytotoxic T lymphocyte-associated antigen 4.* J Exp Med, 2000. **192**(2): p. 303–310.

84. Thompson, C.B. and J.P. Allison, *The emerging role of CTLA-4 as an immune attenuator.* Immunity, 1997. **7**(4): p. 445–450.

85. Schubert, D., et al., *Autosomal dominant immune dysregulation syndrome in humans with CTLA4 mutations.* Nat Med, 2014. **20**(12): p. 1410–1416.

86. Kuehn, H.S., et al., *Immune dysregulation in human subjects with heterozygous germline mutations in CTLA4.* Science, 2014. **345**(6204): p. 1623–1627.

87. Kouki, T., et al., *CTLA-4 gene polymorphism at position 49 in exon 1 reduces the inhibitory function of CTLA-4 and contributes to the pathogenesis of Graves' disease.* J Immunol, 2000. **165**(11): p. 6606–6611.

88. Barreto, M., et al., *Evidence for CTLA4 as a susceptibility gene for systemic lupus erythematosus.* Eur J Hum Genet, 2004. **12**(8): p. 620–626.

89. Marron, M.P., et al., *Insulin-dependent diabetes mellitus (IDDM) is associated with CTLA4 polymorphisms in multiple ethnic groups.* Hum Mol Genet, 1997. **6**(8): p. 1275–1282.

90. Tang, M.J. and Z.B. Zhou, *Association of the CTLA-4 +49A/G polymorphism with rheumatoid arthritis in Chinese Han population.* Mol Biol Rep, 2013. **40**(3): p. 2627–2631.

91. Onishi, Y., et al., *Foxp3+ natural regulatory T cells preferentially form aggregates on dendritic cells in vitro and actively inhibit their maturation.* Proc Natl Acad Sci U S A, 2008. **105**(29): p. 10113–10118.

92. Grohmann, U., et al., *CTLA-4-Ig regulates tryptophan catabolism in vivo*. Nat Immunol, 2002. **3**(11): p. 1097–1101.

93. Klocke, K., et al., *Induction of autoimmune disease by deletion of CTLA-4 in mice in adulthood*. Proc Natl Acad Sci U S A, 2016. **113**(17): p. E2383–2392.

94. Chambers, C.A., M.S. Kuhns, and J.P. Allison, *Cytotoxic T lymphocyte antigen-4 (CTLA-4) regulates primary and secondary peptide-specific CD4(+) T cell responses*. Proc Natl Acad Sci U S A, 1999. **96**(15): p. 8603–8608.

95. Waterhouse, P., et al., *Normal thymic selection, normal viability and decreased lymphoproliferation in T cell receptor-transgenic CTLA-4-deficient mice*. Eur J Immunol, 1997. **27**(8): p. 1887–1892.

96. Tai, X., et al., *Induction of autoimmune disease in CTLA-4-/- mice depends on a specific CD28 motif that is required for in vivo costimulation*. Proc Natl Acad Sci U S A, 2007. **104**(34): p. 13756–13761.

97. Herbst, R.S., et al., *Pembrolizumab versus docetaxel for previously treated, PD-L1-positive, advanced non-small-cell lung cancer (KEYNOTE-010): a randomised controlled trial*. Lancet, 2016. **387**(10027): p. 1540–1550.

98. Semper, H., et al., *Drug-induced myocarditis after nivolumab treatment in a patient with PDL1- negative squamous cell carcinoma of the lung*. Lung Cancer, 2016. **99**: p. 117–119.

99. Tadokoro, T., et al., *Acute lymphocytic myocarditis with anti-PD-1 antibody nivolumab*. Circ Heart Fail, 2016. **9**(10).

100. Geisler, B.P., et al., *Apical ballooning and cardiomyopathy in a melanoma patient treated with ipilimumab: a case of takotsubo-like syndrome*. J Immunother Cancer, 2015. **3**: p. 4.

101. Boutros, C., et al., *Safety profiles of anti-CTLA-4 and anti-PD-1 antibodies alone and in combination*. Nat Rev Clin Oncol, 2016. **13**(8): p. 473–486.

102. Eigentler, T.K., et al., *Diagnosis, monitoring and management of immune-related adverse drug reactions of anti-PD-1 antibody therapy*. Cancer Treat Rev, 2016. **45**: p. 7–18.

103. Heinzerling, L., et al., *Cardiotoxicity associated with CTLA4 and PD1 blocking immunotherapy*. J Immunother Cancer, 2016. **4**: p. 50.

104. Yun, S., et al., *Late onset ipilimumab-induced pericarditis and pericardial effusion: a rare but life threatening complication*. Case Reports in Oncological Medicine, 2015. **2015**: p. 794842.

105. Robert, C., et al., *Ipilimumab plus dacarbazine for previously untreated metastatic melanoma*. N Engl J Med, 2011. **364**(26): p. 2517–2526.

106. Larkin, J., et al., *Combined nivolumab and ipilimumab or monotherapy in untreated melanoma*. N Engl J Med, 2015. **373**(1): p. 23–34.

107. Hu, Y.B., et al., *Evaluation of rare but severe immune related adverse effects in PD-1 and PD-L1 inhibitors in non-small cell lung cancer: a meta-analysis*. Transl Lung Cancer Res, 2017. **6**(Suppl 1): p. S8–S20.

108. Brar, G. and M.A. Shah, *The role of pembrolizumab in the treatment of PD-L1 expressing gastric and gastroesophageal junction adenocarcinoma*. Therap Adv Gastroenterol, 2019. **12**: p. 1756284819869767.

109. Grabie, N., et al., *Endothelial programmed death-1 ligand 1 (PD-L1) regulates CD8+ T-cell mediated injury in the heart*. Circulation, 2007. **116**(18): p. 2062–2071.

110. Moslehi, J.J., et al., *Increased reporting of fatal immune checkpoint inhibitor-associated myocarditis*. Lancet, 2018. **391**(10124): p. 933.

111. Norwood, T.G., et al., *Smoldering myocarditis following immune checkpoint blockade*. J Immunother Cancer, 2017. **5**(1): p. 91.

112. Menzies, A.M., et al., *Anti-PD-1 therapy in patients with advanced melanoma and preexisting autoimmune disorders or major toxicity with ipilimumab*. Ann Oncol, 2017. **28**(2): p. 368–376.

113. Johnson, D.B., R.J. Sullivan, and A.M. Menzies, *Immune checkpoint inhibitors in challenging populations*. Cancer, 2017. **123**(11): p. 1904–1911.

114. Sznol, M., et al., *Pooled analysis safety profile of nivolumab and ipilimumab combination therapy in patients with advanced melanoma*. J Clin Oncol, 2017. **35**(34): p. 3815–3822.

115. Khoury, Z.H., et al., *Combination nivolumab/ipilimumab immunotherapy for melanoma with subsequent unexpected cardiac arrest: a case report and review of literature*. Journal of Immunotherapy, 2019. **42**(8): p. 313–317.

116. Arangalage, D., et al., *Survival after fulminant myocarditis induced by immune-checkpoint inhibitors*. Ann Intern Med, 2017. **167**(9): p. 683–684.

117. Roth, M.E., et al., *Left ventricular dysfunction after treatment with ipilimumab for metastatic melanoma*. Am J Ther, 2016. **23**(6): p. e1925–e1928.

118. Salem, J.E., et al., *Abatacept for severe immune checkpoint inhibitor-associated myocarditis*. N Engl J Med, 2019. **380**(24): p. 2377–2379.

119. Martin Huertas, R., et al., *Cardiac toxicity of immune-checkpoint inhibitors: a clinical case of nivolumab-induced myocarditis and review of the evidence and new challenges*. Cancer Manag Res, 2019. **11**: p. 4541–4548.

120. Fazel, M. and P.M. Jedlowski, *Severe myositis, myocarditis, and myasthenia gravis with elevated anti-striated muscle antibody following single dose of ipilimumab-nivolumab therapy in a patient with metastatic melanoma*. Case Reports Immunol, 2019. **2019**: p. 2539493.

121. So, H., et al., *PD-1 inhibitor-associated severe myasthenia gravis with necrotizing myopathy and myocarditis*. J Neurol Sci, 2019. **399**: p. 97–100.

122. Agrawal, N., et al., *Cardiac toxicity associated with immune checkpoint inhibitors: case series and review of the literature*. Case Rep Oncol, 2019. **12**(1): p. 260–276.

123. Yamaguchi, S., et al., *Late-onset fulminant myocarditis with immune checkpoint inhibitor nivolumab*. Can J Cardiol, 2018. **34**(6): p. 812.e1–812.e3.

124. Kimura, H., et al., *A case of heart failure after treatment with Anti-PD-1 antibody followed by adoptive transfer of cytokine-activated killer cells in a recurrent lung cancer patient*. J Thorac Oncol, 2017. **12**(8): p. e128-e130.

125. Esfahani, K., et al., *Alemtuzumab for immune-related myocarditis due to PD-1 therapy*. N Engl J Med, 2019. **380**(24): p. 2375–2376.

126. Dhenin, A., et al., *Cascade of immunologic adverse events related to pembrolizumab treatment*. BMJ Case Rep, 2019. **12**(6).

127. Lindner, A.K., et al., *Rare, but severe: vasculitis and checkpoint inhibitors*. Eur Urol Focus, 2020. **6**(3): p. 609–612.

128. Hsu, C.Y., Y.W. Su, and S.C. Chen, *Sick sinus syndrome associated with anti-programmed cell death-1*. J Immunother Cancer, 2018. **6**(1): p. 72.

129. Liu, S.Y., et al., *Sequential blockade of PD-1 and PD-L1 causes fulminant cardiotoxicity-from case report to mouse model validation*. Cancers (Basel), 2019. **11**(4).

130. Berner, A.M., et al., *Fatal autoimmune myocarditis with anti-PD-L1 and tyrosine kinase inhibitor therapy for renal cell cancer*. Eur J Cancer, 2018. **101**: p. 287–290.

131. Mahmood, S.S., et al., *Myocarditis with tremelimumab plus durvalumab combination therapy for endometrial cancer: a case report*. Gynecol Oncol Rep, 2018. **25**: p. 74–77.

132. Mir, H., et al., *Cardiac complications associated with checkpoint inhibition: a systematic review of the literature in an important emerging area*. Can J Cardiol, 2018. **34**(8): p. 1059–1068.

133. *Neoadjuvant PD-1 blockade in resectable lung cancer; nivolumab and ipilimumab in advanced melanoma; overall survival with combined nivolumab and ipilimumab in advanced melanoma; prolonged survival in stage III melanoma with ipilimumab adjuvant therapy; combined nivolumab and ipilimumab or monotherapy in untreated melanoma; combined nivolumab and ipilimumab or monotherapy in untreated melanoma; nivolumab and ipilimumab versus ipilimumab in untreated melanoma; rapid eradication of a bulky melanoma mass with one dose of immunotherapy; genetic basis for clinical response to CTLA-4 blockade; genetic basis for clinical response to CTLA-4 blockade in melanoma; nivolumab plus ipilimumab in advanced melanoma; safety and tumor responses with lambrolizumab (anti-PD-1) in melanoma; hepatotoxicity with combination of vemurafenib and ipilimumab.* N Engl J Med, 2018. **379**(22): p. 2185.

134. Wolchok, J.D., et al., *Overall survival with combined nivolumab and ipilimumab in advanced melanoma.* N Engl J Med, 2017. **377**(14): p. 1345–1356.

135. Hodi, F.S., et al., *Nivolumab plus ipilimumab or nivolumab alone versus ipilimumab alone in advanced melanoma (CheckMate 067): 4-year outcomes of a multicentre, randomised, phase 3 trial.* Lancet Oncol, 2018. **19**(11): p. 1480–1492.

136. *Correction to Lancet Oncol 2018; 19: 1480–92.* Lancet Oncol, 2018. **19**(11): p. e581.

137. Escudier, M., et al., *Clinical features, management, and outcomes of immune checkpoint inhibitor-related cardiotoxicity.* Circulation, 2017. **136**(21): p. 2085–2087.

138. Salem, J.E., et al., *Cardiovascular toxicities associated with immune checkpoint inhibitors: an observational, retrospective, pharmacovigilance study.* Lancet Oncol, 2018. **19**(12): p. 1579–1589.

139. Laubli, H., et al., *Acute heart failure due to autoimmune myocarditis under pembrolizumab treatment for metastatic melanoma.* J Immunother Cancer, 2015. **3**: p. 11.

140. Wang, D.Y., et al., *Fatal toxic effects associated with immune checkpoint inhibitors: a systematic review and meta-analysis.* JAMA Oncol, 2018. **4**(12): p. 1721–1728.

141. Michot, J.M., et al., *Immune-related adverse events with immune checkpoint blockade: a comprehensive review.* Eur J Cancer, 2016. **54**: p. 139–148.

142. Chen, D.-Y., et al., *Cardiovascular toxicity of immune checkpoint inhibitors in cancer patients: A review when cardiology meets immuno-oncology.* Journal of the Formosan Medical Association, 2019.

143. Jiang, Y., et al., *Risk and incidence of fatal adverse events associated with immune checkpoint inhibitors: a systematic review and meta-analysis.* Ther Clin Risk Manag, 2019. **15**: p. 293–302.

144. Eggermont, A.M., et al., *Adjuvant ipilimumab versus placebo after complete resection of high-risk stage III melanoma (EORTC 18071): a randomised, double-blind, phase 3 trial.* Lancet Oncol, 2015. **16**(5): p. 522–530.

145. Zimmer, L., et al., *Neurological, respiratory, musculoskeletal, cardiac and ocular side-effects of anti-PD-1 therapy.* Eur J Cancer, 2016. **60**: p. 210–225.

146. Koelzer, V.H., et al., *Systemic inflammation in a melanoma patient treated with immune checkpoint inhibitors-an autopsy study.* J Immunother Cancer, 2016. **4**: p. 13.

147. Behling, J., et al., *New-onset third-degree atrioventricular block because of autoimmune-induced myositis under treatment with anti-programmed cell death-1 (nivolumab) for metastatic melanoma.* Melanoma Res, 2017. **27**(2): p. 155–158.

148. Kolla, B.C. and M.R. Patel, *Recurrent pleural effusions and cardiac tamponade as possible manifestations of pseudoprogression associated with nivolumab therapy- a report of two cases.* J Immunother Cancer, 2016. **4**: p. 80.

149. Nghiem, P.T., et al., *PD-1 blockade with pembrolizumab in advanced merkel-cell carcinoma.* N Engl J Med, 2016. **374**(26): p. 2542–2552.

150. Horn, L., et al., *Clinical activity, safety and predictive biomarkers of the engineered antibody MPDL3280A (anti-PDL1) in non-small cell lung cancer (NSCLC): update from a phase Ia study.* Journal of Clinical Oncology, 2015. **33**(15_suppl): p. 8029–8029.

151. Spigel, D.R., et al., *FIR: Efficacy, safety, and biomarker analysis of a phase II open-label study of atezolizumab in PD-L1-selected patients with NSCLC.* J Thorac Oncol, 2018. **13**(11): p. 1733–1742.

152. Lyon, A.R., et al., *Immune checkpoint inhibitors and cardiovascular toxicity.* Lancet Oncol, 2018. **19**(9): p. e447–e458.

153. Michel, L. and T. Rassaf, *Cardio-oncology: need for novel structures.* Eur J Med Res, 2019. **24**(1): p. 1.

154. Upadhrasta, S., et al., *Managing cardiotoxicity associated with immune checkpoint inhibitors.* Chronic Dis Transl Med, 2019. **5**(1): p. 6–14.

155. Altan, M., et al., *Immune checkpoint inhibitor-associated pericarditis.* J Thorac Oncol, 2019. **14**(6): p. 1102–1108.

156. Januzzi, J.L., et al., *NT-proBNP testing for diagnosis and short-term prognosis in acute destabilized heart failure: an international pooled analysis of 1256 patients: the International Collaborative of NT-proBNP Study.* Eur Heart J, 2006. **27**(3): p. 330–337.

157. Januzzi, J.L., Jr., et al., *Utility of amino-terminal pro-brain natriuretic peptide testing for prediction of 1-year mortality in patients with dyspnea treated in the emergency department.* Arch Intern Med, 2006. **166**(3): p. 315–320.

158. Bassan, R., et al., *B-type natriuretic peptide: a novel early blood marker of acute myocardial infarction in patients with chest pain and no ST-segment elevation.* Eur Heart J, 2005. **26**(3): p. 234–240.

159. Ji, C., et al., *Myocarditis in cynomolgus monkeys following treatment with immune checkpoint inhibitors.* Clin Cancer Res, 2019. **25**(15): p. 4735–4748.

160. Bando, S., et al., *Plasma brain natriuretic peptide levels are elevated in patients with cancer.* PLoS One, 2017. **12**(6): p. e0178607.

161. Chen, Q., et al., *Fatal myocarditis and rhabdomyolysis induced by nivolumab during the treatment of type B3 thymoma.* Clin Toxicol (Phila), 2018. **56**(7): p. 667–671.

162. Chang, E., A.L. Sabichi, and Y.H. Sada, *Myasthenia gravis after nivolumab therapy for squamous cell carcinoma of the bladder.* J Immunother, 2017. **40**(3): p. 114–116.

163. Kimura, T., et al., *Myasthenic crisis and polymyositis induced by one dose of nivolumab.* Cancer Sci, 2016. **107**(7): p. 1055–1058.

164. Suzuki, S., et al., *Nivolumab-related myasthenia gravis with myositis and myocarditis in Japan.* Neurology, 2017. **89**(11): p. 1127–1134.

165. Ganatra, S. and T.G. Neilan, *Immune checkpoint inhibitor-associated myocarditis.* Oncologist, 2018. **23**(8): p. 879–886.

166. Neilan, T.G., et al., *Myocarditis associated with immune checkpoint inhibitors: an expert consensus on data gaps and a call to action.* Oncologist, 2018. **23**(8): p. 874–878.

167. Tocchetti, C.G., M.R. Galdiero, and G. Varricchi, *Cardiac toxicity in patients treated with immune checkpoint inhibitors: it is now time for cardio-immuno-oncology.* J Am Coll Cardiol, 2018. **71**(16): p. 1765–1767.

168. Bami, K., et al., *Noninvasive imaging in acute myocarditis.* Curr Opin Cardiol, 2016. **31**(2): p. 217–223.

169. Akuzawa, N., et al., *Myocarditis, hepatitis, and pancreatitis in a patient with coxsackievirus A4 infection: a case report.* Virology Journal, 2014. **11**(1): p. 3.

170. Aquaro, G.D., et al., *Cardiac MR with late gadolinium enhancement in acute myocarditis with preserved systolic function: ITAMY study.* J Am Coll Cardiol, 2017. **70**(16): p. 1977–1987.

171. Friedrich, M.G., et al., *Cardiovascular magnetic resonance in myocarditis: A JACC White Paper.* J Am Coll Cardiol, 2009. **53**(17): p. 1475–1487.

172. Caforio, A.L., et al., *Current state of knowledge on aetiology, diagnosis, management, and therapy of myocarditis: a position statement of the European Society of Cardiology Working Group on Myocardial and Pericardial Diseases.* Eur Heart J, 2013. **34**(33): p. 2636–2648, 2648a–2648d.

173. Leone, O., et al., *2011 consensus statement on endomyocardial biopsy from the Association for European Cardiovascular Pathology and the Society for Cardiovascular Pathology.* Cardiovasc Pathol, 2012. **21**(4): p. 245–274.

174. Kindermann, I., et al., *Update on myocarditis.* J Am Coll Cardiol, 2012. **59**(9): p. 779–792.

175. Sharma, M., G.A. Suero-Abreu, and B. Kim, *A case of acute heart failure due to immune checkpoint blocker nivolumab.* Cardiol Res, 2019. **10**(2): p. 120–123.

176. Gibson, R., et al., *Suspected autoimmune myocarditis and cardiac conduction abnormalities with nivolumab therapy for non-small cell lung cancer.* BMJ Case Rep, 2016. **2016**.

177. Tay, R.Y., et al., *Successful use of equine anti-thymocyte globulin (ATGAM) for fulminant myocarditis secondary to nivolumab therapy.* Br J Cancer, 2017. **117**(7): p. 921–924.

178. Hassel, J.C., et al., *Combined immune checkpoint blockade (anti-PD-1/anti-CTLA-4): Evaluation and management of adverse drug reactions.* Cancer Treat Rev, 2017. **57**: p. 36–49.

179. Choueiri, T.K., et al., *Preliminary results for avelumab plus axitinib as first-line therapy in patients with advanced clear-cell renal-cell carcinoma (JAVELIN Renal 100): an open-label, dose-finding and dose-expansion, phase 1b trial.* Lancet Oncol, 2018. **19**(4): p. 451–460.

180. Neilan, T.G., et al., *The incidence, pattern, and prognostic value of left ventricular myocardial scar by late gadolinium enhancement in patients with atrial fibrillation.* J Am Coll Cardiol, 2013. **62**(23): p. 2205–2214.

181. Thompson, J.A., et al., *Management of immunotherapy-related toxicities, version 1.2019.* J Natl Compr Canc Netw, 2019. **17**(3): p. 255–289.

182. Puzanov, I., et al., *Managing toxicities associated with immune checkpoint inhibitors: consensus recommendations from the Society for Immunotherapy of Cancer (SITC) Toxicity Management Working Group.* J Immunother Cancer, 2017. **5**(1): p. 95.

183. Wang, D.Y., et al., *Cardiovascular toxicities associated with cancer immunotherapies.* Curr Cardiol Rep, 2017. **19**(3): p. 21.

184. Yancy, C.W., et al., *2013 ACCF/AHA guideline for the management of heart failure: a report of the American College of Cardiology Foundation/American Heart Association Task Force on Practice Guidelines.* J Am Coll Cardiol, 2013. **62**(16): p. e147–239.

185. Ponikowski, P., et al., *2016 ESC Guidelines for the diagnosis and treatment of acute and chronic heart failure: The Task Force for the diagnosis and treatment of acute and chronic heart failure of the European Society of Cardiology (ESC) developed with the special contribution of the Heart Failure Association (HFA) of the ESC.* Eur Heart J, 2016. **37**(27): p. 2129–2200.

186. Brahmer, J.R., et al., *Management of immune-related adverse events in patients treated with immune checkpoint inhibitor therapy: American Society of Clinical Oncology Clinical Practice Guideline.* J Clin Oncol, 2018. **36**(17): p. 1714–1768.

8 Neuronal Regulation of the Immune System in Cardiovascular Diseases

Daniela Carnevale, Giuseppe Lembo,
Marialuisa Perrotta, and Lorenzo Carnevale

CONTENTS

INTRODUCTION

In the past century, communicable diseases have significantly reduced their impact in terms of mortality and disability, while noncommunicable diseases have dramatically raised their burden. Cardiovascular diseases dominate the scenario of overall noncommunicable diseases, prevailing for mortality and morbidity worldwide (Leong et al., 2017). Although a wide array of drugs helping to counteract the onset and progression of cardiovascular diseases are available, the global burden of cardiovascular diseases is still elevated, with a consequent high impact on worldwide healthcare systems (Tzoulaki, Elliott, Kontis, & Ezzati, 2016).

DOI: 10.1201/b22824-9

The advancements obtained with basic and translational studies have unraveled new pathophysiological mechanisms involved in cardiovascular diseases, which might not be targeted by the available drugs. Because of this, the increasing awareness that unbalanced immune responses are involved in the etiology and progression of cardiovascular diseases has fueled a new area of investigation.

Cardiovascular function is profoundly affected by the nervous system, which establishes an array of reflexes formed by the autonomic nervous system (Abboud, 2010; Malpas, 2010). The search for pathophysiological roles of the sympathetic and the parasympathetic nervous systems yielded an enormous quantity of data overall, documenting that autonomic neurohumoral imbalance profoundly affects morbidity and mortality from cardiovascular diseases (Esler, 2015; Goldberger, Arora, Buckley, & Shivkumar, 2019).

The concept that the nervous and immune systems continuously interact with each other in health and disease had already been proposed at the beginning of the 1900s (Elenkov, Wilder, Chrousos, & Vizi, 2000; Ishigami, 1918; Loeper & Crouzon, 1904; Métalnikov, 1929; Nance & Sanders, 2007; Ordovas-Montanes et al., 2015). However, only recently have systematic studies described the dense and organized innervation of lymphoid organs (D. L. Felten, Felten, Carlson, Olschowka, & Livnat, 1985; D. L. Felten et al., 1984; S. Y. Felten & Olschowka, 1987; Williams & Felten, 1981) and showed the ability of immune cells to produce and respond to neurotransmitters (Reardon, Murray, & Lomax, 2018). Taken together, these observations furthered the investigation of the role of bilateral neuroimmune communication in cardiovascular homeostasis and pathophysiology.

ANATOMICAL BASIS OF NEUROIMMUNE COMMUNICATION

The brain and the immune system, as major adaptive systems, extensively communicate with each other in order to preserve body homeostasis. The mutual interaction established between the two systems involves (1) unique areas of the brain, (2) the autonomic nervous system, mainly through its sympathetic branch, and (3) the hypothalamus-pituitary-adrenal axis. Basically, these interactions create neuroanatomical and humoral routes connecting the central nervous system (CNS) to the periphery and vice versa.

The circumventricular organs (CVOs), located around the third and fourth ventricles, are particular brain regions characterized by a leaky blood–brain barrier (BBB) and dense vascularization (Ballabh, Braun, & Nedergaard, 2004). These specialized areas are points of communication between the blood, the brain parenchyma, and the cerebrospinal fluid. The peripheral nervous system (PNS) connects the CNS to peripheral tissues and is mainly organized in two branches comprising the somatic and autonomic systems. Each of these systems further consists of two arms of sensory or afferent neurons – transporting the information from the periphery to the CNS – and motor or efferent neurons, delivering responses toward the effector tissues (Reardon et al., 2018). Additionally, the humoral route regulated by the hypothalamus-pituitary-adrenal axis provides further control of neuroimmune communication in health and disease.

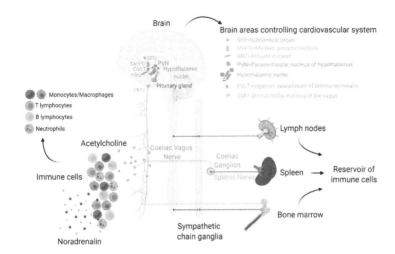

FIGURE 8.1 Neuroanatomical and humoral routes of neuroimmune communication. The peripheral nervous system represents the interface between external stimuli and internal responses by organs of our body. The neural control of the immune system is realized by specific brain regions establishing reflex arcs with arms of the sympathetic and parasympathetic nervous system capable of sensing perturbations in the peripheral environment – the circumventricular organs (CVOs) located in proximity to the cerebral ventricles and the hypothalamic-pituitary-adrenal axis (HPA), including the paraventricular nucleus of the hypothalamus (PVN). In turn, immune cells might establish further routes of neuroimmune communication by releasing neurotrasmitters, like acetylcholine and noradrenalin.

Source: Created with BioRender.com.

TABLE 8.1
The Autonomic Innervation of Lymphoid Organs Mapped Across Different Species

Lymphoid Organ	Innervation	Species	Study Outcome	References
Thymus	Sympathetic and parasympathetic nervous system	Mouse; rat	Thymus innervation originates from the sympathetic chain ganglia	Nance et al., 1987; Tollefson & Bulloch, 1990
	Sympathetic innervation	Mouse; rat	Sympathetic innervation in the thymus enters the vasculature	al-Shawaf et al., 1991; Mignini et al., 2003
	Sympathetic innervation of corticomedullary junctions	Rat	Parasympathetic innervation distributes to both cortex and medulla	al-Shawaf et al., 1991; Cavallotti et al., 1999; Vizi & Elenkov, 2002
	β-adrenergic signaling leads to maturation, proliferation, and differentiation of lymphocytes	Mouse	β-adrenergic signaling induces catecholamine synthesis, which influences T cell differentiation	Leposavić et al., 2011; Madden & Felten, 2001
	Neural control of microcirculation and immune cell dynamics	Mouse	Neuroimmune cross talk in thymus	Al-Shalan et al., 2019

(Continued)

TABLE 8.1
(Continued)

Lymphoid Organ	Innervation	Species	Study Outcome	References
Bone marrow	Parasympathetic innervation of the bone	Mouse	Bone remodeling	Jung et al., 2017; Maryanovich et al., 2018
	Sympathetic innervation leads to osteogenesis suppression, modulation of hematopoietic activity	Mouse; human	Chronic stress and increased sympathetic tone upregulate HSC proliferation and osteogenesis	Heidt et al., 2014; Jan et al., 2017; Takeda et al., 2002
	Sympathetic innervation leads to monocytopoiesis	Mouse	Increased sympathetic tone stimulates monocytopoiesis	Dutta et al., 2015; Swirski et al., 2009
	Cholinergic signaling leads to glucocorticoid-related mediators, leading to HSC mobilization	Mouse	Demonstration of a brain-bone marrow axis mediated by circulating hormones	Pierce et al., 2017
Lymph nodes	Sympathetic innervation	Mouse; rat; guinea pig; cat; pig; human	Study of differential innervation in mammalian lymph nodes	D. L. Felten et al., 1984; Fink & Weihe, 1988
	Innervation of medullary and paracortical structures	Rat	Electron microscopy characterization of rat lymph nodes	Novotny & Kliche, 1986
	Sympathetic nervous system leads to T cell zones, not B cells	Mouse; rat; guinea pig; cat; pig; human	Study of differential innervation in mammalian lymph nodes	D. L. Felten et al., 1984; Fink & Weihe, 1988; Novotny & Kliche, 1986; Sloan et al., 2007
	Sympathetic nerve network leads to fine regulation of immune response	Macaque	Stress induces remodeling of lymph nodes innervation	Sloan et al., 2007; Sloan et al., 2006
	β2-adrenergic signaling leads to regulation of tissue inflammation	Mouse	β2-adrenergic signaling regulates lymphocyte trafficking and inflammation	Druzd et al., 2017; Nakai et al., 2014; Suzuki et al., 2016
Spleen	Mesenteric celiac ganglion leads to sympathetic fibers, leading to the spleen	Mouse; rat	Spleen sympathetic innervation is necessary to elicit the immune response	Bellinger et al., 1989; Carnevale et al., 2014
	Dense sympathetic fibers lead to T, B, and dendritic cells	Rat	Anatomic study of spleen innervation related to the immune germinal centers	Ackerman et al., 1987; Bellinger et al., 1987; D. L. Felten et al., 1987; D. L. Felten et al., 1985
	Sparse sympathetic fibers lead to red pulp	Mouse	Anatomic study of spleen innervation in the red pulp	Williams & Felten, 1981
	Nervous signal leads to regulation of antibodies and adaptive immunity	Mouse	Autonomic splenic innervation is necessary to recruit immune response to various stimuli	Bronte & Pittet, 2013; Carnevale et al., 2014; Carnevale et al., 2016; Cortez-Retamozo et al., 2013; Swirski et al., 2009; Vasamsetti et al., 2018

THE SYSTEM OF CIRCUMVENTRICULAR ORGANS IN THE BRAIN

When perturbations affect peripheral tissues' homeostasis, an alarm message is conveyed to the brain. Blood-borne metabolites, bacteria-derived substances, or host-derived cytokines are perceived by the brain as "danger" or "alarm" signals in those regions where the BBB isolates the CNS less tightly (Ballabh et al., 2004; Banks, 2015). Characterized by an extremely regulated permeability, the BBB ensures that neurons are protected from potentially dangerous substances. Nevertheless, in the CVOs, which are brain regions that monitor the external milieu, the endothelium developed a structural adaptation of the BBB in order to readily detect dangerous substances from the periphery. From the anatomical point of view, the CVOs comprise two groups of brain regions characterized by different functions, principally sensory and secretory roles.

The sensory brain regions comprise the subfornical organ (SFO), the organum vasculosum lamina terminalis (OVLT), and the area postrema (AP), and they have been extensively described as crucial regulators of neuroimmune communication (Reardon et al., 2018). Interestingly, much of the evidence coming from work performed in the last decade underlines a key role of CVOs in cardiovascular diseases (Cancelliere, Black, & Ferguson, 2015; Johnson & Gross, 1993; Siso, Jeffrey, & Gonzalez, 2010). The SFO has been characterized by the abundant expression of angiotensin II (Ang II) receptors, while the OVLT neurons express osmoreceptors that sense extracellular solute concentrations. As an example, sodium/salt load is perceived by this group of neurons. This anatomical architecture allows the SFO, neurons of the OVLT, and the median preoptic nucleus to elaborate the peripheral alterations and transmit information on blood volume, pressure, and extracellular fluid osmolality to the brain (Johnson & Xue, 2018). A further level of control over cardiovascular homeostasis and body fluid is exerted by descending projections of the SFO and OVLT, which innervate the paraventricular nucleus (PVN) of the hypothalamus. Also receiving ascending input from the hindbrain, the PVN establishes an integrative brain station of cardiovascular control. Further neuroanatomical regulation is realized through the axonal projections of the AP, which innervate the nucleus tractus solitarius (NTS) and the dorsal motor nucleus (DMN) of the vagus nerve, known as a crucial regulator of cardiovascular function (Johnson & Xue, 2018).

The brain establishes an additional connection with the periphery by projecting sympathetic premotor neurons from the PVN to the intermediolateral cell column of the spinal cord, either directly or indirectly via the rostral ventrolateral medulla. This latter brain region emerged as an important area controlling the response to various peripheral perturbations – including hypotension, hypoglycemia, hypoxia, hypercapnia, and bacterial infection – by activation of neurons in the locus coeruleus (LC) (Guyenet, 2006; Guyenet et al., 2013). Recognized as the main cluster of noradrenergic neurons in the brain, the LC is characterized by unique functions of setting arousal and attention and controlling noradrenergic firing in various brain areas as well as toward peripheral tissues (D'Andrea et al., 2015; Guyenet, 2006). Additionally, the intermediolateral cell column gives rise to the preganglionic neurons of sympathetic axons leaving the CNS and typically mediating responses to alterations in cardiovascular function and/or fluid balance.

Most of the work done in this field has characterized the neuroanatomical routes and molecular mechanisms underlying the brain's response to peripheral perturbations in cardiovascular function. Nonetheless, a new branch of investigation has started to explore the ways in which psychosocial stressors might affect cardiovascular homeostasis through the modulation of neural reflexes and immune function (Nahrendorf & Swirski, 2015).

NEUROIMMUNE COMMUNICATION THROUGH THE AUTONOMIC NERVOUS SYSTEM

Sensory Routes of the ANS

The periphery signals inflammatory and immune reactions to the brain through afferent neurons of the autonomic and somatosensory peripheral nervous systems comprising receptors for inflammatory and microbial peptides. The two major neural routes achieving the preceding functions are represented by vagal and spinal neurons.

The vagus nerve belongs to the series of cranial nerves and is the longest nerve in the body. Innervating a wide variety of tissues, including the heart, the gastrointestinal tract, and the lungs, the vagus nerve is formed by approximately 70% afferent axons, whose activation can be triggered by a multitude of stimuli, ranging from micronutrients to mechanosensitive receptors in the respiratory and cardiovascular systems (Reardon et al., 2018). The nodose and jugular ganglia engulf cell bodies of the vagus nerve that, once activated in the periphery, regulate synaptic transmission at the central level in the NTS. Hence, the CNS integrates the signals received from the periphery, transmitting neuronal inputs along the DMN, where preganglionic neurons of the efferent neurons reside, and establishing a reflex modulation of target tissues. Besides being one of the major regulators of reflexes involved in cardiovascular function, the vagus nerve is a crucial modulator of reflex responses to peripheral inflammatory and immune challenges. It has been demonstrated that inflammatory mediators like pathogen-associated molecular patterns (PAMPs) (Liu, Xu, Park, Berta, & Ji, 2010; Qi et al., 2011; Tse, Chow, Leung, Wong, & Wise, 2014), danger-associated molecular patterns (DAMPs), ATPs, and cytokines promptly activate the vagus nerve (Reardon et al., 2018). A huge amount of work has utilized the prototype activator of afferent vagus nerve – the endotoxin of gram-negative bacteria, lipopolysaccharide (LPS) – to advance the knowledge of the neuroimmune circuits mediated by the vagus nerve (Reardon et al., 2018). At the molecular level, like other PAMPs, LPS contains a molecular motif with a binding ability to specific Toll-like receptors (TLR). Interestingly, TLRs are expressed both by afferent neurons of the peripheral nervous system and by immune cells, thus suggesting that this molecular pathway might mediate neuroimmune interactions. The TLRs are an ancient family of receptor proteins that has been evolutionarily conserved, and among the multitude of family members, the selective receptor for LPS – TLR4 – has been characterized as being uniquely expressed by vagal afferent neurons with the crucial function of sensing inflammation in the periphery (Hosoi, Okuma, Matsuda, & Nomura, 2005). On this basis, an animal subjected to a subdiaphragmatic vagotomy failed to activate neurons in the NTS in response to a peripheral challenge of LPS (Laye et al., 1995), thus indicating that afferent neurons of the vagus nerve provide a

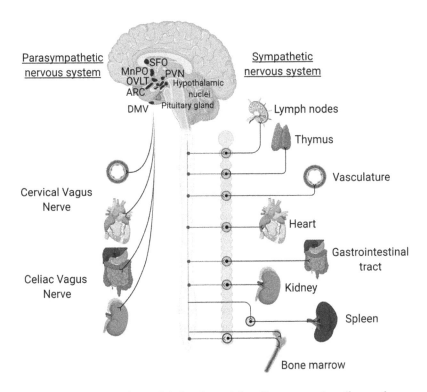

FIGURE 8.2 Neural circuits modulating the activity of immune and cardiovascular organs. The anatomical distribution of the two branches of the autonomic nervous system – sympathetic and parasympathetic – is related to the location of innervated organs. This scheme represents the neural circuits departing from brain nuclei and innervating typical cardiovascular districts and immune organs. Cell bodies of the vagus nerve are located in the dorsal motor nucleus of the vagus (DMV), whereas the sympathetic nervous system extends through the spinal cord to target organs by spinal nerves that synapse with postsynaptic neurons at the level of the ganglia. These neurons project directly onto targeted organs.

Source: Created with BioRender.com.

route for detecting danger in the periphery and signaling to the brain, which in turn integrates immunomodulating reflex functions.

The second major route of afferent neuroimmune communication is represented by neurons whose cell bodies reside in the dorsal root ganglion and respond to various perturbations in the peripheral milieu – like physical, thermal, or chemical stimuli. This somatosensory pathway of the peripheral nervous system comprises afferent neurons passing through the spinal cord and expressing receptors for inflammatory mediators (Reardon et al., 2018). The primary function of these neurons consists in sensing noxious stimuli in the periphery and transferring the related information to the brain. The functions of these neurons as modulators of the local environment through the release of neuropeptides have been described as well. As an example, the peripheral terminals of spinal afferent neurons have been shown to release substance

P and calcitonin gene–related peptide (CGRP) (Baral et al., 2018; Chiu et al., 2013; Riol-Blanco et al., 2014).

Innervation of Immune Organs

Nearly 40 years ago, labeling techniques of anterograde and retrograde neurons were utilized to map the hardwired connections of sympathetic and peptidergic innervation in primary, secondary, and mucosa-associated lymphoid tissues (D. L. Felten et al., 1985; S. Y. Felten & Olschowka, 1987; Williams & Felten, 1981). This work shed light on the potential routes of neural regulation of immune responses. Among of the earliest evidence suggesting the existence of a mutual structural and functional interaction established between nervous and immune systems was the histological observation that primary and secondary lymphoid organs are densely enriched in nerve fibers (D. L. Felten et al., 1985; D. L. Felten et al., 1984; S. Y. Felten & Olschowka, 1987; Williams & Felten, 1981).

Thymus

The autonomic nervous system densely innervates the thymus (Nance, Hopkins, & Bieger, 1987; Tollefson & Bulloch, 1990). Fibers of the sympathetic nervous system penetrate the thymus through the perivascular network, forming branches into the profound cortical region, upper cortical and subcapsular regions, septa, corticomedullary junction, and medulla (al-Shawaf, Kendall, & Cowen, 1991; Mignini, Streccioni, & Amenta, 2003). By using tyrosine hydroxylase (TH) staining, it has been shown that noradrenergic innervation of the thymus consists of a high density of nerve fibers near the corticomedullary junction and fewer in the subcapsule and cortex areas (al-Shawaf et al., 1991; Cavallotti, Artico, & Cavallotti, 1999; Vizi & Elenkov, 2002). The release of norepinephrine by sympathetic nervous system fibers activates β-adrenergic signaling in thymocytes, with inhibitory effects on the maturation, proliferation, and differentiation of thymocytes (Leposavić, Pilipović, & Perišić, 2011; Madden & Felten, 2001). Additionally, a close association of nerve fibers with blood vessels has been observed, indicating that neural signals control blood circulation and immune cell dynamics inside the thymus (Al-Shalan, Hu, Nicholls, Greene, & Ma, 2019).

Bone Marrow

Autonomic nervous system innervation also entangles the bone skeletal structure and penetrates the marrow, entering the deep regions that comprise the hematopoietic stem cell (HSC) niches. Here the innervation participates in the hematopoietic activity involved in the generation of all blood cell lineages. Overall, sympathetic, parasympathetic, and sensory fibers form a dense innervation that spreads through bone and marrow and provides the anatomical basis for the neural regulation of processes like bone formation, hematopoiesis, and immune functions. It is usually reported that parasympathetic and sympathetic innervations control different functions, whereby the parasympathetic nerves are recognized as primary regulators of bone remodeling (Jung, Levesque, & Ruitenberg, 2017; Maryanovich et al., 2018), while sympathetic nerves are more involved in the suppression of bone formation (Takeda et al., 2002) and the fine modulation of hematopoietic activity (Heidt et al., 2014).

Bone marrow innervation is also responsible for the fine-tuning of functions depending on circadian rhythm. It has been observed that, in physiological conditions, HSCs are in a quiescent state. Interestingly, the expression of genes implicated in the retention and egression of HSCs from the bone marrow (Maestroni, 1998; Mendez-Ferrer, Lucas, Battista, & Frenette, 2008) is under the control of noradrenalin, whose release is dependent on circadian oscillations. In pathological conditions, the sympathetic nerves that engulf the bone marrow are recruited to activate HSCs (Katayama et al., 2006). A typical condition known to recruit HSCs through the sympathetic nervous system is the development of hematological malignancies (Jan, Ebert, & Jaiswal, 2017). More recently, it has also been observed that sympathetic nervous system stimulation of hematopoiesis is a crucial process involved in the onset and progression of cardiovascular diseases. In response to stressful stimuli challenging the cardiovascular system, sympathetic innervation primes the mobilization of HSCs that migrate to the spleen to contribute to extramedullary monocytopoiesis, a process recognized as important for guaranteeing the supply of immune cells to the myocardium (Dutta et al., 2015; Swirski et al., 2009). On another note, evidence also highlighted that brain-mediated cholinergic signals might determine HSC mobilization through glucocorticoid-related mediators (Pierce et al., 2017).

Lymph Nodes

The architecture of lymph nodes comprises the vasculature and lymphatic channels, which enter the medulla by branching into parenchymal vessels. The noradrenergic innervation entangles the small vessels of the medulla in a network of nerve fibers (D. L. Felten et al., 1984; Fink & Weihe, 1988). Moreover, nerves entering the medullary and paracortical structures but not associated with blood vessels have also been described (Novotny & Kliche, 1986). On the contrary, no innervation has been observed in the nodular regions or the germinal centers (D. L. Felten et al., 1984). Hence, the fibers of the sympathetic nervous system entangle the T cell zones (D. L. Felten et al., 1984; Fink & Weihe, 1988; Novotny & Kliche, 1986) but do not innervate the B cell–rich germinal centers (D. L. Felten et al., 1984; Sloan et al., 2007). The close contact of noradrenergic neural networks and immune cells provides a route for fine regulation of the immune response (Sloan et al., 2007; Sloan, Tarara, Capitanio, & Cole, 2006). In physiological conditions, it has been observed that noradrenalin release in lymph nodes is dependent on the circadian activation of adrenergic nerves. This phenomenon contributes to the regulation of physiological diurnal recirculation of lymphocytes and is dependent on β2-adrenergic receptor (Druzd et al., 2017; Suzuki, Hayano, Nakai, Furuta, & Noda, 2016). Experiments conducted in animal models of T cell–mediated inflammation showed that neural regulation of immune response is established through β2-adrenergic signals in lymph nodes. In more detail, it was demonstrated that the β2-adrenergic signaling is responsible for the restriction of T cell egress, thus contributing to the regulation of the ensuing tissue inflammation (Nakai, Hayano, Furuta, Noda, & Suzuki, 2014).

Spleen

The spleen is a secondary lymphoid organ exclusively innervated by noradrenergic fibers branching from the splenic nerve, whose cell bodies are engulfed in the superior mesenteric celiac ganglion (Bellinger, Felten, Lorton, & Felten, 1989; Carnevale et al., 2014). This neural network extends to the white and red pulp and the marginal zone, with nerve endings in close proximity to splenic T cells, B cells, and dendritic cells (DCs) (Ackerman, Felten, Bellinger, & Felten, 1987; Bellinger, Felten, Collier, & Felten, 1987; D. L. Felten et al., 1987; D. L. Felten et al., 1985). Red pulp innervation is instead sparse and mainly composed of scattered fibers (Williams & Felten, 1981). Investigations conducted to date have repeatedly shown that no direct cholinergic innervation is present in the spleen (D. L. Felten et al., 1987; S. Y. Felten & Olschowka, 1987; Nance & Sanders, 2007; Straub, 2004; Vida, Peña, Deitch, & Ulloa, 2011; Wang et al., 2003).

Numerous immune functions take place in the spleen, among which the regulation of adaptive immunity and production of antibodies are the most commonly known (Bronte & Pittet, 2013). Additionally, innate immune responses are shaped in the spleen, which has been recognized as a monocyte reservoir that might be recruited in response to tissue injury (Carnevale et al., 2014; Carnevale et al., 2016; Cortez-Retamozo et al., 2013; Swirski et al., 2009; Vasamsetti et al., 2018). The splenic innervation participates as a major regulator of the various immune-related processes by both autonomic efferent and sensory afferent fibers (Andersson & Tracey, 2012). While initially focused on immune and inflammatory processes, researchers in this area have begun to investigate the implications of neural regulation by the spleen in cardiovascular diseases (Carnevale, 2020; Carnevale & Lembo, 2020).

The Hypothalamus-Pituitary-Adrenal Axis

A substantial number of studies have demonstrated that the neuroendocrine and immune systems reciprocally interact to promote mutual regulation in the host organism. One of the earliest observations highlighted the capability of neuroendocrine factors – steroid hormones – to affect the immune system, whereby hormonal alterations influenced the size of the thymus (Butts & Sternberg, 2008; Selye, 1941). Another finding showed that physical stressors, like restraint, or psychological stressors triggered the activation of the hypothalamic-pituitary-adrenal (HPA) axis and resulted in shrinkage of the thymus and other lymphoid organs (Butts & Sternberg, 2008; Selye & Fortier, 1949). It is interesting to note that, several decades later, similar stressors (physical or mental) have been found to have profound effects on the cardiovascular system through immune-mediated functions (Marvar & Harrison, 2012). More specifically, it was shown that mice exposed to chronic stressor conditions develop hypertension and related target organ damage. However, when the same protocol of chronic stress was applied to mice devoid of lymphocytes (*Rag1*⁻⁻ mice), the blood pressure response was significantly attenuated as was target organ damage (Marvar & Harrison, 2012; Marvar et al., 2012), thus indicating that stress-mediated activation of the HPA axis promotes cardiovascular responses by modulating immune function. Interestingly, the effect of chronic stress on the cardiovascular system is not restricted to blood pressure regulation; chronic stress also affects other consequences of increased cardiovascular risk. In fact, another study performed some years later showed that mice experiencing chronic stress are more susceptible to atherosclerosis and myocardial infarction (Heidt et al., 2014). The investigation into the molecular mechanisms of this HPA-cardiac axis further revealed that the effect was mediated by adrenergic signaling in the bone marrow (Heidt et al., 2014), thus indicating that a complex relationship between the HPA axis, immune organs, and the cardiovascular system does exist.

RELEVANCE OF NEUROIMMUNE INTERACTIONS FOR DISEASE

NEUROIMMUNE ACTIVATION AND INFECTIONS: THE CHOLINERGIC INFLAMMATORY REFLEX

The process of neuroimmune interaction is crucial for the establishment of adaptation to challenging stressors for the immune system. One of these situations is represented by infections, during which the splenic neural innervation promptly establishes immune-modulating functions (Chavan, Pavlov, & Tracey, 2017). Sensory neurons situated in the proximity of immune cells perceive peripheral inflammatory stimuli and respond to perturbations in the immune environment, signaling the "danger" to the brain. One of the classical stimuli provoking a reaction of the immune system is the bacterial endotoxin peptide LPS. The spleen plays a crucial role in balancing the acute response to this type of inflammatory and immunological stimulus by mediating neuroimmune functions (Rosas-Ballina et al., 2011). While it is well-known that inflammatory challenges like LPS provoke a storm of pro-inflammatory cytokine production through local and/or systemic immune responses, neural influences have been shown to potently modulate this phenomenon (Borovikova et al., 2000; Chavan et al., 2017), thus revealing new avenues of therapeutic relevance.

Along these lines, a fascinating field of research has begun to investigate the possibility that by modulating the electrical activity of the neural connections reaching the spleen, it might be possible to tune the immune response. With an elegant set of experiments, it has been demonstrated that the electrical stimulation of efferent fibers of the vagus nerve is able to control LPS-induced endotoxemia by contrasting the release of pro-inflammatory cytokines, like tumor necrosis factor (TNF) (Borovikova et al., 2000). The perturbations in peripheral homeostasis induced by LPS recruit afferent activity of the vagus nerve, which in turn signals the danger to the brain. The neural activity of specific brain areas allows the integration of the reflex response established by efferent vagus nerve activity to control peripheral cytokine levels and inflammation (Chavan et al., 2017). The ending effector arm of this neuronal reflex circuit consists of a noradrenergic nerve – the splenic nerve – which branches from the celiac mesenteric ganglion and entangles the spleen, where it potently modulates the functions of splenic immune cells (Rosas-Ballina et al., 2011).

The nerve endings of the splenic nerve, which are catecholaminergic terminals, are strictly intertwined with immune cell areas in close proximity to lymphocytes, regulating a variety of functions. Relevant to the control of infective challenges, a specific subpopulation of T cells expressing choline acetyltransferase (ChAT), the enzyme responsible for acetylcholine biosynthesis, has been identified in the spleen (Rosas-Ballina et al., 2011). When the vagus efferent is electrically stimulated, the splenic nerve discharges the release of noradrenalin in the spleen. In turn, the neurotransmitter binds $\beta2$-adrenergic receptor expressed by the ChAT T cells, promoting the consequent release of acetylcholine (Rosas-Ballina et al., 2011). Interestingly, a unique population of macrophages expressing the $\alpha7$ nicotinic acetylcholine receptor ($\alpha7$nAChR) was discovered, which, once activated, transduces anti-inflammatory intracellular signaling (Wang et al., 2003). Thus, the overall effect of vagus nerve stimulation is transduced by noradrenergic-mediated acetylcholine release from ChAT T cells and, hence, by the anti-inflammatory effect of acetylcholine on α7nAChRs expressed by macrophages. This circuit was termed the "cholinergic inflammatory pathway."

Neuroimmune Activation and Cardiovascular Disease

A general perspective shared by many cardiologists considers the so-called "fight or flight" response coordinated by the autonomic nervous system to be the only reflex regulation of cardiovascular function. Along these lines, a typical hallmark characterizing many cardiovascular diseases is the imbalance between the sympathetic and parasympathetic arms of the autonomic nervous system. Because the renin-angiotensin-aldosterone system (RAAS) represents the other master regulator of cardiovascular functions, the investigation of interactions between the two systems became an object of interest for cardiovascular science (Coffman, 2011). However, for long time, the potential interaction with an additional system – the immune system – was overlooked.

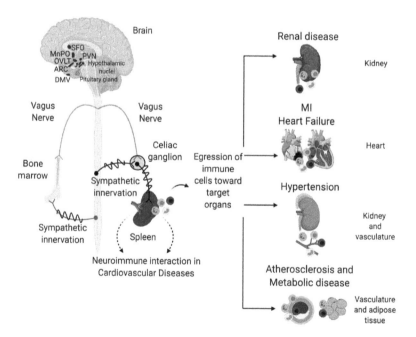

FIGURE 8.3 Neuroimmune interactions in cardiovascular disease. Schematic of the neural modulation of innate and adaptive immune cells, established by the parasympathetic and sympathetic nervous systems, in the setting of major cardiovascular diseases, like renal disease, hypertension, myocardial infarction, heart failure, atherosclerosis, and metabolic disorders. This appears as a newly identified route of regulation of cardiovascular function in health and disease.

Source: Created with BioRender.com.

TABLE 8.2

The Specific Neuroimmune Pathways Associated with Different Cardiovascular Diseases

Cardiovascular Disease	Model	Species	Neuroimmune Mechanism	Study Outcome	References
Hypertension	Chronic peripheral Ang II infusion	Mouse	CD8+ T cell activation	Ang II–induced hypertension is mediated by activation of C8+ T cells, but not B cells	Guzik et al., 2007; Trott et al., 2014
	ICV Ang II infusion	Mouse	Effect on brain circumventricular organs resulting in T cell activation	Ang II hypertensive stimulus response is originated in the brain CVOs	Ganta et al., 2005; Marvar et al., 2010
	Chronic peripheral Ang II infusion	Mouse	Cholinergic inflammatory reflex enhances splenic sympathetic outflow, increases PlGF expression, and mediates T cell activation	PlGF is a key neuroimmune mediator in the Ang II–recruited adrenergic splenic pathway	Carnevale et al., 2014; Carnevale et al., 2016
	Chronic DOCA-salt administration	Mouse	Cholinergic inflammatory reflex enhances splenic sympathetic outflow, increases PlGF expression, and mediates T cell activation	PlGF is a key neuroimmune mediator in the DOCA-salt-recruited adrenergic splenic pathway	Carnevale et al., 2016; Perrotta, 2018
Renal disease	Renal ischemia reperfusion	Rat	Administration of cholinergic agonists reduces inflammation and renal leukocyte infiltrate	Administration of cholinergic agonists reduces renal injury in vagotomized rats	Yeboah et al., 2008
	Renal ischemia reperfusion	Mouse	Ultrasound stimulation reduces circulating and kidney-derived cytokines in IRI	Ultrasound stimulation induces beneficial effects mediated by hematopoietic α7nAChR cells	Gigliotti et al., 2015; Gigliotti et al., 2013
	Sepsis-induced acute kidney injury	Mouse	Cholinergic stimulation	Protective effects on renal damage	Chatterjee et al., 2012
	Chronic peripheral Ang II infusion	Mouse; rat	Bilateral renal denervation	Blunted blood pressure response, no renal inflammation protection	Banek et al., 2018; Xiao et al., 2015

(Continued)

TABLE 8.2
(Continued)

Cardiovascular Disease	Model	Species	Neuroimmune Mechanism	Study Outcome	References
Heart failure	Acute myocardial infarction	Mouse	Sympathetic signaling in bone marrow	Replenishment of splenic monocytes	Dutta et al., 2015; Swirski et al., 2009
	Acute myocardial infarction	Mouse; human	CCR2 signaling in splenic monocytes	CCR2 promotes egression of splenic monocytes involved in the healing of ischemic myocardium	Heidt et al., 2014; Swirski et al., 2009
	Acute myocardial infarction	Mouse	Superior cervical ganglia denervation	No effect on acute ischemic cardiac injury, but reduces the inflammatory infiltrate in long-term remodeling	Ziegler et al., 2018
	Heart failure with preserved ejection fraction	Mouse; human	Cardiac resident and recruited innate immune cells	Balance of local macrophage proliferation and monocyte recruitment	Epelman et al., 2014; Hulsmans et al., 2018
Metabolic disorder	Type 1 diabetes	Mouse	Sympathetic innervation of pancreas	Sympathetic inhibition results in protective effects on pancreatic cells	Christoffersson et al., 2020
	High-fat diet induced obesity	Mouse; human	Neuroimmune regulation of adipose tissue by netrin-1	Netrin-1 guides macrophage infiltration and retention in adipose tissue and insulin resistance	Ramkhelawon et al., 2014
	Types 1 and 2 diabetes	Mouse; human	Sympathetic innervation of the spleen	Sympathetic denervation inhibits myelopoiesis in the spleen and leads to reduced atherosclerotic plaques	Vasamsetti et al., 2018
Atherosclerosis	Ldlr−/− atherosclerosis	Mouse	Netrin-1 in the aorta	Netrin-1 induces plaque macrophage retention	van Gils et al., 2012
	Ldlr−/− atherosclerosis	Mouse; human	Cholinergic α7nAChR signaling in bone marrow	α7nAChR deletion in bone marrow exacerbates atherosclerotic process	Johansson et al., 2014
	ApoE−/−Sleep disorders	Mouse	Hypothalamic hypocretin and leucocytes in atherosclerosis	Increase in Ly6Chi monocytes resulting in larger atherosclerotic lesions, correlated with higher hypothalamic hypocretin and leucocytosis	McAlpine et al., 2019
	ApoE−/−Physical exercise	Mouse; human	Hematopoietic activity and atherosclerosis	Physical exercise decreases hematopoiesis and reduces atherosclerosis	Frodermann et al., 2019

In fact, until recently, the influence of immunity on cardiovascular function was mostly considered to be a peripheral, bystander effect that ensued when tissue damage induced by cardiovascular disease progressed. Only in more recent times has it been recognized that the immune system is an active player implicated in the etiology of cardiovascular disease itself (Drummond, Vinh, Guzik, & Sobey, 2019; Nahrendorf, 2018).

Hypertension

Inflammatory and immune mechanisms have been associated with hypertension for a long time (Ebringer & Doyle, 1970; Hilme, Herlitz, Soderstrom, & Hansson, 1989; Suryaprabha, Padma, & Rao, 1984). Usually, in experimental models of hypertension and in patients, immune and inflammatory reactions have mostly been regarded to be a result of target organ damage ensuing from elevated blood pressure. With the emergence of mechanistic studies investigating the role of immune and inflammatory processes in hypertension, the scenario started to change. *Rag1*$^{-/-}$ mice, which are genetically devoid of T and B lymphocytes, were used to test the hypothesis that the adaptive immune system is involved in the hypertensive response to challenges like angiotensin II and salt-sensitive deoxycorticosterone acetate (DOCA). The finding that mice devoid of lymphocytes (*Rag1*$^{-/-}$) are protected from blood pressure increases in response to various stimuli (Guzik et al., 2007) changed the perspective and paved the way for an intense field of research. In fact, successive studies clarified that CD8 T cells are crucial for hypertension, as CD8 knockout mice, but not CD4 knockout mice, are protected from the typical blood pressure response observed upon chronic infusion of angiotensin II (Trott et al., 2014). Further supporting the involvement of T cells in hypertension, it was shown that severe, combined immunodeficiency protects mice from the development of hypertension (Crowley et al., 2010). The observation that similar effects were present in rats provided information that the involvement of adaptive immunity in hypertension is shared among species (Mattson et al., 2013). Recent provocative findings published by Seniuk and colleagues emphasized that, in their experimental setting, *Rag1*$^{-/-}$ mice surprisingly lost the phenotype of blunted hypertensive response to angiotensin II and a high-salt diet (Seniuk et al., 2020). However, a critical appraisal of these findings (Madhur, Kirabo, Guzik, & Harrison, 2020; Rios, Montezano, & Touyz, 2020; Seniuk et al., 2020) does not deny the notion that the immune system has a role in hypertension, which has been proven by a multitude of published studies (Drummond et al., 2019), but rather it confirms the need for further investigation of immune mechanisms that in some conditions may escape the protection observed in the absence of lymphocytes. In parallel to the investigations of the immune mechanisms involved in hypertension, this field of research was further enriched by interest in the search for potential integration of these new concepts with the traditional mechanisms known to regulate blood pressure.

The autonomic nervous system is a potent regulator of cardiovascular function, and, as such, blood pressure levels are finely tuned by an adequate balance of sympathetic and parasympathetic drives (Esler, 2015; Malpas, 2010). As an example, it has been well described that key physiological parameters important for blood pressure balance – like vascular tone and renal sodium excretion – are under neural control, typically regulated by the sympathetic nervous system (Abboud, 1982;

Coffman, 2011; Johnson & Xue, 2018). Hence, investigation of the interconnections existing between neural regulatory systems, immune mechanisms, and cardiovascular function became an appealing perspective. Following on this, one of the first experiments underlining the existence of neuroimmune-modulating functions of vasoactive agents showed that the intracerebral ventricular infusion of angiotensin II activates the peripheral release of cytokines through the sympathetic nervous system (Abboud, Harwani, & Chapleau, 2012; Ganta et al., 2005). Relevant for hypertensive disease, it has been shown that a selective lesion in brain regions with a permeable BBB – the SFO – hinders the typical hypertensive response to chronic infusion of angiotensin II (Marvar et al., 2010). Interestingly, with a lesioned SFO, mice were unable to prime T cell activation and promote their infiltration into the vasculature (Marvar et al., 2010), thus indicating that neural control of immune activation in hypertension does exist.

Few years later, a series of experiments demonstrated that the brain controls the immune responses in the spleen during hypertensive challenges (Carnevale, 2020). By directly assessing peripheral nerve activity through microneurographic recording of the splenic nerve, it was found that angiotensin II enhances sympathetic outflow in the spleen, in a way similar to that observed in the renal area (Carnevale et al., 2016). Selective denervation of the neural connection existing between the brain and the spleen protected mice from hypertension induced by various stimuli, thus unraveling a crucial role of this neuroimmune reflex in hypertension (Carnevale et al., 2014; Carnevale et al., 2016). By further dissecting this newly identified neural pathway, it was shown that, at odds with expectations, the preganglionic neuron that controls the splenic nerve did not emerge from the spinal cord at the level of the intermediolateral gray column, where the majority of sympathetic nerves involved in cardiovascular regulation are connected to the brain (Guyenet, 2006; Johnson & Xue, 2018). In fact, by combining surgical techniques and microneurographic approaches, it was shown that hypertensive challenges – like angiotensin II and DOCA-salt – activate sympathetic outflow on the splenic nerve through an efferent vagus nerve connection, located in the celiac mesenteric ganglion (Carnevale et al., 2016). Mechanistic studies also uncovered the molecular mediators of the identified neuroimmune connection (Carnevale, 2020). By promoting noradrenalin release in the spleen, the neuroimmune drive recruited by hypertensive stimuli increases the expression of an angiogenic growth factor called placental growth factor (PlGF) (Carnevale et al., 2014; Perrotta et al., 2018), revealing a potential new therapeutic target for hypertension.

Renal Disease

Mechanisms related to the handling of renal sodium, renin secretion, and the renal vasculature are considered a mainstay regulator of the complex balance required for blood pressure regulation (Coffman, 2011). In addition, renal mechanisms interact with the autonomic nervous system to finely tune cardiovascular function. When one of these systems is affected by perturbing challenges, an array of counterregulatory mechanisms is set up to try to maintain balance and to preserve cardiovascular function and blood pressure homeostasis. The persistence of perturbations in these regulatory mechanisms represents one of the most well-known factors contributing to the development of hypertension. In addition, the development of renal failure may ensue from chronic hypertension and is, in fact, recognized as a typical sign of target organ damage. Innervation of the kidneys is made up of afferent and efferent arms belonging to the autonomic nervous system, and together they participate to establish of one of the most studied and well-known reflex systems in our organism (DiBona & Kopp, 1997). Hypertension is often accompanied by enhanced renal sympathetic outflow in experimental models and humans, hence the interest in developing clinical approaches to renal denervation for lowering blood pressure. A recent interesting area of research is the investigation of the mechanisms underlying the neural modulation of renal function and associated inflammatory and immune reactions (Okusa, Rosin, & Tracey, 2017).

Inflammation is an important process involved in the pathophysiology of injury ensuing from renal ischemia reperfusion. Local inflammatory reactions are regulated by vagus nerve–mediated central effects. In fact, it has been shown that electrical or pharmacological stimulation of the vagus-mediated cholinergic inflammatory pathway suppresses the burst of pro-inflammatory cytokine release. Experiments performed in rats subjected to bilateral renal ischemia reperfusion showed that pretreatment with cholinergic agonists dampened the ensuing renal damage (Yeboah et al., 2008). Interestingly, it has also been shown that functional nicotinic acetylcholine receptors are expressed by rat proximal tubule epithelial cells (Yeboah et al., 2008). More recently, it has been shown that ultrasound exposure before renal ischemia reperfusion preserved kidney structure and function by modulating inflammatory and immune response (Gigliotti et al., 2013). Additionally, in mice with α7nAChR blockade or genetic deficiency, beneficial effects of the ultrasound stimulation protocol were abolished (Gigliotti et al., 2013). Further, by utilizing mice generated by bone marrow transplantation between wild-type and α7nAChR$^{-/-}$, it was shown that ultrasound-induced protection required hematopoietic but not parenchymal α7nAChR (Gigliotti et al., 2015). Acute kidney injury can also result from sepsis, and no effective treatment is available for patients. Protective effects of cholinergic stimulation have been observed in this critical health condition as well (Chatterjee et al., 2012), thus suggesting that neural pathways modulate inflammatory processes involved in renal disease from different causes. Taken together, the preceding observations indicate that the cholinergic inflammatory pathway participates in the protective response and is an appealing new therapeutic strategy (Gigliotti et al., 2013).

Future studies will be necessary to untangle the relationships established between the renal system, autonomic nervous system, and immunity. Along these lines, a relevant study that opens new perspectives showed that renal denervation, besides exerting the typical renal effects, modifies previously unidentified immune functions associated with the pathophysiological renal alterations induced by chronic elevated blood pressure (Drummond et al., 2019). As expected, bilateral renal denervation reduced renal norepinephrine levels and blunted blood pressure elevation to chronic infusion of angiotensin II (Xiao et al., 2015). Interestingly, the procedure of renal denervation dampened the accumulation of T cells in the kidney and the ensuing inflammatory response (Xiao et al., 2015). As a consequence, less fibrosis and albuminuria developed (Xiao et al., 2015). By exploring the immune mechanisms underlying this response, the role of renal denervation in promoting the maturation of renal dendritic cells was identified, thus highlighting that renal sympathetic nerves contribute to immune activation, T cell infiltration, and end organ damage in the kidney during hypertension (Xiao et al., 2015). However, more recently, another study showed that, while ameliorating the hypertensive phenotype, renal denervation was ineffective in dampening renal inflammation (Banek et al., 2018), thus raising the need for further investigations aimed at dissecting the mutual neuroimmune interactions in the renal district during hypertension.

Heart Failure

Cardiac function is profoundly influenced by the autonomic nervous system. Sympathetic and parasympathetic innervations tightly control myocardial contractility, conductance and frequency, and vascular tone (Lymperopoulos, Rengo, & Koch, 2013; Triposkiadis et al., 2009). Usually, the preceding functions are ascribed to the effect of the autonomic nervous system on cardiomyocytes. However, it is becoming increasingly clear that neural regulation also modulates the function of nonmyocyte cells in the cardiac tissues. In this regard, the sympathetic nervous system has been identified as a potent modulator of immune cell functions in a multitude of pathophysiological conditions. On the other hand, chronic heart failure usually parallels the presence of enhanced activation of the sympathetic nervous system, regarded as one of the strongest predictors of a negative outcome (Cohn et al., 1984) and, hence, the motivation to investigate the neuroimmune mechanisms that might underlie this pathophysiological relationship.

Inflammatory cells infiltrate the myocardium in response to acute ischemic challenges and during the onset and progression of heart failure (Nahrendorf, 2018). While intense efforts have been dedicated to the identification of specific cell types participating in the process of cardiac remodeling, the interplay established with mechanisms of neural regulation is still the object of investigation.

It has been shown that acute ischemia causes the production of myeloid cells in the spleen through an effect mediated by increased sympathetic signaling in the bone marrow (Dutta et al., 2015; Nahrendorf, 2018; Swirski et al., 2009). The neuroimmune connection established during acute myocardial ischemia allows a reduction in the status of HSCs' quiescence, which in turn promotes C-C chemokine receptor type 2–mediated (CCR2) replenishment of monocytes in the spleen (Heidt et al., 2014; Swirski et al., 2009). Hence, some of the monocytes egress from the spleen and accumulate in the ischemic myocardium, where they participate in the process of cardiac remodeling (Bronte & Pittet, 2013; Nahrendorf, 2018). A successive study investigated the involvement of the cardiosplenic axis in the long-term consequences of myocardial infarction (Ismahil et al., 2014). By studying mice for several weeks after coronary ligation, the researchers observed that, during the development of chronic heart failure, the spleen was subjected to an important process of remodeling (Ismahil et al., 2014).

An additional level of regulation in the complex scenario of the neuroimmune interactions relevant for cardiac remodeling emerges from local cardiac innervation. Fibers of the sympathetic nervous system directly innervate the myocardium by branching from the superior cervical, stellate, and upper thoracic ganglia (Coote & Chauhan, 2016). The projections of these nerves are well-known to entangle cardiomyocytes and vasculature in the myocardium. Whether the nerve terminals can influence the immune cells that populate the myocardium, both at the steady state and upon challenges, is still the object of investigation. Experiments conducted in mice showed that selective denervation of the superior cervical ganglion, performed before inducing myocardial ischemia, had no impact on the acute response to myocardial infarction, despite reducing the sympathetic innervation in the left-ventricular anterior wall (Ziegler et al., 2018). Interestingly, in the long term, cardiac sympathetic denervation impacted the process of chronic remodeling by reducing the inflammatory infiltrate in the myocardium and hampering cardiac dysfunction (Ziegler et al., 2018).

Cardiac remodeling and the associated inflammatory and immune responses are not limited to acute myocardial infarction and the consequent evolution toward heart failure. Also, other chronic challenges, like hypertension and renal failure, impose overload on the myocardium and eventually lead to the development of heart failure, a condition characterized by an increased number of cardiac macrophages. Interestingly, it has been shown that the evolution toward heart failure is associated with elevated circulating levels of pro-inflammatory cytokines and an increased number of cardiac macrophages due to local proliferation and monocyte recruitment (Adamo, Rocha-Resende, Prabhu, & Mann, 2020; Epelman et al., 2014; Hulsmans et al., 2018).

While it is well recognized that a multiplicity of immune cells and pathways infiltrate the failing myocardium, the neuroimmune mechanisms potentially involved are still the object of investigation.

Metabolic Disorders

Lifestyle-related risk factors are well-known to impact cardiovascular function, and it is becoming increasingly clear that immune cells and the inflammatory milieu are affected as well. Interestingly, lifestyle-related risk factors are frequently associated with an impaired autonomic nervous system balance, usually enhancing the sympathetic tone. Uncovering how the neural control of immunity may be implicated in the increased cardiovascular risk ensuing from lifestyle-related comorbidities appears to be fundamental to unraveling new therapeutic targets.

Metabolic derangement ensuing from diabetes is one of the most common causes of increased cardiovascular risk. Interestingly, both the immune system and the autonomic nervous system participate in the onset and progression of type 1 (T1D) and type 2 diabetes (T2D). However, studies investigating the role of neuroimmune communication in metabolic disorders are just beginning.

While various observations had implicated a role for the innervation of pancreatic islets in the development of T1D, evidence of a causal relationship was still missing. A very recent study has highlighted a neuroimmune mechanism underlying the onset of T1D (Christoffersson, Ratliff, & von Herrath, 2020). In order to investigate the potential dependence of immune lesions observed in the pancreas in T1D, a mouse model of autoimmune diabetes was used to study the role of sympathetic signaling (Christoffersson et al., 2020). This T1D model is characterized by CD8+ T cell–mediated attack on pancreatic β cells, resulting in autoreactivity and hyperglycemia within 14 days. As a strategy to inhibit sympathetic signaling in the pancreatic islets of this mouse model, the authors used surgical denervation or chemical ablation of sympathetic innervation by 6-hydroxydopamine (6-OHDA) – a neurotoxin that depletes peripheral sympathetic neurons (Christoffersson et al., 2020). In both cases, they observed a protective effect on the onset of diabetes. Moreover, by using the α1-adrenoceptor inhibitor prazosin or the β-adrenergic blocker propranolol, they also demonstrated that the effect was dependent on α1-adrenergic signaling (Christoffersson et al., 2020). The observation of islet-resident macrophages expressing adrenoceptors highlighted the possibility that neuroimmune-mediated cross talk between innate and adaptive immunity in the pancreas might regulate the onset and progression of T1D.

High-fat diet induced obesity is one of the most common causes of the onset of T2D. Similar to what was observed for T1D, T2D also has profound implications for dysregulation in neural and immune homeostasis. During obesity, the accumulation of macrophages in fat tissue propagates the chronic inflammation and insulin resistance typically associated with T2D. In this regard, fat tissue is critically regulated by neural signals and by immune cells. An interesting study investigated the role of a purely neural signal – netrin-1 – in regulating immune activation in fat tissue. Netrin-1 has been known as a neuroimmune guidance cue that orients axonal growth cones by balancing chemoattractive and chemorepulsive impulses. Interestingly, it was discovered that netrin-1 is also expressed in the adipose tissue of obese mice and humans. This observation led researchers to hypothesize that chemoattractive and chemorepulsive signals might also be relevant for the regulation of immune cell infiltration in fat tissue. In a model of high-fat diet induced obesity, it was found that the expression of netrin-1 controls macrophage infiltration and retention in the adipose tissue, in turn modulating insulin resistance (Ramkhelawon et al., 2014).

However, it is also known that neuroimmune interactions can take place in immune organs – like the spleen – providing a mechanism for controlling inflammatory cell development in disease (Carnevale & Lembo, 2020). A recent study focused on the interactions established by the sympathetic nervous and the immune systems in the spleen in the context of diabetes (Vasamsetti et al., 2018). T1D and T2D experimental models of diabetes were used to investigate the effect of catecholamines released by leukocytes and sympathetic splenic nerve termini on hematopoietic cells, the development of myeloid cells and the recruitment to peripheral tissues. By using denervation techniques obtained by selective surgery on the splenic innervation or by pharmacological disruption of the sympathetic nervous system, this research showed that the ablation of splenic sympathetic innervation hampered the process of myelopoiesis in the spleens of diabetic mice (Vasamsetti et al., 2018). In addition, less inflammatory cells accumulated in the aorta, where this effect determined an overall benefit in the progression of atherosclerotic plaque formation (Vasamsetti et al., 2018).

Atherosclerosis

Accumulation and retention of macrophages engulfing lipid particles in the artery wall characterize the atherosclerotic process, which is dominated by plaque formation. A persistent status of continuous low-grade inflammation and immune activation fuels the plaques with immune cells, leading to disease progression. While a huge amount of work has been done to investigate the mechanisms underlying plaque formation and stability, the role exerted by interactions with neural regulation is just beginning to be identified. In addition, the same neuroimmune cue identified in modulating the retention of macrophages in fat tissue, netrin-1, has been also involved in the process of atherosclerotic plaque formation and progression. In fact, it was discovered that netrin-1 is involved in the process of immune activation in the arterial wall. Produced in the atheromatic macrophages in humans and mice, netrin-1 was shown to inhibit their egression from the plaque through chemokine-driven migration processes (van Gils et al., 2012). According to this observation, the selective deletion of netrin-1 in macrophages led mice to develop less atherosclerosis by favoring the outflow of macrophages from plaques.

Also, the cholinergic inflammatory pathway was involved in the neuroimmune regulation of atherosclerosis. By studying the hypercholesterolemic $Ldlr^{-/-}$ mice, it was revealed that the absence of α7nAChR from bone marrow-derived cells accelerated the atherosclerotic process (Johansson et al., 2014). Interestingly, this observation was translationally relevant because human lesions displayed immune cells positive for α7nAChR (Johansson et al., 2014).

An interesting aspect related to the atherosclerotic process and the well-known consequences in terms of cardiovascular event incidence is related to the increasing awareness that an unhealthy lifestyle potently challenges the homeostasis of the cardiovascular system, increasing the risk of unfavorable events. How lifestyle-related risk factors – like diet, exercise, stress, and sleep – affect chronic inflammatory diseases and impact the cardiovascular and neuroimmune systems is just beginning to be unraveled (Nahrendorf & Swirski, 2015). Along these lines, a fascinating study explained how insufficient and/or disrupted sleep led to increased incidence of cardiovascular diseases (McAlpine et al., 2019). Investigation of the molecular and cellular mechanisms underlying the relationship between sleep and cardiovascular function provided evidence that a mechanism linked to hematopoiesis and residing in the spleen may be the culprit (McAlpine et al., 2019). Mice subjected to sleep disturbances were affected by larger atherosclerotic lesions, characterized by an enhanced number of Ly6Chigh monocytes (McAlpine et al., 2019). When the mechanisms responsible for increased hematopoiesis and Ly6Chigh monocyte production were investigated, a neuroimmune pathway was identified whereby the expression of hypothalamic hypocretin was significantly downregulated by spleen fragmentation (McAlpine et al., 2019). A correlation between hypothalamic hypocretin and increased leukocytosis was found, suggesting that neural control of hematopoiesis regulates monocytes during atherosclerosis (McAlpine et al., 2019).

An additional frequent epidemiological observation reports that regular physical activity counteracts the unfavorable consequences of cardiovascular risk factors. One of the beneficial aspects related to regular exercise derives from improved metabolism, which lowers the cardiovascular risk associated with metabolic derangement and obesity. However, it is interesting to note that another common mediator of physical activity and cardiovascular function is the immune system. In this regard, a recent study showed an intriguing relationship between voluntary running, hematopoietic activity, and atherosclerotic burden in mice and humans (Frodermann et al., 2019). Besides the undoubtable implications of this study in terms of encouraging regular physical exercise to reduce cardiovascular disease, new avenues of investigation emerge. In fact, the experiment performed in this work shows the existence of a molecular mechanism in the adipose tissue recruited by voluntary running to diminish leptin production and stimulates quiescence of the hematopoietic niche in the bone marrow (Frodermann et al., 2019). However, the potential dependence of this pathway on neural control remains to be elucidated.

CLINICAL PERSPECTIVES

Taken together, we have reviewed a series of discoveries that provide compelling evidence that neuroimmune mechanisms participate in cardiovascular homeostasis and, when dysregulated, contribute to the onset and progression of cardiovascular disease.

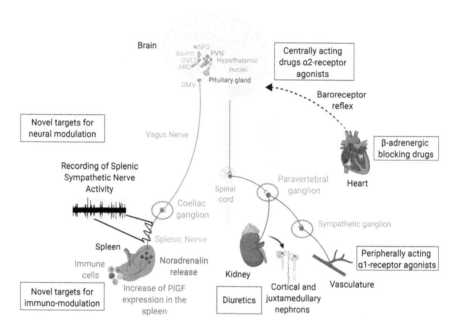

FIGURE 8.4 Translational and clinical implications of neuroimmune interactions in cardiovascular diseases. Hard-wired neural connections are established at the level of cardiovascular organs. The neuroimmune interface established between the brain and the spleen emerged as a crucial neural reflex in cardiovascular diseases. The vagus efferent nerve (in blue) extended from the dorsal motor nucleus (DMV) in the brainstem, interconnecting with sympathetic efferent nerves at the level of the celiac ganglion. Noradrenalin release in the spleen promotes increased expression of placental growth factor (PlGF), which is in turn responsible for the activation of immune cells deployed toward the cardiovascular system. The identification of this neuroimmune pathway, combined with the classical mechanisms regulating cardiovascular system such as baroreceptor reflexes and cardiac, renal, and vascular function, opens the possibility to new therapeutic strategies for counteracting cardiovascular diseases.

Source: Created with BioRender.com.

Nonetheless, the therapeutic implications ensuing from the observations conducted in animal mechanistic studies or deriving from clinical analysis are still extremely limited. In fact, while the data accumulating in the literature would support the concept that inflammatory and immune dysregulation accompanies cardiovascular disease and is tightly associated with alterations in the neural regulation of cardiovascular function, the prospect of introducing therapies targeting neuroimmune interactions is far away. An undoubtable problem is related to the still unknown balance between risks and benefits. Indeed, therapies modulating the immune system have unavoidable potential side effects. In this perspective, the search for innovative strategies that might modulate the neural control of immune responses with targeted interventions, instead of generalized immunosuppression, appears as an interesting possibility. Also, new insights into the molecular mechanisms underlying neuroimmune communication in cardiovascular disease would probably uncover potential therapeutic targets.

BIBLIOGRAPHY

Abboud, F. M. (1982). The sympathetic system in hypertension. State-of-the-art review. *Hypertension, 4*(3 Pt 2), 208–225.

Abboud, F. M. (2010). The Walter B. Cannon Memorial Award Lecture, 2009. Physiology in perspective: The wisdom of the body. In search of autonomic balance: the good, the bad, and the ugly. *Am J Physiol Regul Integr Comp Physiol, 298*(6), R1449–1467. doi:10.1152/ajpregu.00130.2010

Abboud, F. M., Harwani, S. C., & Chapleau, M. W. (2012). Autonomic neural regulation of the immune system: implications for hypertension and cardiovascular disease. *Hypertension, 59*(4), 755–762. doi:10.1161/HYPERTENSIONAHA.111.186833

Ackerman, K. D., Felten, S. Y., Bellinger, D. L., & Felten, D. L. (1987). Noradrenergic sympathetic innervation of the spleen: III. Development of innervation in the rat spleen. *J Neurosci Res, 18*(1), 49–54, 123–125. doi:10.1002/jnr.490180109

Adamo, L., Rocha-Resende, C., Prabhu, S. D., & Mann, D. L. (2020). Reappraising the role of inflammation in heart failure. *Nat Rev Cardiol, 17*(5), 269–285. doi:10.1038/s41569-019-0315-x

Al-Shalan, H. A. M., Hu, D., Nicholls, P. K., Greene, W. K., & Ma, B. (2019). Immunofluorescent characterization of innervation and nerve-immune cell neighborhood in mouse thymus. *Cell Tissue Res, 378*(2), 239–254. doi:10.1007/s00441-019-03052-4

al-Shawaf, A. A., Kendall, M. D., & Cowen, T. (1991). Identification of neural profiles containing vasoactive intestinal polypeptide, acetylcholinesterase and catecholamines in the rat thymus. *J Anat, 174*, 131–143.

Andersson, U., & Tracey, K. J. (2012). Reflex principles of immunological homeostasis. *Annu Rev Immunol, 30*, 313–335. doi:10.1146/annurev-immunol-020711-075015

Ballabh, P., Braun, A., & Nedergaard, M. (2004). The blood-brain barrier: an overview: structure, regulation, and clinical implications. *Neurobiol Dis, 16*(1), 1–13. doi:10.1016/j.nbd.2003.12.016

Banek, C. T., Gauthier, M. M., Baumann, D. C., Van Helden, D., Asirvatham-Jeyaraj, N., Panoskaltsis-Mortari, A., . . . Osborn, J. W. (2018). Targeted afferent renal denervation reduces arterial pressure but not renal inflammation in established DOCA-salt hypertension in the rat. *Am J Physiol-Regul Integr Comp Physiol, 314*(6), R883–R891.

Banks, W. A. (2015). The blood-brain barrier in neuroimmunology: tales of separation and assimilation. *Brain, behavior, and immunity, 44*, 1–8.

Baral, P., Umans, B. D., Li, L., Wallrapp, A., Bist, M., Kirschbaum, T., . . . Chiu, I. M. (2018). Nociceptor sensory neurons suppress neutrophil and gammadelta T cell responses in bacterial lung infections and lethal pneumonia. *Nat Med, 24*(4), 417–426. doi:10.1038/nm.4501

Bellinger, D. L., Felten, S. Y., Collier, T. J., & Felten, D. L. (1987). Noradrenergic sympathetic innervation of the spleen: IV. Morphometric analysis in adult and aged F344 rats. *J Neurosci Res, 18*(1), 55–63, 126–129. doi:10.1002/jnr.490180110

Bellinger, D. L., Felten, S. Y., Lorton, D., & Felten, D. L. (1989). Origin of noradrenergic innervation of the spleen in rats. *Brain Behav Immun, 3*(4), 291–311. doi:10.1016/0889-1591(89)90029-9

Borovikova, L. V., Ivanova, S., Zhang, M., Yang, H., Botchkina, G. I., Watkins, L. R., . . . Tracey, K. J. (2000). Vagus nerve stimulation attenuates the systemic inflammatory response to endotoxin. *Nature, 405*(6785), 458–462. doi:10.1038/35013070

Bronte, V., & Pittet, M. J. (2013). The spleen in local and systemic regulation of immunity. *Immunity, 39*(5), 806–818. doi:10.1016/j.immuni.2013.10.010

Butts, C. L., & Sternberg, E. M. (2008). Neuroendocrine factors alter host defense by modulating immune function. *Cell Immunol, 252*(1–2), 7–15. doi:10.1016/j.cellimm.2007.09.009

Cancelliere, N. M., Black, E. A., & Ferguson, A. V. (2015). Neurohumoral integration of cardiovascular function by the lamina terminalis. *Curr Hypertens Rep, 17*(12), 93. doi:10.1007/s11906-015-0602-9

Carnevale, D. (2020). Neural control of immunity in hypertension: council on hypertension mid career award for research excellence, 2019. *Hypertension, 76*(3), 622–628. doi:10.1161/HYPERTENSIONAHA.120.14637

Carnevale, D., & Lembo, G. (2020). Neuroimmune interactions in cardiovascular diseases. *Cardiovasc Res.* doi:10.1093/cvr/cvaa151

Carnevale, D., Pallante, F., Fardella, V., Fardella, S., Iacobucci, R., Federici, M., . . . Lembo, G. (2014). The angiogenic factor PlGF mediates a neuroimmune interaction in the spleen to allow the onset of hypertension. *Immunity, 41*(5), 737–752. doi:10.1016/j.immuni.2014.11.002

Carnevale, D., Perrotta, M., Pallante, F., Fardella, V., Iacobucci, R., Fardella, S., . . . Lembo, G. (2016). A cholinergic-sympathetic pathway primes immunity in hypertension and mediates brain-to-spleen communication. *Nat Commun, 7*, 13035. doi:10.1038/ncomms13035

Cavallotti, C., Artico, M., & Cavallotti, D. (1999). Occurrence of adrenergic nerve fibers and of noradrenaline in thymus gland of juvenile and aged rats. *Immunol Lett, 70*(1), 53–62. doi:10.1016/s0165-2478(99)00127-3

Chatterjee, P. K., Yeboah, M. M., Dowling, O., Xue, X., Powell, S. R., Al-Abed, Y., & Metz, C. N. (2012). Nicotinic acetylcholine receptor agonists attenuate septic acute kidney injury in mice by suppressing inflammation and proteasome activity. *PLoS One, 7*(5), e35361. doi:10.1371/journal.pone.0035361

Chavan, S. S., Pavlov, V. A., & Tracey, K. J. (2017). Mechanisms and therapeutic relevance of neuro-immune communication. *Immunity, 46*(6), 927–942. doi:10.1016/j.immuni.2017.06.008

Chiu, I. M., Heesters, B. A., Ghasemlou, N., Von Hehn, C. A., Zhao, F., Tran, J., . . . Woolf, C. J. (2013). Bacteria activate sensory neurons that modulate pain and inflammation. *Nature, 501*(7465), 52–57. doi:10.1038/nature12479

Christoffersson, G., Ratliff, S. S., & von Herrath, M. G. (2020). Interference with pancreatic sympathetic signaling halts the onset of diabetes in mice. *Science Advances, 6*(35), eabb2878. doi:10.1126/sciadv.abb2878

Coffman, T. M. (2011). Under pressure: the search for the essential mechanisms of hypertension. *Nat Med, 17*(11), 1402–1409. doi:10.1038/nm.2541

Cohn, J. N., Levine, T. B., Olivari, M. T., Garberg, V., Lura, D., Francis, G. S., . . . Rector, T. (1984). Plasma norepinephrine as a guide to prognosis in patients with chronic congestive heart failure. *N Engl J Med, 311*(13), 819–823. doi:10.1056/NEJM198409273111303

Coote, J. H., & Chauhan, R. A. (2016). The sympathetic innervation of the heart: Important new insights. *Auton Neurosci, 199*, 17–23. doi:10.1016/j.autneu.2016.08.014

Cortez-Retamozo, V., Etzrodt, M., Newton, A., Ryan, R., Pucci, F., Sio, S. W., . . . Pittet, M. J. (2013). Angiotensin II drives the production of tumor-promoting macrophages. *Immunity, 38*(2), 296–308. doi:10.1016/j.immuni.2012.10.015

Crowley, S. D., Song, Y. S., Lin, E. E., Griffiths, R., Kim, H. S., & Ruiz, P. (2010). Lymphocyte responses exacerbate angiotensin II-dependent hypertension. *Am J Physiol Regul Integr Comp Physiol, 298*(4), R1089–1097. doi:10.1152/ajpregu.00373.2009

D'Andrea, I., Fardella, V., Fardella, S., Pallante, F., Ghigo, A., Iacobucci, R., . . . Carnevale, D. (2015). Lack of kinase-independent activity of PI3Kgamma in locus coeruleus induces ADHD symptoms through increased CREB signaling. *EMBO Mol Med, 7*(7), 904–917. doi:10.15252/emmm.201404697

DiBona, G. F., & Kopp, U. C. (1997). Neural control of renal function. *Physiol Rev, 77*(1), 75–197.

Drummond, G. R., Vinh, A., Guzik, T. J., & Sobey, C. G. (2019). Immune mechanisms of hypertension. *Nat Rev Immunol, 19*(8), 517–532. doi:10.1038/s41577-019-0160-5

Druzd, D., Matveeva, O., Ince, L., Harrison, U., He, W., Schmal, C., . . . Scheiermann, C. (2017). Lymphocyte circadian clocks control lymph node trafficking and adaptive immune responses. *Immunity, 46*(1), 120–132. doi:10.1016/j.immuni.2016.12.011

Dutta, P., Hoyer, F. F., Grigoryeva, L. S., Sager, H. B., Leuschner, F., Courties, G., . . . Nahrendorf, M. (2015). Macrophages retain hematopoietic stem cells in the spleen via VCAM-1. *J Exp Med, 212*(4), 497–512. doi:10.1084/jem.20141642

Ebringer, A., & Doyle, A. E. (1970). Raised serum IgG levels in hypertension. *Br Med J, 2*(5702), 146–148. doi:10.1136/bmj.2.5702.146

Elenkov, I. J., Wilder, R. L., Chrousos, G. P., & Vizi, E. S. (2000). The sympathetic nerve—an integrative interface between two supersystems: the brain and the immune system. *Pharmacol Rev, 52*(4), 595–638.

Epelman, S., Lavine, K. J., Beaudin, A. E., Sojka, D. K., Carrero, J. A., Calderon, B., . . . Mann, D. L. (2014). Embryonic and adult-derived resident cardiac macrophages are maintained through distinct mechanisms at steady state and during inflammation. *Immunity, 40*(1), 91–104. doi:10.1016/j.immuni.2013.11.019

Esler, M. (2015). The sympathetic nervous system in hypertension: back to the future? *Curr Hypertens Rep, 17*(2), 11. doi:10.1007/s11906-014-0519-8

Felten, D. L., Felten, S. Y., Bellinger, D. L., Carlson, S. L., Ackerman, K. D., Madden, K. S., . . . Livnat, S. (1987). Noradrenergic sympathetic neural interactions with the immune system: structure and function. *Immunol Rev, 100*(1), 225–260. doi:10.1111/j.1600-065x.1987.tb00534.x

Felten, D. L., Felten, S. Y., Carlson, S. L., Olschowka, J. A., & Livnat, S. (1985). Noradrenergic and peptidergic innervation of lymphoid tissue. *J Immunol, 135*(2 Suppl), 755s-765s.

Felten, D. L., Livnat, S., Felten, S. Y., Carlson, S. L., Bellinger, D. L., & Yeh, P. (1984). Sympathetic innervation of lymph nodes in mice. *Brain Res Bull, 13*(6), 693–699. doi:10.1016/0361-9230(84)90230-2

Felten, S. Y., & Olschowka, J. (1987). Noradrenergic sympathetic innervation of the spleen: II. Tyrosine hydroxylase (TH)-positive nerve terminals form synapticlike contacts on lymphocytes in the splenic white pulp. *J Neurosci Res, 18*(1), 37–48. doi:10.1002/jnr.490180108

Fink, T., & Weihe, E. (1988). Multiple neuropeptides in nerves supplying mammalian lymph nodes: messenger candidates for sensory and autonomic neuroimmunomodulation? *Neurosci Lett, 90*(1–2), 39–44. doi:10.1016/0304-3940(88)90783-5

Frodermann, V., Rohde, D., Courties, G., Severe, N., Schloss, M. J., Amatullah, H., . . . Nahrendorf, M. (2019). Exercise reduces inflammatory cell production and cardiovascular inflammation via instruction of hematopoietic progenitor cells. *Nat Med, 25*(11), 1761–1771. doi:10.1038/s41591-019-0633-x

Ganta, C. K., Lu, N., Helwig, B. G., Blecha, F., Ganta, R. R., Zheng, L., . . . Kenney, M. J. (2005). Central angiotensin II-enhanced splenic cytokine gene expression is mediated by the sympathetic nervous system. *Am J Physiol Heart Circ Physiol, 289*(4), H1683–1691. doi:10.1152/ajpheart.00125.2005

Gigliotti, J. C., Huang, L., Bajwa, A., Ye, H., Mace, E. H., Hossack, J. A., . . . Okusa, M. D. (2015). Ultrasound modulates the splenic neuroimmune axis in attenuating AKI. *J Am Soc Nephrol, 26*(10), 2470–2481. doi:10.1681/ASN.2014080769

Gigliotti, J. C., Huang, L., Ye, H., Bajwa, A., Chattrabhuti, K., Lee, S., . . . Okusa, M. D. (2013). Ultrasound prevents renal ischemia-reperfusion injury by stimulating the splenic cholinergic anti-inflammatory pathway. *J Am Soc Nephrol, 24*(9), 1451–1460. doi:10.1681/ASN.2013010084

Goldberger, J. J., Arora, R., Buckley, U., & Shivkumar, K. (2019). Autonomic nervous system dysfunction: JACC focus seminar. *J Am Coll Cardiol, 73*(10), 1189–1206. doi:10.1016/j. jacc.2018.12.064

Guyenet, P. G. (2006). The sympathetic control of blood pressure. *Nat Rev Neurosci, 7*(5), 335–346. doi:10.1038/nrn1902

Guyenet, P. G., Stornetta, R. L., Bochorishvili, G., Depuy, S. D., Burke, P. G., & Abbott, S. B. (2013). C1 neurons: the body's EMTs. *Am J Physiol Regul Integr Comp Physiol, 305*(3), R187–204. doi:10.1152/ajpregu.00054.2013

Guzik, T. J., Hoch, N. E., Brown, K. A., McCann, L. A., Rahman, A., Dikalov, S., . . . Harrison, D. G. (2007). Role of the T cell in the genesis of angiotensin II induced hypertension and vascular dysfunction. *J Exp Med, 204*(10), 2449–2460. doi:10.1084/jem.20070657

Heidt, T., Sager, H. B., Courties, G., Dutta, P., Iwamoto, Y., Zaltsman, A., . . . Nahrendorf, M. (2014). Chronic variable stress activates hematopoietic stem cells. *Nat Med, 20*(7), 754–758. doi:10.1038/nm.3589

Hilme, E., Herlitz, H., Soderstrom, T., & Hansson, L. (1989). Increased secretion of immunoglobulins in malignant hypertension. *J Hypertens, 7*(2), 91–95.

Hosoi, T., Okuma, Y., Matsuda, T., & Nomura, Y. (2005). Novel pathway for LPS-induced afferent vagus nerve activation: possible role of nodose ganglion. *Auton Neurosci, 120*(1–2), 104–107. doi:10.1016/j.autneu.2004.11.012

Hulsmans, M., Sager, H. B., Roh, J. D., Valero-Munoz, M., Houstis, N. E., Iwamoto, Y., . . . Nahrendorf, M. (2018). Cardiac macrophages promote diastolic dysfunction. *J Exp Med, 215*(2), 423–440. doi:10.1084/jem.20171274

Ishigami, T. (1918). The influence of psychic acts on the progress of pulmonary tuberculosis. *American Review of Tuberculosis, 2*(8), 470–484.

Ismahil, M. A., Hamid, T., Bansal, S. S., Patel, B., Kingery, J. R., & Prabhu, S. D. (2014). Remodeling of the mononuclear phagocyte network underlies chronic inflammation and disease progression in heart failure: critical importance of the cardiosplenic axis. *Circ Res, 114*(2), 266–282. doi:10.1161/CIRCRESAHA.113.301720

Jan, M., Ebert, B. L., & Jaiswal, S. (2017). Clonal hematopoiesis. *Semin Hematol, 54*(1), 43–50. doi:10.1053/j.seminhematol.2016.10.002

Johansson, M. E., Ulleryd, M. A., Bernardi, A., Lundberg, A. M., Andersson, A., Folkersen, L., . . . Hansson, G. K. (2014). alpha7 Nicotinic acetylcholine receptor is expressed in human atherosclerosis and inhibits disease in mice—brief report. *Arterioscler Thromb Vasc Biol, 34*(12), 2632–2636. doi:10.1161/ATVBAHA.114.303892

Johnson, A. K., & Gross, P. M. (1993). Sensory circumventricular organs and brain homeostatic pathways. *FASEB J, 7*(8), 678–686. doi:10.1096/fasebj.7.8.8500693

Johnson, A. K., & Xue, B. (2018). Central nervous system neuroplasticity and the sensitization of hypertension. *Nat Rev Nephrol, 14*(12), 750–766. doi:10.1038/s41581-018-0068-5

Jung, W. C., Levesque, J. P., & Ruitenberg, M. J. (2017). It takes nerve to fight back: The significance of neural innervation of the bone marrow and spleen for immune function. *Semin Cell Dev Biol, 61*, 60–70. doi:10.1016/j.semcdb.2016.08.010

Katayama, Y., Battista, M., Kao, W. M., Hidalgo, A., Peired, A. J., Thomas, S. A., & Frenette, P. S. (2006). Signals from the sympathetic nervous system regulate hematopoietic stem cell egress from bone marrow. *Cell, 124*(2), 407–421. doi:10.1016/j.cell.2005.10.041

Laye, S., Bluthe, R. M., Kent, S., Combe, C., Medina, C., Parnet, P., . . . Dantzer, R. (1995). Subdiaphragmatic vagotomy blocks induction of IL-1 beta mRNA in mice brain in response to peripheral LPS. *Am J Physiol, 268*(5 Pt 2), R1327–1331. doi:10.1152/ajpregu.1995.268.5.R1327

Leong, D. P., Joseph, P. G., McKee, M., Anand, S. S., Teo, K. K., Schwalm, J.-D., & Yusuf, S. (2017). Reducing the global burden of cardiovascular disease, part 2: prevention and treatment of cardiovascular disease. *Circ Res, 121*(6), 695–710.

Leposavić, G., Pilipović, I., & Perišić, M. (2011). Cellular and nerve fibre catecholaminergic thymic network: steroid hormone dependent activity. *Physiological research.*

Liu, T., Xu, Z. Z., Park, C. K., Berta, T., & Ji, R. R. (2010). Toll-like receptor 7 mediates pruritus. *Nat Neurosci, 13*(12), 1460–1462. doi:10.1038/nn.2683

Loeper, M., & Crouzon, O. (1904). L'action de l'adrenaline sur le sang. *Arch Med Exp Anat Pathol, 16*, 83–108.

Lymperopoulos, A., Rengo, G., & Koch, W. J. (2013). Adrenergic nervous system in heart failure: pathophysiology and therapy. *Circ Res, 113*(6), 739–753. doi:10.1161/CIRCRESAHA.113.300308

Madden, K. S., & Felten, D. L. (2001). Beta-adrenoceptor blockade alters thymocyte differentiation in aged mice. *Cell Mol Biol (Noisy-le-grand), 47*(1), 189–196.

Madhur, M. S., Kirabo, A., Guzik, T. J., & Harrison, D. G. (2020). From rags to riches: moving beyond RAG1 in studies of hypertension. *Hypertension, 75*, 930–934.

Maestroni, G. J. (1998). Catecholaminergic regulation of hematopoiesis in mice. *Blood, 92*(8), 2971; author reply 2972–2973.

Malpas, S. C. (2010). Sympathetic nervous system overactivity and its role in the development of cardiovascular disease. *Physiol Rev, 90*(2), 513–557. doi:10.1152/physrev.00007.2009

Marvar, P. J., & Harrison, D. G. (2012). Stress-dependent hypertension and the role of T lymphocytes. *Exp Physiol, 97*(11), 1161–1167. doi:10.1113/expphysiol.2011.061507

Marvar, P. J., Thabet, S. R., Guzik, T. J., Lob, H. E., McCann, L. A., Weyand, C., . . . Harrison, D. G. (2010). Central and peripheral mechanisms of T-lymphocyte activation and vascular inflammation produced by angiotensin II-induced hypertension. *Circ Res, 107*(2), 263–270. doi:10.1161/CIRCRESAHA.110.217299

Marvar, P. J., Vinh, A., Thabet, S., Lob, H. E., Geem, D., Ressler, K. J., & Harrison, D. G. (2012). T lymphocytes and vascular inflammation contribute to stress-dependent hypertension. *Biol Psychiatry, 71*(9), 774–782. doi:10.1016/j.biopsych.2012.01.017

Maryanovich, M., Zahalka, A. H., Pierce, H., Pinho, S., Nakahara, F., Asada, N., . . . Frenette, P. S. (2018). Adrenergic nerve degeneration in bone marrow drives aging of the hematopoietic stem cell niche. *Nat Med, 24*(6), 782–791. doi:10.1038/s41591-018-0030-x

Mattson, D. L., Lund, H., Guo, C., Rudemiller, N., Geurts, A. M., & Jacob, H. (2013). Genetic mutation of recombination activating gene 1 in Dahl salt-sensitive rats attenuates hypertension and renal damage. *Am J Physiol Regul Integr Comp Physiol, 304*(6), R407–414. doi:10.1152/ajpregu.00304.2012

McAlpine, C. S., Kiss, M. G., Rattik, S., He, S., Vassalli, A., Valet, C., . . . Swirski, F. K. (2019). Sleep modulates haematopoiesis and protects against atherosclerosis. *Nature, 566*(7744), 383–387. doi:10.1038/s41586-019-0948-2

Mendez-Ferrer, S., Lucas, D., Battista, M., & Frenette, P. S. (2008). Haematopoietic stem cell release is regulated by circadian oscillations. *Nature, 452*(7186), 442–447. doi:10.1038/nature06685

Métalnikov, S. I. (1929). *Le rôle des réflexes conditionnels dans l'immunite.* éditeur inconnu.

Mignini, F., Streccioni, V., & Amenta, F. (2003). Autonomic innervation of immune organs and neuroimmune modulation. *Auton Autacoid Pharmacol, 23*(1), 1–25. doi:10.1046/j.1474-8673.2003.00280.x

Nahrendorf, M. (2018). Myeloid cell contributions to cardiovascular health and disease. *Nat Med, 24*(6), 711–720. doi:10.1038/s41591-018-0064-0

Nahrendorf, M., & Swirski, F. K. (2015). Lifestyle effects on hematopoiesis and atherosclerosis. *Circ Res, 116*(5), 884–894. doi:10.1161/CIRCRESAHA.116.303550

Nakai, A., Hayano, Y., Furuta, F., Noda, M., & Suzuki, K. (2014). Control of lymphocyte egress from lymph nodes through beta2-adrenergic receptors. *J Exp Med, 211*(13), 2583–2598. doi:10.1084/jem.20141132

Nance, D. M., Hopkins, D. A., & Bieger, D. (1987). Re-investigation of the innervation of the thymus gland in mice and rats. *Brain Behav Immun, 1*(2), 134–147. doi:10.1016/0889-1591(87)90016-x

Nance, D. M., & Sanders, V. M. (2007). Autonomic innervation and regulation of the immune system (1987–2007). *Brain Behav Immun, 21*(6), 736–745. doi:10.1016/j.bbi.2007.03.008

Novotny, G. E., & Kliche, K. O. (1986). Innervation of lymph nodes: a combined silver impregnation and electron-microscopic study. *Acta Anat (Basel), 127*(4), 243–248. doi:10.1159/000146293

Okusa, M. D., Rosin, D. L., & Tracey, K. J. (2017). Targeting neural reflex circuits in immunity to treat kidney disease. *Nat Rev Nephrol, 13*(11), 669–680. doi:10.1038/nrneph.2017.132

Ordovas-Montanes, J., Rakoff-Nahoum, S., Huang, S., Riol-Blanco, L., Barreiro, O., & von Andrian, U. H. (2015). The regulation of immunological processes by peripheral neurons in homeostasis and disease. *Trends Immunol, 36*(10), 578–604. doi:10.1016/j.it.2015.08.007

Perrotta, M., Lori, A., Carnevale, L., Fardella, S., Cifelli, G., Iacobucci, R., . . . Carnevale, D. (2018). Deoxycorticosterone acetate-salt hypertension activates placental growth factor in the spleen to couple sympathetic drive and immune system activation. *Cardiovasc Res, 114*(3), 456–467. doi:10.1093/cvr/cvy001

Pierce, H., Zhang, D., Magnon, C., Lucas, D., Christin, J. R., Huggins, M., . . . Frenette, P. S. (2017). Cholinergic signals from the CNS regulate G-CSF-mediated HSC mobilization from bone marrow via a glucocorticoid signaling relay. *Cell Stem Cell, 20*(5), 648–658 e644. doi:10.1016/j.stem.2017.01.002

Qi, J., Buzas, K., Fan, H., Cohen, J. I., Wang, K., Mont, E., . . . Howard, O. M. (2011). Painful pathways induced by TLR stimulation of dorsal root ganglion neurons. *J Immunol, 186*(11), 6417–6426. doi:10.4049/jimmunol.1001241

Ramkhelawon, B., Hennessy, E. J., Menager, M., Ray, T. D., Sheedy, F. J., Hutchison, S., . . . Moore, K. J. (2014). Netrin-1 promotes adipose tissue macrophage retention and insulin resistance in obesity. *Nat Med, 20*(4), 377–384. doi:10.1038/nm.3467

Reardon, C., Murray, K., & Lomax, A. E. (2018). Neuroimmune communication in health and disease. *Physiol Rev, 98*(4), 2287–2316. doi:10.1152/physrev.00035.2017

Riol-Blanco, L., Ordovas-Montanes, J., Perro, M., Naval, E., Thiriot, A., Alvarez, D., . . . von Andrian, U. H. (2014). Nociceptive sensory neurons drive interleukin-23-mediated psoriasiform skin inflammation. *Nature, 510*(7503), 157–161. doi:10.1038/nature13199

Rios, F. J., Montezano, A. C., & Touyz, R. M. (2020). Lessons learned from RAG-1-deficient mice in hypertension. *Hypertension, 75*, 935–937.

Rosas-Ballina, M., Olofsson, P. S., Ochani, M., Valdes-Ferrer, S. I., Levine, Y. A., Reardon, C., . . . Tracey, K. J. (2011). Acetylcholine-synthesizing T cells relay neural signals in a vagus nerve circuit. *Science, 334*(6052), 98–101. doi:10.1126/science.1209985

Selye, H. (1941). Variations in organ size caused by chronic treatment with adrenal cortical compounds: An example of a dissociated adaptation to a hormone. *J Anat, 76*(Pt 1), 94–99.

Selye, H., & Fortier, C. (1949). Adaptive reactions to stress. *Res Publ Assoc Res Nerv Ment Dis, 29*, 3–18.

Seniuk, A., Thiele, J. L., Stubbe, A., Oser, P., Rosendahl, A., Bode, M., . . . Ehmke, H. (2020). B6.Rag1 knockout mice generated at the Jackson Laboratory in 2009 show a robust wild-type hypertensive phenotype in response to Ang II (Angiotensin II). *Hypertension, 75*(4), 1110–1116. doi:10.1161/HYPERTENSIONAHA.119.13773

Siso, S., Jeffrey, M., & Gonzalez, L. (2010). Sensory circumventricular organs in health and disease. *Acta Neuropathol, 120*(6), 689–705. doi:10.1007/s00401-010-0743-5

Sloan, E. K., Capitanio, J. P., Tarara, R. P., Mendoza, S. P., Mason, W. A., & Cole, S. W. (2007). Social stress enhances sympathetic innervation of primate lymph nodes: mechanisms and implications for viral pathogenesis. *J Neurosci, 27*(33), 8857–8865. doi:10.1523/JNEUROSCI.1247-07.2007

Sloan, E. K., Tarara, R. P., Capitanio, J. P., & Cole, S. W. (2006). Enhanced replication of simian immunodeficiency virus adjacent to catecholaminergic varicosities in primate lymph nodes. *J Virol, 80*(9), 4326–4335. doi:10.1128/JVI.80.9.4326-4335.2006

Straub, R. H. (2004). Complexity of the bi-directional neuroimmune junction in the spleen. *Trends Pharmacol Sci, 25*(12), 640–646. doi:10.1016/j.tips.2004.10.007

Suryaprabha, P., Padma, T., & Rao, U. B. (1984). Increased serum IgG levels in essential hypertension. *Immunol Lett, 8*(3), 143–145. doi:10.1016/0165-2478(84)90067-1

Suzuki, K., Hayano, Y., Nakai, A., Furuta, F., & Noda, M. (2016). Adrenergic control of the adaptive immune response by diurnal lymphocyte recirculation through lymph nodes. *J Exp Med, 213*(12), 2567–2574. doi:10.1084/jem.20160723

Swirski, F. K., Nahrendorf, M., Etzrodt, M., Wildgruber, M., Cortez-Retamozo, V., Panizzi, P., . . . Pittet, M. J. (2009). Identification of splenic reservoir monocytes and their deployment to inflammatory sites. *Science, 325*(5940), 612–616. doi:10.1126/science.1175202

Takeda, S., Elefteriou, F., Levasseur, R., Liu, X., Zhao, L., Parker, K. L., . . . Karsenty, G. (2002). Leptin regulates bone formation via the sympathetic nervous system. *Cell, 111*(3), 305–317. doi:10.1016/s0092-8674(02)01049-8

Tollefson, L., & Bulloch, K. (1990). Dual-label retrograde transport: CNS innervation of the mouse thymus distinct from other mediastinum viscera. *J Neurosci Res, 25*(1), 20–28. doi:10.1002/jnr.490250104

Triposkiadis, F., Karayannis, G., Giamouzis, G., Skoularigis, J., Louridas, G., & Butler, J. (2009). The sympathetic nervous system in heart failure physiology, pathophysiology, and clinical implications. *J Am Coll Cardiol, 54*(19), 1747–1762. doi:10.1016/j.jacc.2009.05.015

Trott, D. W., Thabet, S. R., Kirabo, A., Saleh, M. A., Itani, H., Norlander, A. E., . . . Harrison, D. G. (2014). Oligoclonal CD8+ T cells play a critical role in the development of hypertension. *Hypertension, 64*(5), 1108–1115. doi:10.1161/HYPERTENSIONAHA.114.04147

Tse, K. H., Chow, K. B., Leung, W. K., Wong, Y. H., & Wise, H. (2014). Primary sensory neurons regulate Toll-like receptor-4-dependent activity of glial cells in dorsal root ganglia. *Neuroscience, 279*, 10–22. doi:10.1016/j.neuroscience.2014.08.033

Tzoulaki, I., Elliott, P., Kontis, V., & Ezzati, M. (2016). Worldwide Exposures to Cardiovascular Risk Factors and Associated Health Effects: Current Knowledge and Data Gaps. *Circulation, 133*(23), 2314–2333. doi:10.1161/CIRCULATIONAHA.115.008718

van Gils, J. M., Derby, M. C., Fernandes, L. R., Ramkhelawon, B., Ray, T. D., Rayner, K. J., . . . Moore, K. J. (2012). The neuroimmune guidance cue netrin-1 promotes atherosclerosis by inhibiting the emigration of macrophages from plaques. *Nat Immunol, 13*(2), 136–143. doi:10.1038/ni.2205

Vasamsetti, S. B., Florentin, J., Coppin, E., Stiekema, L. C. A., Zheng, K. H., Nisar, M. U., . . . Dutta, P. (2018). Sympathetic neuronal activation triggers myeloid progenitor proliferation and differentiation. *Immunity, 49*(1), 93–106 e107. doi:10.1016/j.immuni.2018.05.004

Vida, G., Peña, G., Deitch, E. A., & Ulloa, L. (2011). α7-cholinergic receptor mediates vagal induction of splenic norepinephrine. *The Journal of Immunology, 186*(7), 4340–4346.

Vizi, E. S., & Elenkov, I. J. (2002). Nonsynaptic noradrenaline release in neuro-immune responses. *Acta Biol Hung, 53*(1–2), 229–244. doi:10.1556/ABiol.53.2002.1-2.21

Wang, H., Yu, M., Ochani, M., Amella, C. A., Tanovic, M., Susarla, S., . . . Tracey, K. J. (2003). Nicotinic acetylcholine receptor alpha7 subunit is an essential regulator of inflammation. *Nature, 421*(6921), 384–388. doi:10.1038/nature01339

Williams, J. M., & Felten, D. L. (1981). Sympathetic innervation of murine thymus and spleen: a comparative histofluorescence study. *Anat Rec, 199*(4), 531–542. doi:10.1002/ar.1091990409

Xiao, L., Kirabo, A., Wu, J., Saleh, M. A., Zhu, L., Wang, F., . . . Harrison, D. G. (2015). Renal denervation prevents immune cell activation and renal inflammation in angiotensin II-induced hypertension. *Circ Res, 117*(6), 547–557. doi:10.1161/CIRCRESAHA.115.306010

Yeboah, M., Xue, X., Duan, B., Ochani, M., Tracey, K., Susin, M., & Metz, C. (2008). Cholinergic agonists attenuate renal ischemia—reperfusion injury in rats. *Kidney international, 74*(1), 62–69.

Ziegler, K. A., Ahles, A., Wille, T., Kerler, J., Ramanujam, D., & Engelhardt, S. (2018). Local sympathetic denervation attenuates myocardial inflammation and improves cardiac function after myocardial infarction in mice. *Cardiovasc Res, 114*(2), 291–299. doi:10.1093/cvr/cvx227

9 Immune Responses Regulated by Exosomal Mechanisms in Cardiovascular Disease

Brooke Lee, Ioannis D. Kyriazis, Ruturaj Patil, Syed Baseeruddin Alvi, Amit Kumar Rai, Mahmood Khan, and Venkata Naga Srikanth Garikipati

CONTENTS

EXOSOME BIOGENESIS

Recently denoted as the smallest group of extracellular vesicles (EVs), exosomes play a vital role in cell-to-cell communication (Kanno, Hirano et al. 2020; Xie, Xiong et al. 2020). Exosomes are constructed by forming an early endosome, which occurs when the lumen undergoes inward budding (Klumperman and Raposo 2014; Garikipati, Shoja-Taheri et al. 2018; Xie, Xiong et al. 2020). The early endosome (number 1 in Figure 9.1) contains membrane-bound structures of the designated area of engulfment. Upon fusion with a new cell, the EV encounters a disruption of its intraluminal vesicles (ILVs), further forcing its cargo to be released from the late endosome (number 2 in Figure 9.1) (Wu, Gao et al. 2019). Once the components of the EV are released, they can be degraded by lysosomes (number 3 in Figure 9.1), or the contents will fuse with the plasma membrane to be secreted toward the extracellular space (number 4 in Figure 9.1) (Garikipati, Shoja-Taheri et al. 2018; Wu, Gao et al. 2019; Xie, Xiong et al. 2020).

EVs can bind to specific receptors on a target cell, where they then fuse with the cell membrane. Suppose the target cell is an antigen-presenting cell (APC); in that case, the EVs' components will be degraded and taken up by the complement system, which then binds to receptors of specific major histocompatibility complexes (MHCs), either class I or class II (Kowal, Arras et al. 2016; Garikipati, Shoja-Taheri et al. 2018). This function is driven by a well-orchestrated, but complicated cascade of signaling pathways that initiate an adequate immune system response against the presented proteins by MHC class I or II (Raposo and Stoorvogel 2013). The specific location of the lumen's inward budding depends on the endosomal sorting complex required for transport (ESCRT), which is composed of proteins Hrs, Tsg101, Alix, and Vsg4. This protein collection selects which surface proteins will be taken in by the cell in order to form an early endosome (Trajkovic, Hsu et al. 2008). Ceramides are formed in microdomains with upregulated sphingolipids,

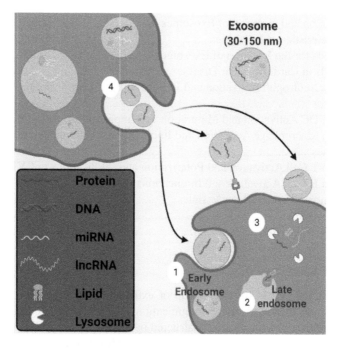

FIGURE 9.1 Biogenesis of exosomes. (1) Early endosome forms when the membrane's inward budding occurs. (2) Late endosomes will release their cargo into the intracellular space. (3) Lysosomes can potentially degrade the late endosome cargo, or (4) the cargo will be released from the cell into the extracellular space.

Source: Created with BioRender.com.

and they are essential to induce the budding of EVs (Gulbins and Kolesnick 2003). Limited information exists concerning the EVs' function despite an understanding of their biogenesis, and the current methods used to characterize them are specific and time-consuming.

CHARACTERIZATION AND ISOLATION OF EXOSOMES

CHARACTERISTICS OF EXOSOMES

EVs have been found to use the paracrine system for cell-to-cell communication (Raposo and Stoorvogel 2013; Garikipati, Shoja-Taheri et al. 2018; Martin-Rufino, Espinosa-Lara et al. 2019; Kang, Nasr et al. 2020; Xie, Xiong et al. 2020). Exosomes are, on average, 30–150 nm in diameter, have a lipid bilayer, and consist of membrane-bound structures: lipids (Colombo, Raposo et al. 2014), proteins (Nguyen, Lewis et al. 2018), DNA (Phinney, Di Giuseppe et al. 2015), messenger RNA (mRNA) (Zhou, Ghoroghi et al. 2016), noncoding RNA (ncRNA) (Phinney, Di Giuseppe et al. 2015), and other organelles (Wu, Gao et al. 2019; Kanno, Hirano et al. 2020; Xie, Xiong et al. 2020). The components within exosomes have increasingly been identified in various diseases, as many have been categorized as biomarkers (Feng, Huang et al. 2014; Lee, Chen et al. 2017; Wang, Zhang et al. 2017; Dragomir, Chen et al. 2018; Brook, Jenkins et al. 2019; Chen, Zhou et al. 2019; Dai, Wang et al. 2020). Recently, studies have uncovered that ncRNA, RNA that does not encode for proteins, makes up approximately 98% of the complex human transcriptome (Djebali, Davis et al. 2012; Huang, Kafert-Kasting et al. 2020). The intriguing ncRNA is further characterized as long, non-coding RNA (lncRNA) (Dinger, Amaral et al. 2008), ribosomal RNA (rRNA) (Noller 1984), microRNA (miRNA or miR) (Bushati and Cohen 2007), circular RNA (circRNA) (Salzman, Gawad et al. 2012), and small nucleolar RNA (snoRNA) (Bachellerie, Cavaillé et al. 2002). Exosomes have been found in a variety of human specimens, including blood (van der Laan, Döpp et al. 1999), saliva (Gallo, Tandon et al. 2012), milk (Manca, Upadhyaya et al. 2018), and bronchoalveolar lavage fluid (Kim, Eom et al. 2018; Kanno, Hirano et al. 2020), allowing them to travel throughout the body. Their ability to communicate has sparked interest in investigating whether exosomes possess therapeutic properties in immune and cardiovascular conditions (Garikipati, Shoja-Taheri et al. 2018; Martin-Rufino, Espinosa-Lara et al. 2019; Wu, Gao et al. 2019; Xie, Xiong et al. 2020). EVs mirror the parent cell from which they are derived; furthermore, they reflect the level of stress to which the parent cell is exposed (Ribeiro-Rodrigues, Laundos et al. 2017). Exosomes have been found to impact target cells' gene expression (Valadi, Ekström et al. 2007; Xie, Xiong et al. 2020). Recent findings show that two types of exosomes have therapeutic capabilities when isolated *in vitro*. Naïve EVs are derived from parental cells and hold immune-modulating effects, protective qualities, and regenerative traits (Batrakova and Kim 2016). Interestingly, gene and drug delivery has been displayed in genetically modified immunocytes in a Parkinson's disease model, but not yet in CVD (Haney, Zhao et al. 2013).

Multiple investigative techniques have the ability to characterize exosomes. The most common methods used are electron microscopy, mass spectrometry, flow cytometry, and Western blot assays. Sophisticated techniques like nanoparticle tracking analysis, nanoplasmonic exosome assays, resistive pulse sensing, and dynamic light scattering can also be used for characterization (Garikipati, Shoja-Taheri et al. 2018). The urgency to uncover a quicker, highly efficient, and economical method to characterize exosomes increases with each discovery made about them. EVs' ability to influence the profile of noncoding RNA and various proteins needs to be further explored to understand their parent cells' physiological state, as this may potentially hold the ability to further understand the role of exosomes (Zhang, Hu et al. 2017; Zhang, Liu et al. 2019).

METHODS FOR THE ISOLATION OF EXOSOMES

EVs are nanoparticles and, when precise methods are used, can be isolated and purified. One characteristic that plays a vital role in EVs' ability to be isolated is their susceptibility to degradation by ribonuclease (RNase) (Mitchell, Parkin et al. 2008; Wu, Gao et al. 2019). The gold standard technique to isolate exosomes is ultracentrifugation (100,000 g) (Théry, Amigorena et al. 2006). The high-speed centrifuge separates dead cells, debris, and proteins from the exosomes, yielding highly purified exosomes. Despite the level of purity this approach achieves, it is lengthy, it requires substantial labor, the equipment is expensive, and it generates a limited amount of exosomes because of the high potential for EV destruction during the process (Théry, Amigorena et al. 2006; Wu, Gao et al. 2019). Size-based techniques can also be used to isolate exosomes (Li, Kaslan et al. 2017). The two most common size-based methods that are used are ultrafiltration and size exclusion chromatography (SEC) (Baranyai, Herczeg et al. 2015; Li, Kaslan et al. 2017). Ultrafiltration is a technique comparable to membrane filtration that is dependent on a particle's size and weight. SEC utilizes a porous, stationary-phase mechanism that separates small and large particles (Feng, Huang et al. 2014; Baranyai, Herczeg et al. 2015; Li, Kaslan et al. 2017). Though both procedures do have their drawbacks, ultrafiltration produces a fair amount of pure, isolated exosomes only, while the SEC technique can result in vesicle trapping and isolation of lipoproteins, along with very low-density lipoprotein (VLDL) remnants that are similar in size (Askeland, Borup et al. 2020). Unfortunately, they generate a moderate amount of isolated EVs. Even though the SEC method precisely preserves EVs' integrity and functionality (Liangsupree, Multia et al. 2020), it is time-consuming and does not produce an extravagant amount of purified EVs (Feng, Huang et al. 2014; Li, Kaslan et al. 2017). By changing the EVs' solubility in water, exosome precipitation is another method that can be used to isolate EVs without polymers. This procedure does not require special measures to be taken and yields a large sample. However, it is laborious and produces impure EVs, because nonexosomal components, such as proteins, are also precipitated (Baranyai, Herczeg et al. 2015; Li, Kaslan et al. 2017).

Furthermore, by using an immunoaffinity capture–based approach, exosomes can be explicitly isolated by targeting of specific surface antigens on EVs with immobile antibodies. This method has been shown to generate the highest level of purified exosomes. However, it should be noted that the reagents used for this method are expensive, targets need to be identified, and epitopes of the antigens can potentially be compromised. Furthermore, even though a high level of pure EVs is generated, the mechanism yields a small sample size (Zarovni, Corrado et al. 2015; Li, Kaslan et al. 2017). Last, a microfluidics-based method is a technique that separates EVs on the basis of their size or immunoaffinity (Meng, Asghari et al. 2021). This allows researchers to yield EVs from fluids on a microscale, avoiding complications such as purity, cost, and laborious and complicated workflows, which further enables them to be utilized in drug delivery studies.

IMMUNE CELLS IN CARDIOVASCULAR DISEASE

Globally, in 2017, the number of deaths related to CVD was approximately 17.8 million (95% CI, 17.5–18.0 million) (Virani, Alonso et al. 2020). Inflammation is a natural response within the heart when an injury is enacted upon, but excessive inflammation leads to myocardial remodeling and worsens cardiovascular disease. Different immune cells are implicated in cardiac inflammation. For instance, Figure 9.2 represents the time line in which various immune cells react within the heart following a myocardial infarction (MI) event. Different cells have unique roles, depending on whether they belong to the innate or adaptive immune system. Recently, EVs' role within the heart has been investigated (Chen, Xu et al. 2017; Dragomir, Chen et al. 2018; Martin-Rufino, Espinosa-Lara et al. 2019; Dai, Wang et al. 2020; Liu, Chen et al. 2020). Therefore, it is essential to better understand immune cell kinetics and how they cross talk via cell secretory factors such as exosomes. Further, this concept has the potential to identify promising therapeutic targets in CVD. The cargo within exosomes can determine whether a pro-inflammatory or an anti-inflammatory response is generated; this depends on the immune cell type from which the EV is derived.

EVs derived from immune cells are unique, as they can affect the pathophysiology of CVD. EVs hold specific constitutive immune system proteins and nucleic acids that assist in the phenotypical functions occurring in different diseases (Dragomir, Chen et al. 2018). For example, exosomes can safeguard the heart by palliating myocardial ischemic reperfusion injury, promoting angiogenesis, inhibiting myocardial fibrosis, and inducing cardiac regeneration (Chen, Xu et al. 2017; Wu, Gao et al. 2019). Additionally, EVs demonstrate guided tropism, as they have been shown to be shuttled to the spleen and liver, where immune cells reside. Thus, EVs can be packaged within immune cells that are recruited to the site of injury within the heart (Wei, Jie et al. 2017; Zheng, Li et al. 2018). Haney et al. have demonstrated this by using EVs as a drug delivery system, in which EVs are injected with specific drugs. EVs can also be loaded with therapeutic agents via physical entrapment or chemical conjugation to achieve desired therapeutic effects (Sun, Zhuang et al. 2010; Wu, Gao et al. 2019). For instance, EVs loaded with curcumin (from rhizomes of turmeric) can deliver it to $CD11b^+Gr-1^+$ cells, induce cell apoptosis, and enhance the solubility and stability of curcumin inside the cell (Sun, Zhuang et al. 2010). It is also suggested that the use of EVs derived from host immune cells may be a futuristic drug delivery mechanism, as they can avoid triggering an immune response within the host (Sun, Zhuang et al. 2010).

EXOSOMES IN NEUTROPHIL ACTIVATION AND
IMPLICATIONS FOR CARDIOVASCULAR DISEASES

Neutrophils are the first-responder phagocytes of the innate immune system that secrete various cytokines and chemokines. Recently, it has been uncovered that neutrophils can release their DNA into the extracellular space, forming neutrophil extracellular traps (NETs) that protect against infection, induce an immune or auto-immune response, and may trigger vaso-occlusion when formed inside the circulatory blood vessels (Papayannopoulos 2018). Neutrophils are known to have a short life span, and via their ROS-mediated scavenging ability, which retains all of the toxic components used within itself, the neutrophil undergoes apoptosis assisted by macrophages (MACs) (Savill, Wyllie et al. 1989). This apoptotic "getaway" has been described as therapeutic in inflammatory diseases (van Rees, Szilagyi et al. 2016). Although neutrophils are the great foot soldiers of the immune system, they can initiate an unwanted inflammatory response that damages tissues (Abram, Roberge et al. 2013; Kaplan 2013; van Rees, Szilagyi et al. 2016). In addition, neutrophils have been shown to act as APCs and produce cytokines and chemokines (Savill, Wyllie et al. 1989).

Neutrophil-derived EVs were first recorded in 1991 by Stein and Luzio (Stein and Luzio 1991). Like other cell-derived exosomes, neutrophil-derived EVs inherit characteristics of the parent cell, including their receptors, adhesion molecules (Slater, Finkielsztein et al. 2017), and complement receptors (Gasser and Schifferli 2005). Since then, a subtype known as neutrophil-derived EV trails has been uncovered to mediate intercellular communication and directly impact immune function (Hong 2018). The contents of neutrophil-derived exosomes have been revealed to be proteins involved in the innate immune response (Vargas, Roux-Dalvai et al. 2016). EVs from neutrophils are stimulated by lipid polysaccharides (LPSs) to transfer proteins that facilitate an immune response to suppress smooth muscle airway cell proliferation. This feature provides reason to investigate further whether neutrophil-derived EVs are associated with cardiac remolding (Vargas, Roux-Dalvai et al. 2016). Recently, neutrophil-derived EVs enriched in neutrophil elastase have been reported to be involved in the progression of inflammation and tissue damage when targeting the alveolar extracellular matrix (Li, Zuo et al. 2020). Our understanding of neutrophil-derived exosomes and their contents in relation to CVD still has a long way to go. It has been reported that miRNA and lncRNA are derived from neutrophils in other diseases (Brook, Jenkins et al. 2019; Li, Zuo et al. 2020).

miRNA has 21–25 nucleotides and is loaded within EVs. Additionally, it has been reported to function as a gene regulator (Beermann, Piccoli et al. 2016). On the other hand, lncRNA has over 200 nucleotides; hence, they are named "long" (Bär, Chatterjee et al. 2016). Further, lncRNA is tissue-specific, making it a prospect for targeted drug therapies (Sarropoulos, Marin et al. 2019). MiR-223 is a biomarker associated with the differentiation of an inflammatory response and a pathogenic inflammatory reaction in non-cardiac-related diseases (Brook, Jenkins et al. 2019). These findings serve as evidence to prompt researchers to investigate the roles ncRNA may have in bacterial endocarditis, as individuals who have had cardiac valve complications or congenital heart issues have an increased risk of developing the condition (Cabell, Abrutyn et al. 2003). Li et al. uncovered lncRNA-miRNA-mRNA pairs from neutrophil-derived exosomes that utilize the adenosine monophosphate–activated protein kinase (AMPK) signaling pathway, Wnt signaling pathway, and NOTCH signaling pathway and may contain biomarkers for angiogenesis and fibrosis in diffuse cutaneous systemic sclerosis. lncRNA-miRNA-mRNA pairs may hold vital information regarding fibrotic and angiogenic pathways in diseased states and may very well be linked to the immune response in CVD.

Like most of the aforementioned immune system cells, neutrophils have also been found to exert protective and destructive CVD qualities. When neutrophils are activated in the bone marrow by a stimulant (stress, irregular sleep, malnutrition), it can promote an inflammatory response within the cardiac tissue (Silvestre-Roig, Braster et al. 2020). Alternatively, neutrophils can induce angiogenesis and endothelial growth to restore tissue function following myocardial infarction (Silvestre-Roig, Braster et al. 2020). Post-MI, neutrophils infiltrate into the infarcted area, which allows them to engulf and destroy dying cardiac cells or to induce apoptosis in healthy ones (Epelman, Liu et al. 2015). Neutrophils can use their intracellular components (mitochondrial DNA that resembles bacterial DNA), to induce Toll-like receptor-9 (TLR-9) to mediate inflammation within cardiomyocytes (Oka, Hikoso et al. 2012).

Additionally, formylated peptides resemble bacterial DNA and can be detected by formyl peptide receptor 1, a chemoattractant that can also activate neutrophils (Oka, Hikoso et al. 2012). Neutrophil activation may be induced by the state of cardiac endothelial cells, which allow neutrophils to pass through their barrier to treat the injured cell (Singh and Saini 2003). It has recently been identified that activated neutrophils release exosomes that express neutrophil elastase extracellularly and that have the ability to attach to the extracellular matrix to further provoke the development of chronic obstructive pulmonary disease (COPD) (Genschmer, Russell et al. 2019). The work done by Genschmer et al. can serve as a platform for investigating the pathophysiological correlation between COPD and CVD, as they commonly coexist (Rabe, Hurst et al. 2018).

The potential therapeutic techniques for neutrophils are long from being completely comprehended. The apoptotic process that is involved should be further investigated as it has shown the ability to be therapeutic. In addition, a better understanding of neutrophils' involvement in the adaptive immune system will help us understand their complexity. Recent discoveries of neutrophil-derived EV effects on different types of endothelial cells also support the need for investigations into their impact on cardiac endothelial cells.

EXOSOMES IN DC ACTIVATION AND MATURATION AND IMPLICATIONS FOR CVDs

Recent studies have mainly explored how exosomes derived from dendritic cells (DCs) can activate other immune cell types. Only a few studies have focused on DCs as an exosome target cell type. Because DC-derived exosomes contain all of the molecules for proper antigen presentation (Zitvogel, Regnault et al. 1998; Wu, Gao et al. 2019), such as MHC-II (signal 1), co-stimulatory factors (signal 2), and cytokines (signal 3), they presumably represent small and fully functional presenting units that can promote a cellular immune response (Segura and Théry 2010; Lindenbergh and Stoorvogel 2018). EVs that contain MHC-II molecules are responsible for T-cell activation and proliferation (Qazi, Gehrmann et al. 2009; Liu, Gao et al. 2016; Leone, Peschel et al. 2017), while other studies have indicated that DC-derived EVs do not contain adequate co-stimulatory molecules and require additional support from naïve DCs (Théry, Duban et al. 2002), therefore indicating the need for further exploration.

DCs are shown to play a vital part in regulating the immune system post-MI (Nagai, Honda et al. 2014; Dieterlen, John et al. 2016). DCs can uptake myocardial peptides, leading to T-cell activation and subsequent recruitment of mature DCs (CD11c[+] and CD11b[+]) to the damaged cardiac tissue (Hawiger, Inaba et al. 2001; Naito, Anzai et al. 2008). It has been demonstrated that DCs exert protective effects in the heart post-MI because they can regulate monocytes and macrophages (Anzai, Anzai et al. 2012). Additionally, cardiac dysfunction progression has been reported in mice when EVs are released from bone marrow DCs (Liu, Gao et al. 2016). EVs derived from DCs may trigger regulatory T-cells (Tregs) to protect cardiomyocytes post-MI (Hofmann, Beyersdorf et al. 2012; Liu, Gao et al. 2016; Wu, Gao et al. 2019).

Recently, interest has sparked around understanding how EVs derived from DCs affect cardiomyocytes, cardiac function, and cardiac remodeling. DC-derived exosomes have been primarily found in the spleen and liver (Wei, Jie et al. 2017; Wu, Gao et al. 2019), although large quantities of DC-derived EVs are present in the heart post-MI. DC-derived EVs can improve mouse cardiac function post-MI and deliver antigen-specific signals while also expressing immune-stimulatory molecules. When exosomes were injected into mice, cardiac function was significantly improved on day 7 following MI compared with the control (Liu, Gao et al. 2016). As mentioned earlier, exosomes derived from DCs can be fully functional, possessing features similar to those of DCs, such as MHC complexes, co-stimulatory molecules, and cytokines. Their ability to modulate the immune system responses has drawn investigators' interest to uncover whether DC-derived EVs have a role in the development or the progression of cardiovascular pathophysiologies. EVs derived from dendritic cells have also shown significant promise in cancer treatment because of the EVs' ability to mediate anti-tumor immune responses along with immunostimulatory traits (Pitt, André et al. 2016).

DCs have also been found to dispatch exosomes and receive information from other cells through their exosomal cargo, thus activating the DCs. This could be driven by cross talk, where DCs endocytose and present intact and functional MHC-antigen complexes found within EVs (Campana, De Pasquale et al. 2015). Exosomal intercellular communication is one of the three ways a donor cell can activate DCs apart from trogocytosis and tunneling nanotubes. For example, heart allograft rejection is mediated by exosomes from the donor DCs that are processed via the host in the adjacent lymph nodes (Liu, Rojas-Canales et al. 2016). Endothelial cell-derived

EVs that exhibit elevated CXCR1 chemokine expression can increase DC migration (Brown, Johnson et al. 2018).

Additionally, circulatory EVs not only present antigens to DCs but also stimulate them using the nuclear factor kappa light chain enhancer of activated B-cell (NF-kB) signaling pathway in Hashimoto thyroiditis patients (Cui, Liu et al. 2019). This route of DC activation has been studied extensively within tumor-derived exosomes. Tumor-specific or highly expressed proteins in cancer cells are transferred to DCs, promoting their maturation and a robust anti-tumor immune response. This indicates that DCs activated by the tumor-derived exosomes can serve as the driving force for specific anti-tumor cytotoxic T-lymphocyte (CTL) responses, representing a novel approach of tumor immunotherapy (Liu, Chen et al. 2018). Experiments using DCs that were stimulated with glioma-derived EVs showed enhanced T-cell response via an increase in CD80 protein, CD86 protein, and MHC-II molecules in DCs.

Studies on pancreatic tumor cells revealed that exosomes containing miR-212-3p lead to a reduced expression of MHC-II molecules in DCs through the downregulation of the regulatory factor X–associated protein (RFXAP) transcription factor (Ding, Zhou et al. 2015). Similarly, miR-203 decreased TLR4 (Toll-like receptor 4) expression in immature DCs when treated with exosomes derived from human pancreatic cancer (PANC-1) cells (Zhou, Chen et al. 2014). Additionally, a detailed study from Montecalvo et al. revealed that exosomes contain miRNA not present in the parent DCs, hinting that EV miRNA may be released at different maturation stages that require unique enrichment factors (Montecalvo, Larregina et al. 2012). Of these miRNAs, miR-148a and miR-451 were found in mature DCs and specifically regulated the unspecified reporter gene used (Montecalvo, Larregina et al. 2012). It was uncovered that the maturation stage of parental DCs affects an exosome's cargo and the exosome acceptor DCs' function. miR-155 and miR146a are associated with the inflammatory response to endotoxins (Alexander, Hu et al. 2015). These two miRNAs are negatively correlated with respect to their effects on the severity of the inflammatory response affecting gene expression; miR-155 promotes inflammation, while miR-146a reduces inflammation (Alexander, Hu et al. 2015). The level of inflammation induced by endotoxins was examined and showed that miR-155 promoted endotoxin-induced inflammation, while miR-146a inhibited inflammation (Alexander, Hu et al. 2015).

While numerous investigations have examined the pathophysiological role of DCs in cardiovascular disease, scientists are only in the beginning stages of understanding DC-derived exosomes. Table 9.1 displays the roles of the noncoding RNA types discussed within this chapter and their association to the noted immune cells from which exosomes are derived. A comprehensive understanding of the involvement of EVs and noncoding RNA in communication between immune cells will be crucial in enhancing therapeutics for CVD treatment. In addition, more insight into the relationship between T-cells and DCs is another potential research avenue to understanding whether specific DC-derived exosomes will trigger an inflammatory or anti-inflammatory response.

TABLE 9.1
Role of Immune Cell-Derived Exosomes in Cardiovascular Disease

Cell Derived from	Noncoding RNA	Target	Outcome	Reference
Dendritic cell	miR-155	BACH1*, SHIP1	Promotes inflammation when responding to endotoxin	Alexander, Hu et al. 2015
Dendritic cell	miR-146	IRAK1, TRAF6	Represses inflammation when responding to endotoxin	Alexander, Hu et al. 2015
Dendritic cell	Multiple microRNAs, including miR-148a and miRNA-451	N/A	Transfer of exosomal microRNA between dendritic cells	Montecalvo, Larregina et al. 2012
Macrophage	miR-155	SOS1	Suppression of fibroblast proliferation while increasing fibroblast inflammation	Wang, Zhang et al. 2017
Macrophage	miR-181b	Prkcd, Cpd, Cnr1, Ncoa2, Map4k4	Cardioprotection	de Couto 2019
Macrophage	lncRNA-ASLNCS5088	miR-200c-3p OR GLS and α-SMA expression	Suppress fibroblast activation	Chen, Zhou et al. 2019
T-cell	miR-155	PRI1	Prevents human cardiomyocyte necrotic cell death post-MI	Liu, van Mil et al. 2011
T-cell	miR-142-3p	RAB11RIP2	Impairs endothelial cell physiology and vascular integrity	Sukma Dewi, Celik et al. 2017
T-cell	miR-29a-3p	IFN-γ	Induction of IFN-γ in T-helper cells	Steiner, Thomas et al. 2011
T-cell	LNA-miR-29	miR-29	Reduced lesion size in aortic roots and brachiocephalic arteries neutralizes miR-29 isoforms	Ulrich, Rotllan et al. 2016
T-cell	miR-29	Col1A, Col3A	Enhances fibrous cap thickness, reduces lesion size and necrotic zones	Ulrich, Rotllan et al. 2016
T-cell	miR-19	Pten, SOCS1, deubiquitinase A20	Enhances Th2 inflammatory signaling	Kuo, Wu et al. 2019
T-cell	miR-19	Pten	Represses proliferation and apoptosis	Gao, Kataoka et al. 2019
B-cell	miR-23a	ND	Inhibits B lymphopoiesis *in vitro* and *in vivo*	Kong, Owens et al. 2010
B-cell	miR-23a	MuRF1	Enhances cardiomyocyte hypertrophy	Lin, Murtaza et al. 2009

*Abbreviations: BACH1, BTB and CNC homology 1; SHIP1, SH2-containing inositol 5-phosphatase 1; IRAK1, interleukin-1 receptor-associated kinase-1; TRAF6, TNF receptor–associated factor 6; SOS1, son of sevenless homolog 1; PRKCD, protein kinase C delta type; CPD, carboxypeptidase D precursor; Crn1, cannabinoid receptor 1; Ncoa2, nuclear receptor coactivator 2; 3., mitogen-activated protein kinase kinase kinase kinase 4; GLS, glutaminase; PRI1, receptor-interacting protein 1; Col1, collagen type 1; Col3A, collagen type III alpha 1; Pten, phosphatase and tensin homolog; SOCS1, suppressor of cytokine signaling 1; ND, not determined; MuRF1, muscle RING-finger protein-1.

EXOSOMES IN MACROPHAGE ACTIVATION AND IMPLICATIONS FOR CARDIOVASCULAR DISEASES

MACs, like DCs and neutrophils, are also professional APCs of the innate immune system and are a part of the first line of defense against foreign or pathogenic antigens (Munn, Sharma et al. 2004; Sancho, Joffre et al. 2009; Shortman and Heath 2010; Wu, Gao et al. 2019). MACs modify their transcriptional signature by using a polarization mechanism that divides them into two distinct subtypes, macrophage type 1 (M1) and macrophage type 2 (M2) (Buscher, Ehinger et al. 2017; Orecchioni, Ghosheh et al. 2019). Class M1-MACs (displayed in Figure 9.2) on days 0–4 have pro-inflammatory machinery that degrades pathogens, dying cells, or cell debris when presented to M1 (Mills, Kincaid et al. 2000; Italiani and Boraschi 2014; Orecchioni, Ghosheh et al. 2019). Alternatively, M2-MACs during days 5–14 (Figure 9.2) are shown to be equipped with anti-inflammatory elements that enable them to endorse tissue repair and cell proliferation when partnered with T-helper cells (Mills, Kincaid et al. 2000; Italiani and Boraschi 2014; Orecchioni, Ghosheh et al. 2019). Interestingly, the microRNA miR-21 from MAC-derived EVs has been revealed to trigger a pro-inflammatory response, upregulating the M1 phenotype (Madhyastha, Madhyastha et al. 2021). Alternatively, miR-21 has demonstrated the ability to downregulate the MAC target gene programmed cell death protein 4 (PDCD4) (Madhyastha, Madhyastha et al. 2021). When PDCD4 is downregulated

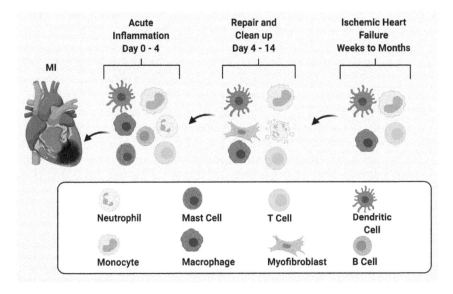

FIGURE 9.2 Immune cells in myocardial infarction. Immune cells are deployed at different time points following injury. Immune cells work together to combat cleaning up the damage and debris with a pro-inflammatory response, while also healing the injury with an anti-inflammatory response.

Source: Created with BioRender.com.

by miR-21, it prevents the apoptotic functions of cytokine NF-κB, which is found within islet β-cells and can help prevent the development of type 1 diabetes (Ruan, Wang et al. 2011). This may be translatable to CVD, as a recent study has found a life expectancy reduction of approximately 12 years among individuals with diabetes mellitus and CVD (Pennells, Kaptoge et al. 2019). Essentially, MACs' responsibility is to govern immune responses in inflammatory and reparative states, a crucial switch during myocardial repair post-MI (Wynn and Barron 2010; Cao 2018; Cao, Schiattarella et al. 2018).

The contributions of exosomes derived from MACs to immune responses are becoming more apparent, leaving researchers curious about their role and function. *In vivo* and *in vitro* studies have confirmed that EVs released from macrophages in a diseased state have a stimulatory role during pro-inflammatory responses (Bhatnagar, Shinagawa et al. 2007). Since this discovery, MAC-derived exosomes have been recorded in the exacerbation of various diseases, cell death, tissue repair, and pathogen supervision, and they have been used to administer drugs. Additionally, MAC-derived EVs have demonstrated the ability to alter endothelial cell function and genes associated with endothelial cells during angiogenesis by distorting the endothelial basement membrane (Potente, Gerhardt et al. 2011; Weis and Cheresh 2011; Baer, Squadrito et al. 2013). This insinuates that MACs found in the perivascular space during angiogenesis may secrete EVs to endothelial cells, altering the vascular membranes (Baer, Squadrito et al. 2013).

Recent studies have investigated the components within macrophage-derived EVs. M2-derived EVs have been reported to contain miR-148, which blocks the thioredoxin-interacting protein signaling pathway and the NF-κB/NLRP3 (NOD-, LRR-, and pyrin domain–containing protein 3) inflammasome signaling pathway, palliating the trauma caused by MI (Dai, Wang et al. 2020). The upregulation of miR-155 in injured hearts has sparked interest in its characteristics. Macrophage-derived EVs with miR-155 have been found to inhibit fibroblast proliferation when suppressing son of sevenless 1 (*Sos1*), while also to promote fibroblast inflammation by inhibiting suppressor of cytokine signaling 1 (*Socs1*) (Wang, Zhang et al. 2017). Further understanding of the function and mechanisms of miR-155 within MAC-derived EVs is needed to clarify its features. MiR-181b present in MAC-derived EVs has also been shown to exert cardioprotective abilities and mediate polarization of MACs post-MI (de Couto, Gallet et al. 2017). M2-derived EVs were observed to contain the lncRNA lnrNCS5088, which potentially plays a role in scar tissue formation because it can inhibit fibroblast function by sponging miR-200c-3p found within fibroblasts (Chen, Zhou et al. 2019). Interestingly, MAC-derived EV participation has been reported to induce matrix metalloproteinase-2 found in vascular smooth muscle via c-jun N-terminal kinase (JNK) and p38 MAPK (mitogen-activated protein kinase), promoting the development of abdominal aortic aneurysms (Wang, Jia et al. 2019). M1s have been recently shown to release pro-inflammatory EVs post-MI that expedite MI damage (Liu, Chen et al. 2020). Moreover, anti-angiogenic and cardiac restorative characteristics were also recorded when M1-derived miR-155 enters endothelial cells, targeting various pathways simultaneously (Liu, Chen et al. 2020).

Macrophage-derived EVs have been habitually involved in cancer, as discoveries of their interactions continue to surface. Recently, a link between CVD and the risk of cancer development has been proposed (Lau, Paniagua et al. 2021). Lau et al. used a 10-year risk estimation tool for atherosclerotic CVD that uncovered a 6.5% increased risk in cancer incidence compared to no cancer in participants with CVD. Additionally, natriuretic peptides, which are CVD biomarkers, were also associated with cancer among participants (Lau, Paniagua et al. 2021). Still, this proposal is in its initial phase, as translational research will be needed to confirm the concept. In the future, researchers should strive to make connections among the contents within exosomes and to attempt to find a link between ncRNA involved in cancer and CVD.

EXOSOMES IN T-CELL ACTIVATION AND POLARIZATION AND IMPLICATIONS IN CVD

T-cells have been heavily involved with the development of CVD (Blanton, Carrillo-Salinas et al. 2019). It is already well-known that T-cells are driven by several cardiovascular pathophysiologies, for instance, ischemia reperfusion (I/R) and MI, and T-cell reactions contribute to the end-point phenotype. T-cells are also responsible for orchestrating the development of several cardiovascular conditions, such as heart transplant rejection (Ingulli 2010), myocarditis (Vdovenko and Eriksson 2018), and atherosclerosis (Saigusa, Winkels et al. 2020). T-cells are recruited via chemotaxis during cardiac tissue injury. Here, it is their job to induce remodeling by promoting inflammation or by hindering other resident or recruited leukocytes (Stephenson, Savvatis et al. 2017). The release of cytokines (TNFα, IFNγ, IL-10, and IL-17) dictates the immune response during heart failure, with a restrictive or preserved ejection fraction (Blanton, Carrillo-Salinas et al. 2019). After an infection or ischemic condition, T-cells are also involved in cardiac remodeling as they induce fibroblast differentiation into myofibroblasts to occupy the space left following cardiomyocyte death (Bradshaw and DeLeon-Pennell 2020). This is again caused by cytokine or chemokine release from CD8[+], CD4[+], or Treg cells. T-cells and B-cells have been reported to be associated with myocardial recovery and immune regulation post-MI (Hofmann, Beyersdorf et al. 2012; Kang, Nasr et al. 2020). T-cells additionally play a vital role in cardiac conditions such as heart failure (Hofmann, Beyersdorf et al. 2012; Kang, Nasr et al. 2020). Extensive research has been conducted concerning the contribution of T-cells to atherosclerosis formation. CD4[+] helper T-cells and Tregs have been found in atherosclerotic plaque, although they perform various functions (Pastrana, Sha et al. 2012). T-helper cells have a clear, pro-atherogenic contribution through a sustained inflammatory response, whereas Tregs suppress atherogenesis; despite this, the contribution of CD8[+] cells in atherosclerosis remains unclear (van Duijn, Kuiper et al. 2018).

Apart from the cross-presentation or cross talk described in the respective DC section, T-cells can be directly activated by fully functional exosomes containing MHC complexes. Further, EVs modulated the T-cell-related adaptive immune response, regardless of whether they were derived from T-cells

(Raposo, Nijman et al. 1996; Théry, Duban et al. 2002). Additionally, vast literature in cancer biology reveals that exosomes could contain several antigens that will modulate the activation or polarization of T-cells. Even though cancer-derived exosomes may be expected to dispatch information to suppress immune cell activity, dodging their control, several studies also found that EVs carry signaling molecules activate T-cells, without knowing the exact mechanisms that govern the inhibitory or stimulatory outcome. Exosomes can affect T-cell differentiation or proliferation bidirectionally. More specifically, transforming growth factor-β-enriched (TGF-β) exosomes can immunosuppress T-cells, converting them into Tregs (Rong, Li et al. 2016). They even can affect T-cells' proliferation ability (Lazarova and Steinle 2019). In line with the previous studies, it has been found that the cytokines or proteins present in exosomal cargo, such as TNF-related apoptosis-inducing ligand (TRAIL), Fas ligand (FasL), and programmed death-ligand 1 (PD-L1), can halt CD8+ CTL proliferation. Mechanistic analyses revealed that activation of pro-apoptotic Bcl-2-associated X protein (Thygesen, Alpert et al. 2007) via the Akt/PKB pathway is responsible for cellular apoptosis of CD8+ T-cells. Furthermore, culturing of tumor-derived EVs with CD4+ Treg cells, conventional CD4+ T-cells, or CD8+ T-cells increased the expression of TGF-β, IL-10, the COX-2 enzyme, the CD39 enzyme, and the CD73 enzyme, further dictating immunosuppression (Muller, Mitsuhashi et al. 2016). The CD39 and CD73 enzymes induce adenosine secretion, an immunosuppressive factor that negatively regulates the immune response (Schuler, Saze et al. 2014; Muller, Mitsuhashi et al. 2016). Conversely, EVs carry heat-shock proteins or the synthetic glycolipid α-galactosylceramide, which has potent anti-tumor effects, combined with a tumor antigen that can induce T-cell activation. Furthermore, DCs that tumor antigens have compromised secrete EVs that transfer MHC complexes to stimulate naïve CD4+ T-cells. T-cell-derived exosomal function follows the phenotypically differentiated and activated effector T-cell characteristics. Tregs secrete extensive EVs, compared to any other T-cell type. These Tregs mainly deploy immunosuppressive functions that mostly express CD25 and CTLA-4 molecules (Okoye, Coomes et al. 2014). It has also been found that Treg-derived exosomes carry several enclosed or surface molecules, such as miRNA-155, RAB family proteins, IL-35, IL-10, TGF-β, and CD73, that allow Tregs to increase tolerance and suppress autoimmune Th1 response (Okoye, Coomes et al. 2014). Immunosuppression is also promoted via exosome delivery when T-cells interact with the DCs (Mittelbrunn, Gutiérrez-Vázquez et al. 2011). FasL-carrying exosomes induce apoptosis in mature DCs and other activated T-cells, favoring immune response inhibition (Zhang, Xie et al. 2011) and protecting from autoimmunity. CD8+ cytotoxic T-cells can secrete exosomes that inhibit APCs' function (Xie, Zhang et al. 2010), further supporting tumor progression or cell-mediated contact hypersensitivity (Nazimek, Ptak et al. 2015). Additionally, T-cell-derived EVs can modulate humoral responses by interacting with B-cells via CD40 ligand (Dustin 2017). Moreover, CD4+ T-cells, upon activation, have the expertise of dispatching exosomes to modulate and activate distant naïve T-cells (van der Vlist, Arkesteijn et al. 2012).

Numerous studies have examined the role of noncoding RNAs in the development or progression of cardiovascular diseases, while only a few have managed to implicate their presence in exosomes derived from T-cells that affect different cardiovascular pathophysiology.

The majority of the studies examining miRNA's role in T-cell functional regulation have involved cancerous diseases. Briefly, EVs derived from nasopharyngeal carcinoma cells possess elevated amounts of miRNA (hsa-miR-24-3p, hsa-miR-891a, hsa-miR-106a-5p, hsa-miR-20a-5p, and hsa-miR-1908), which inhibited T-cell differentiation and proliferation via the MAPK pathway (Ye, Li et al. 2014). This action shifts Th1 and Th17 subtypes into Th2 and Tregs, respectively. Additionally, in mice, lung cancer and sarcomas show that miR-214 drives Treg differentiation through the phosphatase and tensin homolog (Pten) (Walsh, Buckler et al. 2006). Conversely, the lack of miR-155 expression inhibits Treg and Th17 cell development, affecting $CD4^+$-mediated immunosuppression (Chen, Gao et al. 2020). miR-155 has been found to block cellular necrosis post-myocardial injury, further supporting cardiomyocyte survival (Liu, van Mil et al. 2011). miR-142-3p, packaged inside of EVs derived from activated $CD4^+$ T-cells following MI, has been found to deteriorate cardiac remodeling through the molecular fibrosis process via the wingless-related integration site (WNT) pathway (Pontis, Costa et al. 2014). Additionally, a decrease in miR-142-3p exhibited decreased $CD4^+$ T-cell recruitment in atherosclerotic plaque, due to alterations to cytoskeleton dynamics (Pontis, Costa et al. 2014). Furthermore, miR-142-3p upregulation in the exosomes of activated T-cells increases endothelial permeability, which may be implicated in acute cellular rejection in heart transplantations (Sukma Dewi, Celik et al. 2017). Also, miR-29 plays a role in promoting CVD through T-cells. MiR29a-3p and miR-29b-3p can modulate the target genes, T-box transcription factor 21 (Tbx21) and eomesodermin (EOMES). These genes are master transcriptional regulators of $CD4^+$ Th1 cells and can alleviate atherosclerosis development when quenching Th1 progression and stabilizing atherosclerotic plaque (Steiner, Thomas et al. 2011). Conversely, LNA-miR-29 can be administered to silence miR-29 possessing the same qualities by reducing plaque formation (Ulrich, Rotllan et al. 2016). miR-19 is highly expressed during T-cell and B-cell development, promoting lymphocyte survival (Kuo, Wu et al. 2019). Alternatively, it may be a promising target to enhance treatment of an ischemic injury, as it enhances cardiomyocyte proliferation and is found to be upregulated in cardiomyocytes (Gao, Kataoka et al. 2019).

Conclusively, exosomes derived from activated T-cells can transfer biological information similar to that of the "mothership cell" and seem to be a supportive arm of T-cell-mediated immune response contributing to the inflammatory phenotype in cardiovascular diseases. Thus far, noncoding RNA enclosed within EVs has been investigated more frequently in T-lymphocytes than in any other immune cell, as shown in Figure 9.3. To better assess the unique characteristics of noncoding RNA in T-cells, further investigative research and uniform databases are demanded.

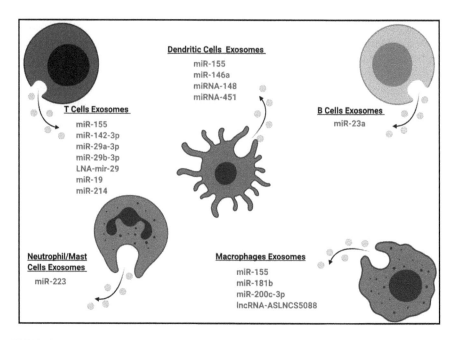

FIGURE 9.3   Immune cell exosomal cargo. Exosomes are being released from each immune cell, where they cross talk with different cells. Depending on the cargo within the exosome, different responses can arise.

Source: Created with BioRender.com

EXOSOMES IN B-CELL ACTIVATION AND IMPLICATIONS FOR CVDs

The role of B-cells has also been studied extensively in cardiovascular diseases, but it is essential to state that B-cells seem to have both detrimental and beneficial effects. B-cell contribution in acute cardiomyopathy is mainly due to the binding of antibodies. These antibodies can recognize specific cardiomyocyte antigens that further promote programmed cell death (Kaya, Leib et al. 2012; Nussinovitch and Shoenfeld 2013). This effect is detrimental for cardiomyocytes because they cannot regenerate (Steinhauser and Lee 2011). Apart from that, antibodies against Na$^+$/K$^+$-ATPase or intracellular structural proteins seem to cause arrhythmias or autoimmune myocarditis (Neu, Rose et al. 1987; Baba, Yoshikawa et al. 2002; Doesch, Mueller et al. 2011). Even though B-cells seem to infiltrate after 3 days in ischemic models (Santos-Zas, Lemarié et al. 2018; Rusinkevich, Huang et al. 2019), they contribute to the recruitment of Ly6C$^+$ monocytes from bone marrow via a chemokine-dependent mechanism (Zouggari, Ait-Oufella et al. 2013). It has been established that B-cell depletion may alleviate myocardial injury outcomes. It has been reported that bone marrow-derived B-cells beneficially participate in the injured myocardium (Goodchild, Robinson et al. 2009); this discrepancy is also evident in other pathological models, like pressure overload. B-cell depletion showed reduced inflammatory cytokines, causing minimal remodeling (Cordero-Reyes, Youker et al. 2016), while IL-10-producing B-cells can protect the hypertrophic phenotype through an immunosuppressive effect on T-cells (Kallikourdis, Martini et al. 2017). In other cases, B-cell cytokine release, following a T-cell/B-cell interaction, establishes a biochemical environment that promotes unfavorable inflammatory responses in the failing myocardium (Cappuzzello, Di Vito et al. 2011). Apart from the critical role that B-cell-derived antibodies play against cardiomyocyte-specific antigens, memory B-cells' chronic secondary reaction can exacerbate severe cellular damage. B-cells have an atheroprotective effect via IgM antibodies that block oxidized low-density lipoprotein (oxLDL) (Srikakulapu and McNamara 2017). Conversely, B-cells can aggravate atherosclerosis through monocyte and T-cell stimulation. Finally, B-cells are also implicated in the development of an abdominal aortic aneurysm (Forester, Cruickshank et al. 2005; Schaheen, Downs et al. 2016).

Following established knowledge that B-cell differentiation and proliferation rely on DCs or T-cell interaction, EVs that are derived from mature DCs or activated T-cells play a regulatory role in B-cell immune responses. In a sophisticated study, DC-derived EVs can promote the Th1 immune response, in which T-cell activation is driven through B-cells (Qazi, Gehrmann et al. 2009). This confirms that exosomes can serve as a tool for complicated communications among various immune cells. Additionally, exosomes, not microvesicles, from activated DCs can increase the B-cell population in the germinal center, indicating the unique feature that exosomes possess that assists in intracellular communication (Wahlund, Güclüler et al. 2017). It has been shown that $CD4^+$ T-cell-derived EVs can stimulate B-cell activation, proliferation, and differentiation through CD40L (Lu, Wu et al. 2019). CD40L seems to be crucial in mast cell and B-cell communication. Hence, EVs derived from mast cells stimulate the maturation of B-cells that produce IL-10 (Imai, Imai et al. 2015). Furthermore, mast cell-derived EVs possessing CD40 can also promote B-cell differentiation (Imai, Imai et al. 2015). Finally, other studies have reported that prostaglandins loaded in EVs have been associated with suppression of B-cell activation (Murn, Alibert et al. 2008; Subra, Grand et al. 2010).

B-cell-derived EVs contain the same proteins that the B-cells' plasma membrane possesses, explaining why B-cell-derived exosomes have similar cell-to-cell communication features. In addition, EVs can contain co-stimulatory factors, adhesion molecules, and antigen-presenting MHC class I and II molecules on their surface to facilitate T-cell immune responses (Raposo, Nijman et al. 1996) that help to exert their antigen-presenting role, respectively. Further, the presence of MHC characteristics drives B-cell-derived EVs to impact the T-cell-mediated adaptive immune response, as previously mentioned (Raposo, Nijman et al. 1996). Detailed studies from Saunderson et al. have found that B-cell-derived EVs are responsible for inducing an adequate cytotoxic T-cell response when communicating with other T-cells and NK (natural killer) cells (Saunderson, Schuberth et al. 2008; Saunderson and McLellan 2017). For that reason, B-cell-derived exosomes may be an exciting target to halt carotid artery disease and potentially myocardial infarction in which $CD8^+$ cells have been implicated (Kolbus, Ljungcrantz et al. 2013).

Although B-cells represent a significant "arm" of adaptive immunity, limited information exists on noncoding RNAs freighted in exosomes that contribute to cardiovascular diseases. miR-23a is highly expressed in B-cells and contributes to their maturation and differentiation processes (Kong, Owens et al. 2010). In addition, miR-23a can suppress the anti-hypertrophic muscle RING-finger protein-1 (MuRF1) in cardiomyocytes and is associated with cardiac pathophysiologies, rendering it an attractive target (Lin, Murtaza et al. 2009).

Regarding CD4$^+$ T-cells, B-cell-derived exosomes can promote their cell death through FasL (Klinker, Lizzio et al. 2014). This shows that B-cells manipulate T-cell responses (Lundy, Klinker et al. 2015) and uncovers targeting potential in instances of cardiovascular diseases in which CD4$^+$ cells have been implicated, such as myocarditis (Opavsky, Penninger et al. 1999), atherosclerosis (Grönberg, Nilsson et al. 2017), or cardiomyopathy after ischemic conditions (Hofmann and Frantz 2016).

TRANSPLANTATION OF EXTRACELLULAR VESICLES

Targeted exosomes' delivery to the infarcted cardiac region is a challenge due to the nonspecific uptake of injected exosomes by the reticuloendothelial system (Wiklander, Nordin et al. 2015). Despite the efficacy of exosomes, their inability to target the tissue of interest has spurred researchers to engineer hybrid EVs with homing peptides. To target and retain the exosomes within the ischemic myocardium, ischemic myocardium peptide targeted (IMPT) has been explored; the EVs were engineered by tagging IMPT on the exosomal surface by following simple click chemistry via dibenzocyclooctyne (DBCO) and azide at physiological conditions. These exosomes displayed localization within the ischemic region 24 hours post intravenous (IV) administration compared with unmodified EVs (Zhu, Tian et al. 2018). Similarly, cardiac stem cell-derived EVs were tagged with a cardiac homing peptide (CHP) by the phospholipid DOPE-NHS linker; these exosomes improved cardiac functionality and inhibited scar formation upon IV administration (Vandergriff, Huang et al. 2018).

Researchers have developed bioengineered exosomes by integrating cardiomyocyte-specific peptide (CSP) with the exosomal protein Lamp2b. The fusion of these proteins has led to the biogenesis of hybrid exosomes with inherent targeting capacity. Results have demonstrated that cardiomyocytes, rather than cardiac fibroblasts, specifically took up these EVs; upon intramyocardial delivery, these exosomes could be retained at the injected site compared with nontargeted exosomes (Mentkowski and Lang 2019). Similarly, the Lamp2b protein was fused with IMTP, which exhibited superior cellular uptake via hypoxia-injured cardiac cells compared to unmodified EVs. In addition, the modified exosomes showed specific accumulation in the infarcted region and were retained for 72 hours post IV injection.

Significant inflammation inhibition was also observed (Wang, Chen et al. 2018). However, the use of various targeting peptides may enhance its targeting efficacy, resulting in its clearance from the system. For that reason, repeated dosing with EVs is warranted to achieve a therapeutic outcome. Alternatively, hydrogels are being used to avoid multiple doses and improve the availability of exosomes because of their ability to be retained at the injected site.

Exosomes were derived from mesenchymal stem cells (MSCs) and encapsulated in a peptide-based hydrogel, and the self-assembled peptides were able to retain the exosomes for 22 days while exhibiting enzyme-triggered localized release of EVs (Han, Zhou et al. 2019). EVs derived from induced pluripotent stem cells (iPSCs) have also been encapsulated in a light-responsive hyaluronic acid–based hydrogel. These hydrogels reveal UV-based cross-linking and display localized retention for 14 days upon pericardial administration. Furthermore, the *in vivo* studies demonstrated significant cardiac function enhancement post-treatment (Zhu, Li et al. 2021). A shear-thinning hydrogel, made of gelatin and silicate nanoparticles, has been explored for the localized delivery of stem cell secretomes (including exosomes) for cardiac repair. The *in vivo* study demonstrated a significant improvement in cardiac function and suppressed inflammation (Waters, Alam et al. 2018). In another instance, a ureidopyrimidinone-based hydrogel was fabricated by incorporating cardiac progenitor cell-derived EVs. The hydrogel retained exosomes within the matrix for 4 days, and the released EVs were functionally viable (Mol, Lei et al. 2019). However, further research is warranted to develop hydrogels for exosome delivery that can accommodate large doses and exhibit sustained release with superior ability to be injected.

FUTURE PERSPECTIVES

Exosomes contain surface molecules that have the characteristics of the "mothership" immune cell, and because of that, they are primarily able to exert similar activities. Conversely, their content is so heterogenic that opposing results are reported, especially in cardiovascular diseases. Over the last decades, research efforts have extensively described the functions of the different immune cell types and their contributions to plastic phenotypes or cardiovascular pathophysiologies. The discovery of EVs complicated the mechanistic approach that scientists initially proposed and opened new avenues to intervene in or diagnose CVD. This is because exosomes have been used to immunosuppress undesired inflammatory responses or to carry molecules that reflect the existing pathological condition. This technological improvement allows scientists to perform more sophisticated experiments that will further the description of exosome functions, which, per se, are complex due to their motile nature and the cell from which they originated. The topics discussed in this chapter have started to generate targeted interventions as exosomes can modulate the immune response in favor of cardiac healing and immune cells can process their cargo and comply with it (Sun, Wang et al. 2020; Tu, Wang et al. 2020; Xia, Chen et al. 2020; Yu, Qin et al. 2020). Still, little is known about the restorative properties of immune cells' EVs, and there is great potential for developing immune therapies. Understanding the functional differences between different cell subtypes of neutrophils, DCs, T-cells, B-cells, and MACs has progressed therapeutic understanding. Future work on the bioengineering of immune cell-derived exosomes and their delivery methods will give us more insights on developing novel therapeutics to treat CVD. This will be reinforced by identifying the exosomes' cargo derived from the immune cells to comprehend cardiac inflammation and repair.

BIBLIOGRAPHY

Abram, C. L., et al. (2013). "Distinct roles for neutrophils and dendritic cells in inflammation and autoimmunity in motheaten mice." *Immunity* **38**(3): 489–501.

Alexander, M., et al. (2015). "Exosome-delivered microRNAs modulate the inflammatory response to endotoxin." *Nature Communications* **6**(1): 1–16.

Anzai, A., et al. (2012). "Regulatory role of dendritic cells in postinfarction healing and left ventricular remodeling." *Circulation* **125**(10): 1234–1245.

Askeland, A., et al. (2020). "Mass-spectrometry based proteome comparison of extracellular vesicle isolation methods: comparison of ME-kit, size-exclusion chromatography, and high-speed centrifugation." *Biomedicines* **8**(8): 246.

Baba, A., et al. (2002). "Autoantibodies produced against sarcolemmal Na-K-ATPase: possible upstream targets of arrhythmias and sudden death in patients with dilated cardiomyopathy." *Journal of the American College of Cardiology* **40**(6): 1153–1159.

Bachellerie, J.-P., et al. (2002). "The expanding snoRNA world." *Biochimie* **84**(8): 775–790.

Baer, C., et al. (2013). "Reciprocal interactions between endothelial cells and macrophages in angiogenic vascular niches." *Experimental Cell Research* **319**(11): 1626–1634.

Bär, C., et al. (2016). "Long noncoding RNAs in cardiovascular pathology, diagnosis, and therapy." *Circulation* **134**(19): 1484–1499.

Baranyai, T., et al. (2015). "Isolation of exosomes from blood plasma: qualitative and quantitative comparison of ultracentrifugation and size exclusion chromatography methods." *PLoS ONE* **10**(12): e0145686.

Batrakova, E. V. and M. S. Kim (2016). "Development and regulation of exosome-based therapy products." *Wiley Interdisciplinary Reviews: Nanomedicine and Nanobiotechnology* **8**(5): 744–757.

Beermann, J., et al. (2016). "Non-coding RNAs in development and disease: background, mechanisms, and therapeutic approaches." *Physiological Reviews* **96**(4): 1297–1325.

Bhatnagar, S., et al. (2007). "Exosomes released from macrophages infected with intracellular pathogens stimulate a proinflammatory response in vitro and in vivo." *Blood* **110**(9): 3234–3244.

Blanton, R. M., et al. (2019). "T-cell recruitment to the heart: friendly guests or unwelcome visitors?" *The American Journal of Physiology-Heart and Circulatory Physiology* **317**(1): H124–H140.

Bradshaw, A. D. and K. Y. DeLeon-Pennell (2020). "T-cell regulation of fibroblasts and cardiac fibrosis." *Matrix Biology* **91–92**: 167–175.

Brook, A. C., et al. (2019). "Neutrophil-derived miR-223 as local biomarker of bacterial peritonitis." *Scientific Reports* **9**(1): 1–12.

Brown, M., et al. (2018). "Lymphatic exosomes promote dendritic cell migration along guidance cues." *Journal of Cell Biology* **217**(6): 2205–2221.

Buscher, K., et al. (2017). "Natural variation of macrophage activation as disease-relevant phenotype predictive of inflammation and cancer survival." *Nature Communications* **8**(1): 1–10.

Bushati, N. and S. M. Cohen (2007). "microRNA functions." *Annual Review of Cell and Developmental Biology* **23**: 175–205.

Cabell, C. H., et al. (2003). "Bacterial endocarditis: the disease, treatment, and prevention." *Circulation* **107**(20): e185–e187.

Campana, S., et al. (2015). "Cross-dressing: an alternative mechanism for antigen presentation." *Immunology Letters* **168**(2): 349–354.

Cao, D. J. (2018). "Macrophages in cardiovascular homeostasis and disease." *Circulation* **138**(22): 2452–2455.

Cao, D. J., et al. (2018). "Cytosolic DNA sensing promotes macrophage transformation and governs myocardial ischemic injury." *Circulation* **137**(24): 2613–2634.

Cappuzzello, C., et al. (2011). "Increase of plasma IL-9 and decrease of plasma IL-5, IL-7, and IFN-γ in patients with chronic heart failure." *Journal of Translational Medicine* **9**: 28.

Chen, G.-H., et al. (2017). "Exosomes: promising sacks for treating ischemic heart disease?" *American Journal of Physiology-Heart and Circulatory Physiology* **313**(3): H508–H523.

Chen, J., et al. (2019). "Blockade of lncRNA-ASLNCS5088—enriched exosome generation in M2 macrophages by GW4869 dampens the effect of M2 macrophages on orchestrating fibroblast activation." *The FASEB Journal* **33**(11): 12200–12212.

Chen, L., et al. (2020). "miR-155 indicates the fate of CD4." *Immunology Letters* **224**: 40–49.

Colombo, M., et al. (2014). "Biogenesis, secretion, and intercellular interactions of exosomes and other extracellular vesicles." *Annual Review of Cell and Developmental Biology* **30**: 255–289.

Cordero-Reyes, A. M., et al. (2016). "Full expression of cardiomyopathy is partly dependent on b-cells: a pathway that involves cytokine activation, immunoglobulin deposition, and activation of apoptosis." *Journal of the American Heart Association* **5**(1).

Cui, X., et al. (2019). "Circulating exosomes activate dendritic cells and induce unbalanced CD4+ T cell differentiation in hashimoto thyroiditis." *The Journal of Clinical Endocrinology & Metabolism* **104**(10): 4607–4618.

Dai, Y., et al. (2020). "M2 macrophage-derived exosomes carry microRNA-148a to alleviate myocardial ischemia/reperfusion injury via inhibiting TXNIP and the TLR4/NF-κB/NLRP3 inflammasome signaling pathway." *Journal of Molecular and Cellular Cardiology* **142**: 65–79.

de Couto, G. (2019). "Macrophages in cardiac repair: environmental cues and therapeutic strategies." *Experimental & Molecular Medicine* **51**(12): 1–10.

de Couto, G., et al. (2017). "Exosomal microRNA transfer into macrophages mediates cellular postconditioning." *Circulation* **136**(2): 200–214.

Dieterlen, M.-T., et al. (2016). "Dendritic cells and their role in cardiovascular diseases: a view on human studies." *Journal of Immunology Research* **2016**.

Ding, G., et al. (2015). "Pancreatic cancer-derived exosomes transfer miRNAs to dendritic cells and inhibit RFXAP expression via miR-212–3p." *Oncotarget* **6**(30): 29877.

Dinger, M. E., et al. (2008). "Long noncoding RNAs in mouse embryonic stem cell pluripotency and differentiation." *Genome Research* **18**(9): 1433–1445.

Djebali, S., et al. (2012). "Landscape of transcription in human cells." *Nature* **489**(7414): 101–108.

Doesch, A. O., et al. (2011). "Impact of troponin I-autoantibodies in chronic dilated and ischemic cardiomyopathy." *Basic Research in Cardiology* **106**(1): 25–35.

Dragomir, M., et al. (2018). "Exosomal lncRNAs as new players in cell-to-cell communication." *Translational Cancer Research* **7**(Suppl 2): S243.

Dustin, M. L. (2017). "Help to go: T cells transfer CD40L to antigen-presenting B cells." *European Journal of Immunology* **47**(1): 31–34.

Epelman, S., et al. (2015). "Role of innate and adaptive immune mechanisms in cardiac injury and repair." *Nature Reviews Immunology* **15**(2): 117–129.

Feng, Y., et al. (2014). "Ischemic preconditioning potentiates the protective effect of stem cells through secretion of exosomes by targeting Mecp2 via miR-22." *PLoS ONE* **9**(2): e88685.

Forester, N. D., et al. (2005). "Functional characterization of T cells in abdominal aortic aneurysms." *Immunology* **115**(2): 262–270.

Gallo, A., et al. (2012). "The majority of microRNAs detectable in serum and saliva is concentrated in exosomes." *PLoS ONE* **7**(3): e30679.

Gao, F., et al. (2019). "Therapeutic role of miR-19a/19b in cardiac regeneration and protection from myocardial infarction." *Nature Communications* **10**(1): 1–15.

Garikipati, V. N. S., et al. (2018). "Extracellular vesicles and the application of system biology and computational modeling in cardiac repair." *Circulation Research* **123**(2): 188–204.

Gasser, O. and J. A. Schifferli (2005). "Microparticles released by human neutrophils adhere to erythrocytes in the presence of complement." *Experimental Cell Research* **307**(2): 381–387.

Genschmer, K. R., et al. (2019). "Activated PMN exosomes: pathogenic entities causing matrix destruction and disease in the lung." *Cell* **176**(1–2): 113–126, e115.

Goodchild, T. T., et al. (2009). "Bone marrow-derived B cells preserve ventricular function after acute myocardial infarction." *JACC: Cardiovascular Interventions* **2**(10): 1005–1016.

Grönberg, C., et al. (2017). "Recent advances on CD4." *European Journal of Pharmacology* **816**: 58–66.

Gulbins, E. and R. Kolesnick (2003). "Raft ceramide in molecular medicine." *Oncogene* **22**(45): 7070–7077.

Han, C., et al. (2019). "Human umbilical cord mesenchymal stem cell derived exosomes encapsulated in functional peptide hydrogels promote cardiac repair." *Biomaterials Science* **7**(7): 2920–2933.

Haney, M. J., et al. (2013). "Specific transfection of inflamed brain by macrophages: a new therapeutic strategy for neurodegenerative diseases." *PLoS ONE* **8**(4): e61852.

Hawiger, D., et al. (2001). "Dendritic cells induce peripheral T cell unresponsiveness under steady state conditions in vivo." *The Journal of Experimental Medicine* **194**(6): 769–780.

Hofmann, U., et al. (2012). "Activation of CD4+ T lymphocytes improves wound healing and survival after experimental myocardial infarction in mice." *Circulation* **125**(13): 1652–1663.

Hofmann, U. and S. Frantz (2016). "Role of T-cells in myocardial infarction." *European Heart Journal* **37**(11): 873–879.

Hong, C.-W. (2018). "Extracellular vesicles of neutrophils." *Immune Network* **18**(6).

Huang, C.-K., et al. (2020). "Preclinical and clinical development of noncoding RNA therapeutics for cardiovascular disease." *Circulation Research* **126**(5): 663–678.

Imai, Y., et al. (2015). "Evaluation of postoperative pregabalin for attenuation of postoperative shoulder pain after thoracotomy in patients with lung cancer, a preliminary result." *General Thoracic and Cardiovascular Surgery* **63**(2): 99–104.

Ingulli, E. (2010). "Mechanism of cellular rejection in transplantation." *Pediatric Nephrology* **25**(1): 61–74.

Italiani, P. and D. Boraschi (2014). "From monocytes to M1/M2 macrophages: phenotypical vs. functional differentiation." *Frontiers in Immunology* **5**: 514.

Kallikourdis, M., et al. (2017). "T cell costimulation blockade blunts pressure overload-induced heart failure." *Nat Commun* **8**: 14680.

Kang, Y., et al. (2020). "Administration of cardiac mesenchymal cells modulates innate immunity in the acute phase of myocardial infarction in mice." *Scientific Reports* **10**(1): 1–13.

Kanno, S., et al. (2020). "Scavenger receptor MARCO contributes to cellular internalization of exosomes by dynamin-dependent endocytosis and macropinocytosis." *Scientific Reports* **10**(1): 1–12.

Kaplan, M. J. (2013). "Role of neutrophils in systemic autoimmune diseases." *Arthritis Research & Therapy* **15**(5): 1–9.

Kaya, Z., et al. (2012). "Autoantibodies in heart failure and cardiac dysfunction." *Circulation Research* **110**(1): 145–158.

Kim, J. E., et al. (2018). "Diagnostic value of microRNAs derived from exosomes in bronchoalveolar lavage fluid of early-stage lung adenocarcinoma: a pilot study." *Thoracic Cancer* **9**(8): 911–915.

Klinker, M. W., et al. (2014). "Human B cell-derived lymphoblastoid cell lines constitutively produce fas ligand and secrete MHCII(+)FasL(+) killer exosomes." *Front Immunol* **5**: 144.

Klumperman, J. and G. Raposo (2014). "The complex ultrastructure of the endolysosomal system." *Cold Spring Harbor Perspectives in Biology* **6**(10): a016857.

Kolbus, D., et al. (2013). "Association between CD8+ T-cell subsets and cardiovascular disease." *Journal of Internal Medicine* **274**(1): 41–51.

Kong, K. Y., et al. (2010). "MIR-23A microRNA cluster inhibits B-cell development." *Experimental Hematology* **38**(8): 629–640.e621.

Kowal, J., et al. (2016). "Proteomic comparison defines novel markers to characterize heterogeneous populations of extracellular vesicle subtypes." *Proceedings of the National Academy of Sciences* **113**(8): E968–E977.

Kuo, G., et al. (2019). "MiR-17–92 cluster and immunity." *Journal of the Formosan Medical Association* **118**(1 Pt 1): 2–6.

Lau, E. S., et al. (2021). "Cardiovascular risk factors are associated with future cancer." *Cardio Oncology* **3**(1): 48–58.

Lazarova, M. and A. Steinle (2019). "Impairment of NKG2D-mediated tumor immunity by TGF-β." *Frontiers in Immunology* **10**: 2689.

Lee, W. H., et al. (2017). "Comparison of non-coding RNAs in exosomes and functional efficacy of human embryonic stem cell-versus induced pluripotent stem cell-derived cardiomyocytes." *Stem Cells* **35**(10): 2138–2149.

Leone, D. A., et al. (2017). "Surface LAMP-2 is an endocytic receptor that diverts antigen internalized by human dendritic cells into highly immunogenic exosomes." *The Journal of Immunology* **199**(2): 531–546.

Li, L., et al. (2020). "The profiles of miRNAs and lncRNAs in peripheral blood neutrophils exosomes of diffuse cutaneous systemic sclerosis." *Journal of Dermatological Science* **98**(2): 88–97.

Li, P., et al. (2017). "Progress in exosome isolation techniques." *Theranostics* **7**(3): 789.

Liangsupree, T., et al. (2020). "Modern isolation and separation techniques for extracellular vesicles." *Journal of Chromatography A*: 461773.

Lin, Z., et al. (2009). "miR-23a functions downstream of NFATc3 to regulate cardiac hypertrophy." *Proceedings of the National Academy of Sciences* **106**(29): 12103–12108.

Lindenbergh, M. F. and W. Stoorvogel (2018). "Antigen presentation by extracellular vesicles from professional antigen-presenting cells." *Annual Review of Immunology* **36**: 435–459.

Liu, H., et al. (2016). "Exosomes derived from dendritic cells improve cardiac function via activation of CD4+ T lymphocytes after myocardial infarction." *Journal of Molecular and Cellular Cardiology* **91**: 123–133.

Liu, H., et al. (2018). "Dendritic cells loaded with tumor derived exosomes for cancer immunotherapy." *Oncotarget* **9**(2): 2887.

Liu, J., et al. (2011). "MicroRNA-155 prevents necrotic cell death in human cardiomyocyte progenitor cells via targeting RIP1." *Journal of Cellular and Molecular Medicine* **15**(7): 1474–1482.

Liu, Q., et al. (2016). "Donor dendritic cell—derived exosomes promote allograft-targeting immune response." *The Journal of Clinical Investigation* **126**(8): 2805–2820.

Liu, S., et al. (2020). "M1-like macrophage-derived exosomes suppress angiogenesis and exacerbate cardiac dysfunction in a myocardial infarction microenvironment." *Basic Research in Cardiology* **115**(2): 1–17.

Lu, J., et al. (2019). "CD4+ T Cell-released extracellular vesicles potentiate the efficacy of the HBsAg vaccine by enhancing B Cell responses." *Advanced Science* **6**(23): 1802219.

Lundy, S. K., et al. (2015). "Killer B lymphocytes and their fas ligand positive exosomes as inducers of immune tolerance." *Front Immunol* **6**: 122.

Madhyastha, R., et al. (2021). "MicroRNa 21 elicits a pro-inflammatory response in macrophages, with exosomes functioning as delivery vehicles." *Inflammation*: 1–14.

Manca, S., et al. (2018). "Milk exosomes are bioavailable and distinct microRNA cargos have unique tissue distribution patterns." *Scientific Reports* **8**(1): 1–11.

Martin-Rufino, J. D., et al. (2019). "Targeting the immune system with mesenchymal stromal cell-derived extracellular vesicles: what is the cargo's mechanism of action?" *Frontiers in Bioengineering and Biotechnology* **7**: 308.

Meng, Y., et al. (2021). "Microfluidics for extracellular vesicle separation and mimetic synthesis: recent advances and future perspectives." *Chemical Engineering Journal* **404**: 126110.

Mentkowski, K. I. and J. K. Lang (2019). "Exosomes engineered to express a cardiomyocyte binding peptide demonstrate improved cardiac retention in vivo." *Scientific Reports* **9**(1): 10041–10041.

Mills, C. D., et al. (2000). "M-1/M-2 macrophages and the Th1/Th2 paradigm." *The Journal of Immunology* **164**(12): 6166–6173.

Mitchell, P. S., et al. (2008). "Circulating microRNAs as stable blood-based markers for cancer detection." *Proceedings of the National Academy of Sciences* **105**(30): 10513–10518.

Mittelbrunn, M., et al. (2011). "Unidirectional transfer of microRNA-loaded exosomes from T cells to antigen-presenting cells." *Nature Communications* **2**: 282.

Mol, E. A., et al. (2019). "Injectable supramolecular ureidopyrimidinone hydrogels provide sustained release of extracellular vesicle therapeutics." *Advanced Healthcare Materials* **8**(20): e1900847.

Montecalvo, A., et al. (2012). "Mechanism of transfer of functional microRNAs between mouse dendritic cells via exosomes." *Blood* **119**(3): 756–766.

Muller, L., et al. (2016). "Tumor-derived exosomes regulate expression of immune function-related genes in human T cell subsets." *Scientific Reports* **6**(1): 1–13.

Munn, D. H., et al. (2004). "Expression of indoleamine 2, 3-dioxygenase by plasmacytoid dendritic cells in tumor-draining lymph nodes." *The Journal of Clinical Investigation* **114**(2): 280–290.

Murn, J., et al. (2008). "Prostaglandin E2 regulates B cell proliferation through a candidate tumor suppressor, Ptger4." *The Journal of Experimental Medicine* **205**(13): 3091–3103.

Nagai, T., et al. (2014). "Decreased myocardial dendritic cells is associated with impaired reparative fibrosis and development of cardiac rupture after myocardial infarction in humans." *Journal of the American Heart Association* **3**(3): e000839.

Naito, K., et al. (2008). "Differential effects of GM-CSF and G-CSF on infiltration of dendritic cells during early left ventricular remodeling after myocardial infarction." *The Journal of Immunology* **181**(8): 5691–5701.

Nazimek, K., et al. (2015). "Macrophages play an essential role in antigen-specific immune suppression mediated by T CD8+ cell-derived exosomes." *Immunology* **146**(1): 23–32.

Neu, N., et al. (1987). "Cardiac myosin induces myocarditis in genetically predisposed mice." *Journal of Immunology* **139**(11): 3630–3636.

Nguyen, D. C., et al. (2018). "Extracellular vesicles from bone marrow-derived mesenchymal stromal cells support ex vivo survival of human antibody secreting cells." *Journal of Extracellular Vesicles* **7**(1): 1463778.

Noller, H. F. (1984). "Structure of ribosomal RNA." *Annual Review of Biochemistry* **53**(1): 119–162.

Nussinovitch, U. and Y. Shoenfeld (2013). "The clinical significance of anti-beta-1 adrenergic receptor autoantibodies in cardiac disease." *Clinical Reviews in Allergy & Immunology* **44**(1): 75–83.

Oka, T., et al. (2012). "Mitochondrial DNA that escapes from autophagy causes inflammation and heart failure." *Nature* **485**(7397): 251–255.

Okoye, I. S., et al. (2014). "MicroRNA-containing T-regulatory-cell-derived exosomes suppress pathogenic T helper 1 cells." *Immunity* **41**(1): 89–103.

Opavsky, M. A., et al. (1999). "Susceptibility to myocarditis is dependent on the response of alphabeta T lymphocytes to coxsackieviral infection." *Circulation Research* **85**(6): 551–558.

Orecchioni, M., et al. (2019). "Macrophage polarization: different gene signatures in M1 (LPS+) vs. classically and M2 (LPS—) vs. alternatively activated macrophages." *Frontiers in Immunology* **10**: 1084.

Papayannopoulos, V. (2018). "Neutrophil extracellular traps in immunity and disease." *Nature Reviews Immunology* **18**(2): 134.

Pastrana, J. L., et al. (2012). "Regulatory T cells and Atherosclerosis." *Journal of Clinical and Experimental Cardiology* **2012**(Suppl 12): 2.

Pennells, L., et al. (2019). "Equalization of four cardiovascular risk algorithms after systematic recalibration: individual-participant meta-analysis of 86 prospective studies." *European Heart Journal* **40**(7): 621–631.

Phinney, D. G., et al. (2015). "Mesenchymal stem cells use extracellular vesicles to outsource mitophagy and shuttle microRNAs." *Nature Communications* **6**(1): 1–15.

Pitt, J. M., et al. (2016). "Dendritic cell—derived exosomes for cancer therapy." *The Journal of Clinical Investigation* **126**(4): 1224–1232.

Pontis, J. A., et al. (2014). "Color, phenolic and flavonoid content, and antioxidant activity of honey from Roraima, Brazil." *Food Science and Technology* **34**: 69–73.

Potente, M., et al. (2011). "Basic and therapeutic aspects of angiogenesis." *Cell* **146**(6): 873–887.

Qazi, K. R., et al. (2009). "Antigen-loaded exosomes alone induce Th1-type memory through a B cell—dependent mechanism." *Blood* **113**(12): 2673–2683.

Rabe, K. F., et al. (2018). "Cardiovascular disease and COPD: dangerous liaisons?" *European Respiratory Review* **27**(149).

Raposo, G., et al. (1996). "B lymphocytes secrete antigen-presenting vesicles." *Journal of Experimental Medicine* **183**(3): 1161–1172.

Raposo, G. and W. Stoorvogel (2013). "Extracellular vesicles: exosomes, microvesicles, and friends." *Journal of Cell Biology* **200**(4): 373–383.

Ribeiro-Rodrigues, T. M., et al. (2017). "Exosomes secreted by cardiomyocytes subjected to ischaemia promote cardiac angiogenesis." *Cardiovascular Research* **113**(11): 1338–1350.

Rong, L., et al. (2016). "Immunosuppression of breast cancer cells mediated by transforming growth factor-β in exosomes from cancer cells." *Oncology Letters* **11**(1): 500–504.

Ruan, Q., et al. (2011). "The microRNA-21– PDCD4 axis prevents type 1 diabetes by blocking pancreatic β cell death." *Proceedings of the National Academy of Sciences* **108**(29): 12030–12035.

Rusinkevich, V., et al. (2019). "Temporal dynamics of immune response following prolonged myocardial ischemia/reperfusion with and without cyclosporine A." *The Acta Pharmacologica Sinica* **40**(9): 1168–1183.

Saigusa, R., et al. (2020). "T cell subsets and functions in atherosclerosis." *Nature Reviews Cardiology* **17**(7): 387–401.

Salzman, J., et al. (2012). "Circular RNAs are the predominant transcript isoform from hundreds of human genes in diverse cell types." *PLoS ONE* **7**(2): e30733.

Sancho, D., et al. (2009). "Identification of a dendritic cell receptor that couples sensing of necrosis to immunity." *Nature* **458**(7240): 899–903.

Santos-Zas, I., et al. (2018). "Adaptive immune responses contribute to post-ischemic cardiac remodeling." *Frontiers in Cardiovascular Medicine* **5**: 198.

Sarropoulos, I., et al. (2019). "Developmental dynamics of lncRNAs across mammalian organs and species." *Nature* **571**(7766): 510–514.

Saunderson, S. C. and A. D. McLellan (2017). "Role of lymphocyte subsets in the immune response to primary B cell-derived exosomes." *Journal of Immunology* **199**(7): 2225–2235.

Saunderson, S. C., et al. (2008). "Induction of exosome release in primary B cells stimulated via CD40 and the IL-4 receptor." *The Journal of Immunology* **180**(12): 8146–8152.

Savill, J. S., et al. (1989). "Macrophage phagocytosis of aging neutrophils in inflammation. Programmed cell death in the neutrophil leads to its recognition by macrophages." *The Journal of Clinical Investigation* **83**(3): 865–875.

Schaheen, B., et al. (2016). "B-Cell depletion promotes aortic infiltration of immunosuppressive cells and is protective of experimental aortic aneurysm." *Arteriosclerosis, Thrombosis, and Vascular Biology* **36**(11): 2191–2202.

Schuler, P., et al. (2014). "Human CD 4+ CD 39+ regulatory T cells produce adenosine upon co-expression of surface CD 73 or contact with CD 73+ exosomes or CD 73+ cells." *Clinical & Experimental Immunology* **177**(2): 531–543.

Segura, E. and C. Théry (2010). "Exosomes: naturally occurring minimal antigen-presenting units." *Allergy Frontiers: Future Perspectives*: 305–319.

Shortman, K. and W. R. Heath (2010). "The CD8+ dendritic cell subset." *Immunological Reviews* **234**(1): 18–31.

Silvestre-Roig, C., et al. (2020). "Neutrophils as regulators of cardiovascular inflammation." *Nature Reviews Cardiology*: 1–14.

Singh, M. and H. K. Saini (2003). "Resident cardiac mast cells and ischemia-reperfusion injury." *Journal of Cardiovascular Pharmacology and Therapeutics* **8**(2): 135–148.

Slater, T. W., et al. (2017). "Neutrophil microparticles deliver active myeloperoxidase to injured mucosa to inhibit epithelial wound healing." *The Journal of Immunology* **198**(7): 2886–2897.

Srikakulapu, P. and C. A. McNamara (2017). "B cells and atherosclerosis." *The American Journal of Physiology-Heart and Circulatory Physiology* **312**(5): H1060–H1067.

Stein, J. M. and J. P. Luzio (1991). "Ectocytosis caused by sublytic autologous complement attack on human neutrophils. The sorting of endogenous plasma-membrane proteins and lipids into shed vesicles." *Biochemical Journal* **274**(2): 381–386.

Steiner, D. F., et al. (2011). "MicroRNA-29 regulates T-box transcription factors and interferon-γ production in helper T cells." *Immunity* **35**(2): 169–181.

Steinhauser, M. L. and R. T. Lee (2011). "Regeneration of the heart." *EMBO Molecular Medicine* **3**(12): 701–712.

Stephenson, E., et al. (2017). "T-cell immunity in myocardial inflammation: pathogenic role and therapeutic manipulation." *British Journal of Pharmacology* **174**(22): 3914–3925.

Subra, C., et al. (2010). "Exosomes account for vesicle-mediated transcellular transport of activatable phospholipases and prostaglandins." *Journal of Lipid Research* **51**(8): 2105–2120.

Sukma Dewi, I., et al. (2017). "Exosomal miR-142–3p is increased during cardiac allograft rejection and augments vascular permeability through down-regulation of endothelial RAB11FIP2 expression." *Cardiovascular Research* **113**(5): 440–452.

Sun, D., et al. (2010). "A novel nanoparticle drug delivery system: the anti-inflammatory activity of curcumin is enhanced when encapsulated in exosomes." *Molecular Therapy* **18**(9): 1606–1614.

Sun, P., et al. (2020). "Circulating exosomes control CD4." *Molecular Therapy* **28**(12): 2605–2620.

Théry, C., et al. (2002). "Indirect activation of naïve CD4+ T cells by dendritic cell—derived exosomes." *Nature Immunology* **3**(12): 1156–1162.

Théry, C., et al. (2006). "Isolation and characterization of exosomes from cell culture supernatants and biological fluids." *Current Protocols in Cell Biology* **30**(1): 3.22.21–23.22.29.

Thygesen, K., et al. (2007). "Universal definition of myocardial infarction." *Circulation* **116**(22): 2634–2653.

Trajkovic, K., et al. (2008). "Ceramide triggers budding of exosome vesicles into multivesicular endosomes." *Science* **319**(5867): 1244–1247.

Tu, F., et al. (2020). "Novel role of endothelial derived exosomal HSPA12B in regulating macrophage inflammatory responses in polymicrobial sepsis." *Front Immunol* **11**: 825.

Ulrich, V., et al. (2016). "Chronic miR-29 antagonism promotes favorable plaque remodeling in atherosclerotic mice." *EMBO Molecular Medicine* **8**(6): 643–653.

Valadi, H., et al. (2007). "Exosome-mediated transfer of mRNAs and microRNAs is a novel mechanism of genetic exchange between cells." *Nature Cell Biology* **9**(6): 654–659.

Vandergriff, A., et al. (2018). "Targeting regenerative exosomes to myocardial infarction using cardiac homing peptide." *Theranostics* **8**(7): 1869–1878.

van der Laan, L. J., et al. (1999). "Regulation and functional involvement of macrophage scavenger receptor MARCO in clearance of bacteria in vivo." *The Journal of Immunology* **162**(2): 939–947.

van der Vlist, E. J., et al. (2012). "CD4(+) T cell activation promotes the differential release of distinct populations of nanosized vesicles." *Journal of Extracellular Vesicles* **1**.

van Duijn, J., et al. (2018). "The many faces of CD8+ T cells in atherosclerosis." *Current Opinion in Lipidology* **29**(5): 411–416.

van Rees, D. J., et al. (2016). "Immunoreceptors on neutrophils." *Seminars in Immunology*, **28**(2): 94–108. Elsevier.

Vargas, A., et al. (2016). "Neutrophil-derived exosomes: a new mechanism contributing to airway smooth muscle remodeling." *American Journal of Respiratory Cell and Molecular Biology* **55**(3): 450–461.

Vdovenko, D. and U. Eriksson (2018). "Regulatory role of CD4." *Journal of Immunology Research* **2018**: 4396351.

Virani, S. S., et al. (2020). "Heart disease and stroke statistics—2020 update: a report from the American Heart Association." *Circulation* **141**(9): e139–e596.

Wahlund, C. J., et al. (2017). "Exosomes from antigen-pulsed dendritic cells induce stronger antigen-specific immune responses than microvesicles in vivo." *Scientific Reports* **7**(1): 1–9.

Walsh, P. T., et al. (2006). "PTEN inhibits IL-2 receptor—mediated expansion of CD4+ CD25+ Tregs." *The Journal of Clinical Investigation* **116**(9): 2521–2531.

Wang, C., et al. (2017). "Macrophage-derived mir-155-containing exosomes suppress fibroblast proliferation and promote fibroblast inflammation during cardiac injury." *Molecular Therapy* **25**(1): 192–204.

Wang, X., et al. (2018). "Engineered exosomes with ischemic myocardium-targeting peptide for targeted therapy in myocardial infarction." *Journal of the American Heart Association* **7**(15): e008737.

Wang, Y., et al. (2019). "Involvement of macrophage-derived exosomes in abdominal aortic aneurysms development." *Atherosclerosis* **289**: 64–72.

Waters, R., et al. (2018). "Stem cell-inspired secretome-rich injectable hydrogel to repair injured cardiac tissue." *Acta Biomater* **69**: 95–106.

Wei, G., et al. (2017). "Dendritic cells derived exosomes migration to spleen and induction of inflammation are regulated by CCR7." *Scientific Reports* **7**(1): 1–9.

Weis, S. M. and D. A. Cheresh (2011). "Tumor angiogenesis: molecular pathways and thera-peutic targets." *Nature Medicine* **17**(11): 1359–1370.

Wiklander, O. P., et al. (2015). "Extracellular vesicle in vivo biodistribution is determined by cell source, route of administration and targeting." *Journal of Extracellular Vesicles* **4**: 26316.

Wu, R., et al. (2019). "Roles of exosomes derived from immune cells in cardiovascular dis-eases." *Frontiers in Immunology* **10**: 648.

Wynn, T. A. and L. Barron (2010). Macrophages: master regulators of inflammation and fibrosis. *Seminars in Liver Disease*, NIH Public Access.

Xia, W., et al. (2020). "PD-1 inhibitor inducing exosomal miR-34a-5p expression mediates the cross talk between cardiomyocyte and macrophage in immune checkpoint inhibitor-related cardiac dysfunction." *Journal for ImmunoTherapy of Cancer* **8**(2).

Xie, M., et al. (2020). "Immunoregulatory effects of stem cell-derived extracellular vesicles on immune cells." *Frontiers in Immunology* **11**.

Xie, Y., et al. (2010). "Dendritic cells recruit T cell exosomes via exosomal LFA-1 leading to inhibition of CD8+ CTL responses through downregulation of peptide/MHC class I and Fas ligand-mediated cytotoxicity." *Journal of Immunology* **185**(9): 5268–5278.

Ye, S.-B., et al. (2014). "Tumor-derived exosomes promote tumor progression and T-cell dys-function through the regulation of enriched exosomal microRNAs in human nasopha-ryngeal carcinoma." *Oncotarget* **5**(14): 5439.

Yu, H., et al. (2020). "Exosomes derived from hypertrophic cardiomyocytes induce inflam-mation in macrophages." *Front Immunol* **11**: 606045.

Zarovni, N., et al. (2015). "Integrated isolation and quantitative analysis of exosome shuttled proteins and nucleic acids using immunocapture approaches." *Methods* **87**: 46–58.

Zhang, H., et al. (2011). "CD4(+) T cell-released exosomes inhibit CD8(+) cytotoxic T-lymphocyte responses and antitumor immunity." *Cellular & Molecular Immunology* **8**(1): 23–30.

Zhang, Y., et al. (2017). "Characteristics and roles of exosomes in cardiovascular disease." *DNA and Cell Biology* **36**(3): 202–211.

Zhang, Y., et al. (2019). "Exosomes: biogenesis, biologic function and clinical potential." *Cell & Bioscience* **9**(1): 1–18.

Zheng, L., et al. (2018). "Exosomes derived from dendritic cells attenuate liver injury by modulating the balance of Treg and Th17 cells after ischemia reperfusion." *Cellular Physiology and Biochemistry* **46**(2): 740–756.

Zhou, J., et al. (2016). "Characterization of induced pluripotent stem cell microvesicle gen-esis, morphology and pluripotent content." *Scientific Reports* **6**(1): 1–10.

Zhou, M., et al. (2014). "Pancreatic cancer derived exosomes regulate the expression of TLR4 in dendritic cells via miR-203." *Cellular Immunology* **292**(1–2): 65–69.

Zhu, D., et al. (2021). "Minimally invasive delivery of therapeutic agents by hydrogel injec-tion into the pericardial cavity for cardiac repair." *Nature Communications* **12**(1): 1412.

Zhu, L. P., et al. (2018). "Hypoxia-elicited mesenchymal stem cell-derived exosomes facili-tates cardiac repair through miR-125b-mediated prevention of cell death in myocardial infarction." *Theranostics* **8**(22): 6163–6177.

Zitvogel, L., et al. (1998). "Eradication of established murine tumors using a novel cell-free vaccine: dendritic cell derived exosomes." *Nature Medicine* **4**(5): 594–600.

Zouggari, Y., et al. (2013). "B lymphocytes trigger monocyte mobilization and impair heart function after acute myocardial infarction." *Nature Medicine* **19**(10): 1273–1280.

10 Ion Channels in Immune Cells

Physiological and Pathophysiological Roles

Devasena Ponnalagu, Shridhar Sanghvi,
Shyam S. Bansal, and Harpreet Singh

CONTENTS

INTRODUCTION

Similar to other cells, immune cells possess ion channels and transporters in the plasma membrane and in intracellular organelles[1]. However, very few of the known ion channels and transporters have been identified in immune cells or demonstrated to regulate their function. This apparent negligence of studying ion channels in immune cells could be attributed to their nonexcitable nature, and therefore the need for ion channels in them is questionable[2]. Nevertheless, the channels and transporters that have been characterized to date are essential in maintaining ionic homeostasis, membrane potential, calcium (Ca^{2+}) signaling, migration, and activation of pro-inflammatory signaling molecules, such as reactive oxygen species (ROS), in immune cells[3]. One of the well-known pathways regulated by ion channels in immune cells

DOI: 10.1201/b22824-11

is the modulation of intracellular Ca^{2+} signaling, which is required for the activation of many enzymes and transcription factors that govern the activation and maturation of immune cells[4]. Ca^{2+} entry into the cells depolarizes the membrane and, if unimpeded, reverses the electrochemical gradient of Ca^{2+}, restricting its further entry. Thus, the potassium (K^+) channels open up and maintain a hyperpolarized state by K^+ efflux, which eventually leads to Ca^{2+} entry via Ca^{2+} release–activated Ca^{2+} (CRAC) channels that are present in the immune cells[5–8]. Of the several K^+ channels present in immune cells, the ones that are well studied are the voltage-activated potassium channel ($K_v1.3$) and the Ca^{2+}-activated intermediate conductance potassium ($K_{Ca}3.1$) channel[9,10]. Ca^{2+} influx in lymphocytes is also regulated by transient receptor potential melastatin (TRPM) cation channel subfamily member 4, which is activated upon Ca^{2+} entry and depolarizes the membrane by triggering sodium (Na^+) influx. This further restrains the Ca^{2+} entry, thereby inducing Ca^{2+} oscillations in lymphocytes[11]. The changes in the intracellular Ca^{2+} are also regulated by chloride (Cl^-) channels[1,3]. The chloride channels that are present in immune cells are volume-regulated anion channels (VRAC) or Cl_{Swell}, cystic fibrosis transmembrane conductance regulator (CFTR), and benzodiazepine-sensitive γ-aminobutyric acid ($GABA_A$) receptor channels[12]. Activation of $GABA_A$ receptor channels has been shown to inhibit the proliferation of T cells. ATP-gated P2X receptor cation channels are also implicated in modulating immune cell function, and any mutations or inhibitory mechanisms in them have been shown to lead to abnormal immune responses[12,13].

It is evident that the functional interplay of these ion channels is important for Ca^{2+} signaling, cell-volume regulation, and activation of immune cells. In the subsequent sections of this chapter, we will be discussing in detail some of the key ion channels that are present in immune cells in the context of their roles in moderating immune response, their pathophysiological consequences, and their therapeutic potential.

ION CHANNELS OF THE ADAPTIVE AND INNATE ARMS OF THE IMMUNE SYSTEM

There is no doubt that ionic homeostasis plays an integral role in maintaining the structural and functional integrity of both adaptive and innate cells of the immune system. There are five prevalent ionic currents corresponding to five distinct channels – $K_v1.3$[10,14–16], $K_{Ca}3.1$[17], CRAC channel[8], TRPM7[18–20], and Cl_{Swell}[21] – recorded in T cells[5] and associated with their activation[5]. Apart from Ca^{2+}, which plays a predominant role in immune cell signaling, many other ions such as Zn^{2+}, Mg^{2+}, K^+, Na^+, and Cl^- have been shown to be essential for B cell development, activation, and differentiation into effector B cells[22]. Knockdown of channels in B cells such as VRAC[23], TRPM7[24], and zinc transporter ZIP10[25] has been shown to inhibit their maturation. Further knockin mutation of zinc transporter ZIP7 showed a lower or nondetectable amount of basal circulating levels of sera IgG and IgM, indicating their role in the generation of antibodies[26]. CRAC channels present in the plasma membrane of dendritic cells (DCs) are responsible for the increase in cytoplasmic Ca^{2+} levels, which is a prerequisite for their activation and maturation as well as triggering their response to any pathogens or foreign stimuli[27,28]. DCs are also conferred with the cardiac isoform of the L-type Ca^{2+} channel ($Ca_V1.2$) in their plasma membrane which, upon activation by membrane depolarization, triggers Ca^{2+} release from ryanodine receptor 1 (RyR1)[29,30]. Activation of RyR1 further increases the expression of MHC class II molecules in DCs for antigen presentation to T cells in the early phase of the immune response[29]. Other channels such as TRP, voltage-gated K^+, and Na^+/Ca^{2+} exchangers present in DCs are shown to be essential for their migration and interaction with T cells[30]. Furthermore, ion channels in NK cells have been well studied in relation to their function of invading cancer cells[31]. Similar to macrophages and DCs, K^+ and Ca^{2+} channels play a key role in invoking the cytotoxic function of NK cells. In fact, modulation of the activities of ion channels in NK cells has been considered as a therapeutic strategy for cancer. In the subsequent subsections, the structure-function properties of some of the key channels of immune cells such as CRAC, K^+, and TRP and chloride channels will be discussed.

CALCIUM RELEASE–ACTIVATED CALCIUM (CRAC) CHANNELS

The intracellular Ca^{2+} concentration in lymphocytes (B and T cells) is around 50–100 nM, which upon antigenic stimulation can rise to 1 μM[3]. Ca^{2+} influx upon antigenic stimulation activates phospholipase C, resulting in the generation of inositol triphosphate 3 (IP3), which further potentiates the release of Ca^{2+} from the endoplasmic reticulum (ER)[3]. The ER Ca^{2+} release triggers Ca^{2+} influx across the plasma membrane through CRAC channels. This whole process is termed store-operated calcium entry (SOCE), which plays a central role in maintaining cellular Ca^{2+} homeostasis[3,32]. The major players in SOCE are ER Ca^{2+} sensor stromal interaction molecule 1 (STIM1) and STIM2 proteins and their interaction with plasma membrane CRAC channel component ORAI[3]. STIM1 is a single-pass transmembrane protein comprising ER Ca^{2+}-sensing EF-hand motif and multiple protein-protein interaction motifs[33]. There are three homologs of ORAI – ORAI1, ORAI2, and ORAI3 – which form Ca^{2+} channels but differ in their pharmacological properties, tissue expression, and inactivation kinetics[3,34].

ORAI1 is the well-established isoform mediating SOCE in lymphocytes. It is a pore-forming subunit of the CRAC channel and constitutes four transmembrane domains with both the amino and carboxyl termini facing the cytoplasmic side of the plasma membrane[3]. The selectivity of the CRAC channel for Ca^{2+} is ~1,000-fold higher than for other monovalent ions[35] such as Na^+ and shows extremely low conductance. In T cells and mast cells, the activity of the CRAC channel indicated a conductance of 9–24 fS and <1 pS, respectively[6,8,19,35,36]. The activation and deactivation kinetics of the CRAC channel are very slow; thus, the high selectivity for Ca^{2+} and very low selectivity for Na^+ avoid membrane depolarization and ensure Ca^{2+} entry over a long period. The major factor that determines the activation of ORAI1 CRAC channels is the STIM proteins[37]. Upon lymphocyte stimulation, once the ER Ca^{2+} store is depleted, the STIM proteins oligomerize and distribute into discrete puncta in ER sites that are in close proximity to the plasma membrane[37,38]. This enables it to interact with the N- and C-termini of ORAI1 and to activate the CRAC channel[39]. The isoform STIM2 also activates the ORAI1 channel in lymphocytes in a similar manner[3].

Autosomal recessive mutations in *ORAI1* and *STIM1* genes inhibited Ca^{2+} influx in NK, B, and T cells via the CRAC channel and increased its susceptibility to bacterial, fungal, and viral infections[3,40,41]. It further causes a decrease in cytokine secretion by $CD4^+$ and $CD8^+$ T cells and NK cells, respectively, likely due to impaired Ca^{2+}-dependent activation of a transcription factor – nuclear factor of activated T cells (NFAT)[42–44]. In addition, defects in the activity of STIM1 and ORAI1 have been shown to inhibit the proliferation of B and T cells after antigenic stimulation[45,46]. It has also been established that actin rearrangement at the synapse between T cells and antigen-presenting cells is required for T cell receptor (TCR) microcluster assembly, with its downstream signaling leading to T cell activation[47]. Interestingly, Ca^{2+} influx through the CRAC channel was demonstrated to induce actin movements, which is essential for orienting the CRAC channel at the immune synapse for activating T cells[47]. Furthermore, mice with B cell–specific knockout of STIM1 and STIM2 proteins showed decreased anti-inflammatory cytokine secretion by regulatory B cells, which aggravated autoimmune inflammation in the encephalomyelitis (EAE) model of multiple scelorosis[48]. Moreover, STIM1 deficiency in patients has also resulted in a reduction of $CD25^+FOXP3^+$ regulatory T cells[49]. Ca^{2+} is a major intracellular messenger involved in activating cells of the innate immune system as well[50]. In neutrophils, CRAC channel opening is known to stimulate nicotinamide adenine dinucleotide phosphate (NADPH) oxidase activity, leading to ROS generation and activation[50]. In addition, studies using either STIM1- or STIM2-deficient neutrophils have demonstrated the significance of the CRAC channel in the degranulation and phagocytic activity of neutrophils[51–53]. There is limited understanding of the role of the CRAC channel in the function of monocytes and macrophages, probably due to conflicting data regarding their function[50]. On the other hand, it is well established that CRAC channels are extremely important for the function of mast cells[50]. An important role of the CRAC channel was established in FcεR1 cross-linking-induced human lung mast cell activation[54]. Furthermore, it was demonstrated that an inhibitor of the CRAC channel, Synta66, reduced SOCE and resulted in weakened cytokine and histamine release from mast cells[55]. Mice lacking either STIM1 or ORAI1 also exhibited a defect in histamine release and reduced TNFα secretion and leukotriene production in mast cells[50,56]. All of these studies imply an essential role for the CRAC channel in immune cells. Additionally, single nucleotide polymorphisms (SNPs) associated with ORAI1 are reported in allergic and autoimmune disorders like rheumatoid arthritis, Kawasaki's disease, atopic dermatitis, and chronic spontaneous urticaria; thus, much still needs to be understood regarding the regulatory mechanism of CRAC channels in immune cell functions[50].

TRANSIENT RECEPTOR POTENTIAL (TRP) CHANNELS

The mammalian TRP channel superfamily comprises 28 cation-selective channels[57]. On the basis of their sequence and structural homology, TRP channel family members are classified into six main groups, which include canonical (TRPC), melastatin (TRPM), vanilloid (TRPV), mucolipin (TRPM), polycystin (TRPP), and ankyrin (TRPA) channel proteins[57]. All of the members of the TRP channel family of proteins comprise six transmembrane helices that combine as tetramers to form a cation-selective pore[58]. They exhibit polymodal activation properties and, therefore, become activated upon alteration in temperature, pH, and osmolarity[12]. A body of evidence shows their importance not only in the sensory system but also in various physiological and pathophysiological conditions like cancer, neural development, and cardiac and renal physiology.

TRP channels are present in both the adaptive and the innate immune cells and act as mediators to conduct Ca^{2+}, Mg^{2+} (TRPM2, TRPM6, TRPM7), and Na^+ (TRPM4). As described earlier, the major role of some of the TRP channels is to modulate intracellular Ca^{2+} in immune cells and, thus, influence their function. They have been established to play a role in phagocytosis, immune cell migration, and the release of inflammatory cytokines. It is known that, following TCR stimulation, TRPM2 channels become activated probably via release of cyclic ADP ribose (ADPR) from the ER, which is involved in their proliferation and pro-inflammatory cytokine secretion[59,60]. Moreover, TRPM2 deficiency mitigated the development of encephalomyelitis in mice[61]. TRPM2-mediated Ca^{2+} signaling was also shown to be involved in the maturation of DCs through modulation of the processing of MHC class II molecules[62]. The absence of TRPM4 channels in DCs led to impaired migration due to disruption of Ca^{2+} homeostasis[60]. In addition, phagocytic activity and cytokine release by macrophages were diminished in TRPM4-deficient mice[60]. B cells lacking a TRPM7 channel exhibited an inability to proliferate and an increased death rate[60]. In the case of T cells as well, mice lacking T cell–specific TRPM7 showed a defect in T cell development[60]. There are also other members of this channel group that have been studied extensively and shown to be important in modulating immune cell function and development and inflammatory diseases[60]. Due to their key role in immune cell maturation and activation, they are also considered to be a great therapeutic target against autoimmune disorders, like rheumatoid arthritis, type I diabetes, lupus erythematosus, and multiple sclerosis, and thus need to be evaluated clinically.

POTASSIUM (K⁺) CHANNELS

K⁺ channels are important for maintaining cellular physiological functions such as the regulation of membrane potential, cell volume, Ca^{2+} signaling, and generating an action potential[63]. On the basis of their biophysical properties and secondary structure, the K⁺ channels can be divided into different groups: channels; sodium-activated K⁺ channels; inward rectifier K⁺ channels (Kir); two-pore K⁺ channels (K2P); and K_{Ca} channels[64–68]. Among the K⁺ channels, K_v and K_{Ca} channel activity is predominantly observed in immune cells and will be explicitly discussed in this section.

Voltage-Activated K⁺ Channel (K_v)

K_v channels were first discovered and identified in T lymphocytes[69], and since then they have been found to be expressed in many other cell types, including macrophages[70]. The human genome encodes 80 K⁺ channel genes, of which 40 genes code for K_v channels[71]. The K_v channel that was first recorded in the plasma membrane of T cells is identified as $K_v1.3$[72,73]. It is also observed in the mitochondria of T lymphocytes, where it was shown to mediate Bax-induced apoptosis[74,75].

K_v channels are tetramers of pore-forming α subunits, each with six transmembrane helices (S1–S6)[76]. The S1–S4 transmembrane helices comprise the voltage sensor domain (VSD), and the K^+-selective pore is formed by the S5 and S6 transmembrane helices and the linker between them[76]. The S4 segment comprises predominantly positively charged residues that contribute to most of the voltage dependence of the channel gating[76]. The K^+ channel opens upon membrane depolarization, causing K^+ ion efflux down its electrochemical gradient[5]. The membrane depolarization induces a conformational change in the S4 segment that causes the displacement of the S4-S5 linker and, hence, is responsible for activation of the channel[76]. The continuous membrane depolarization can also cause inactivation of the K_v1.3 channel, resulting in channel closure, and contributes to its sigmoid voltage dependence properties[5]. Hence, this sigmoid voltage dependence property of the K_v1.3 channel acts as a mechanism to safeguard against the continuous depolarization of the membrane upon Ca^{2+} entry[5].

The K^+ conductance is enhanced in T cells upon mitogen-mediated activation[14,77,78]. Along with the Cl_{Swell} channel, K_v1.3 regulates cell-volume changes of T lymphocytes[21]. It was also shown that K_v1.3 channels are necessary for the differentiation of CD8[+] T cells into cytotoxic T lymphocytes[79]. K_v1.3 channels stimulate the proliferation of macrophages[80] and of B cells[81] as well. The K_v channels present in DCs are essential for their migration and interaction with T cells[30]. In NK cells and T cells, K^+ and Ca^{2+} channels are known to localize at the immune synapse between the NK cells/cytotoxic T lymphocytes and the target cells to facilitate the killing process[82]. Furthermore, depletion, inhibition, or mutation of K_v1.3 channels has been demonstrated to reduce cytokine production by NK cells, thereby inhibiting their activation[31,44,83–87].

The K_v1.3 channel inhibitors have been used to cope with many autoimmune disorders. Effector memory T cells (T_{EM}), which are prominent in mediating the pathogenesis of multiple sclerosis (MS), have higher expression of K_v1.3 channels, and their antigen-induced activation and proliferation are inhibited by K_v1.3 channel blockers[88]. K_v1.3 channel expression was also upregulated in T_{EM} cells isolated from the synovial fluid of patients with rheumatoid arthritis[89]. Interestingly, K_v1.3 blocking peptide ShK-L5-amide was shown to reduce the severity of erosion of cartilage and bone in the joints of the rat arthritis model, thus decreasing the detrimental effects of the disease[89]. In the type I diabetes model as well, it was observed that blockage of the channel activity of K_v1.3 can delay the onset of diabetes due to its high expression in their T_{EM} cells[89]. Hence, K_v1.3 channels are considered to be a novel therapeutic target in many autoimmune disorders[89,90]. K_v channels also regulate tumor cell proliferation by modulating membrane potential[91]. The expression changes of ion channels are observed in many cancers[91]. In human B cell lymphoma, overexpression of the K_v1.3 channel mediates the cell's resistance to apoptosis, and the antibody-based drug rituximab has a profound role in treating B cell lymphoma by inhibiting the activity of K_v1.3 channels[92].

Calcium-Activated K^+ Channel (K_{Ca})

K_{Ca} channels comprise the small conductance (SK_{Ca}, ~10 pS), the intermediate conductance (IK_{Ca}, ~40 pS), and the large conductance (BK_{Ca}, ~300 pS) K^+ channels[93]. The K_{Ca}3.1 (also known as IK_{Ca}, KCNN4, Gardos channel, K_{Ca}3.1, and human SK4) currents were first observed in erythrocytes in which it was shown to be important for cell-volume regulation[93,94]. Later on, $K_{Ca}3.1$ was observed in many of the immune cells[12,65,95–97].

As the name suggests, the $K_{Ca}3.1$ channel is activated upon an increase in intracellular Ca^{2+} levels. $K_{Ca}3.1$ channels do not bind to Ca^{2+} ions directly like BK_{Ca}[98]; they associate with it indirectly via Ca^{2+}-binding protein calmodulin (CaM)[99]. Therefore, the channel gating is mediated by CaM. CaM was shown to co-purify with $K_{Ca}3.1$ in the presence or absence[99] of Ca^{2+}, suggesting that CaM binding to $K_{Ca}3.1$ is independent of the Ca^{2+} concentration. Both the SK_{Ca} and IK_{Ca} channels possess the CaM-binding domain at their C-terminus region, which contributes to their sensitivity to intracellular Ca^{2+} changes[100–103]. The IK_{Ca} and SK_{Ca} channels also exhibit structural similarities. They consist of six transmembrane domains, as opposed to seven transmembrane domains in BK_{Ca}, and are closely related to the K_v channel[65]. Out of the six transmembrane domains (S1–S6), four alpha-helical transmembrane domains constitute VSD (S1–S4) and a K^+-selective pore region is present between the last two transmembrane domains (S5 and S6)[65]. In comparison to other K_v channels, the fourth transmembrane domain of the SK_{Ca} and IK_{Ca} channels possesses a lower number of positively charged residues and, therefore, is insensitive toward changes in transmembrane voltage.

The major role of the $K_{Ca}3.1$ channel is to hyperpolarize the membrane for Ca^{2+} influx into the immune cells, which results in their activation, cytokine secretion, proliferation, and cell-volume regulation[12]. It has been established that increased cytosolic Ca^{2+} influx generated by the negative membrane potential of the membrane via $K_{Ca}3.1$ channels induces translocation of nuclear factors to the nucleus for the transcription of genes responsible for immune cell activation[103,104]. Both naïve and memory T cells exhibit increased expression of the $K_{Ca}3.1$ channel upon their activation[95]. The expression and activity of the $K_{Ca}3.1$ channel in immune cells are modulated in inflammatory disorders and cancer, and therefore its therapeutic potential has been widely explored. For example, in inflammatory bowel disease, genetic depletion or, via use of the $K_{Ca}3.1$ channel inhibitor, the inflammation associated with the disease was significantly reduced[105]. It was shown that blockage of the $K_{Ca}3.1$ channel reduced the expression of pro-inflammatory genes and thereby inhibited macrophage differentiation into the M1 phenotype[106]. In addition, $K_{Ca}3.1$ channel inhibition increased the cytotoxicity and degranulation of NK cells, resulting in the suppression of tumor growth[87]. Taken together, these studies suggest K^+ channels in immune cells as a potential therapeutic target, but their efficacy in a clinical trial needs to be explored.

ANION (CHLORIDE) CHANNELS OF IMMUNE CELLS

Although chloride channels are important for cell-volume regulation, unfortunately they are often neglected due to their lack of molecular identity and nonselective nature. However, few of the plasma membrane anion channels characterized, such as Cl_{Swell}, $GABA_A$, and CFTR, have been implicated in immune cell activation and function[12,107–115]. The role of chloride channels in the volume regulation of T cells was identified in pioneering research done in the 1980s[21]. They were defined as VRAC or

Cl_{Swell}, as the permeability to anions increased in the peripheral blood mononuclear cells (PBMC) upon osmolarity changes. Later, LRRC8A was identified as a molecular component of Cl_{Swell}[110]. It is predicted to be a hexameric channel with a pannexin-like transmembrane topology comprising hetero multimers of LRRC8A and other LRRC8 (-B, -C, -D, and -E) subunits[12]. Interestingly, a case study demonstrated that a mutation in LRRC8 was responsible for agammaglobulinemia, a congenital syndrome defined by a defect in B cell development[116]. In patients with agammaglobulinemia, translocation of the *LRRC8* gene was observed that led to the truncation of half of the seventh and complete deletion of the eighth and ninth LRR domains located at the C-terminal of the LRRC8 protein, which eventually resulted in the inhibition of B cell development and proliferation[116]. Furthermore, knockdown of the *LRRC8* gene abolished hypotonicity-induced volume regulation in T cells, decreased their proliferation, and induced apoptosis[12]. Similar to neurons, activation of $GABA_A$ receptors in T cells has an inhibitory role. GABA inhibited T cell proliferation and production of IL-2 and IFN-γ in *in vitro* experiments. A possible mechanism that was proposed is that opening of $GABA_A$ receptor channels induces Cl^- efflux, cell depolarization, and decreased Ca^{2+} influx, resulting in inhibition of T cell function[12]. In patients with cystic fibrosis as well, defects in the CFTR gene were suggested to contribute to the impaired immune response, thus strengthening the role of chloride channels in immune response[12].

Even intracellular ion channels localized to mitochondria and other organelles have been established to contribute to immune cell activation by regulating key cellular signaling pathways, including mitochondrial pathways, as summarized in a recent review[1]. A family of anion channel proteins called chloride intracellular channel (CLIC) proteins has been identified in the mitochondria of cardiomyocytes, in which these proteins were shown to be important in maintaining cardiac mitochondrial physiology[117]. Their function is also implicated in macrophage activation and the formation of inflammasome complex[118–120]. CLICs contain glutathione S-transferase (GST) omega fold and are therefore classified under the GST superfamily of proteins[121–124]. CLICs are an evolutionarily conserved unique class of ion channel proteins that can exist in both soluble and integral membrane forms[123–126]. There are six main paralogs of CLIC proteins that are identified in mammals. They are referred to as CLIC1–CLIC6[127–135]. Some of the CLICs, such as CLIC5 and CLIC6, also seem to exhibit splice variation[126]. Other than mammals, CLIC orthologs are also observed in plants[136], invertebrates[137,138], and prokaryotes[139], in which they have been shown to exhibit channel-like activity[139,140]. Similar to GST, some of the CLIC members, CLIC1, CLIC2, and CLIC4, exhibit glutaredoxin-like activity[122]. CLICs, through either their channel activity or other regulatory mechanisms, have been demonstrated to play a role in many of the physiological and pathophysiological processes[125,141].

CLICs autoinsert into lipid membranes and function as ion channels[142,143]. The transition from soluble to integral membrane form requires structural rearrangements in the protein, but the exact mechanism has not yet been deciphered. The most studied CLIC in terms of channel activity is CLIC1. It has been shown that the channel activity of CLIC1 is pH dependent[144,145]. The conformational stability of the CLIC1 protein was found to be altered at lower pH, as it was observed that

CLIC forms partially unfolded intermediates that increase further upon low pH[146] and thereby help in its autoinsertion. The N-terminal sequence between C24 and V46, comprising the putative transmembrane (PTM) domain, has been shown to form a helical structure both at pH 7.4 and at a lower pH of 5.0[146]. It was also shown that the mutation of PTM residue C24 resulted in the inhibition of channel activity, but the channel insertion or formation was not affected[147].

Amid the several cellular processes that they regulate, CLIC channel activity is also considered to be important for immune cell activation. Bone marrow-derived dendritic cells (BMDCs) isolated from *clic1−/−* mice showed diminished antigen presentation due to impaired phagosomal acidification[148]. In DCs, phagocytosis triggered the translocation of cytoplasmic CLIC1 to a phagosomal membrane, where it was shown to regulate phagosomal pH and proteolysis of the antigen[148]. Pharmacological blockage of the DCs isolated from wild-type mice with CLIC inhibitor indanyloxyacetic acid (IAA-94) also showed a similar defect in their antigen presentation ability, indicating that the channel activity of CLICs contributes to this function[148]. CLIC1, CLIC4, and CLIC5, as shown in Figure 10.1, are present in the circulating monocytes of mice as well. It was observed that CLIC1 expression increased

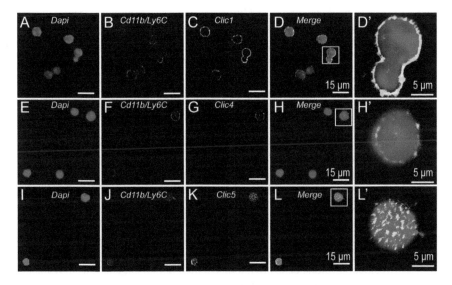

FIGURE 10.1   Localization of CLIC1, CLIC4, and CLIC5 in macrophages. Peripheral blood cells were isolated from 10- to 12-week-old mice; monocytes were labeled with anti-Cd11b/Ly6C antibodies and sorted into homogeneous populating flow sorters. Monocytes were fixed with 4% (v/v) PFA for 10 minutes. Nonspecific labeling was blocked by incubating cells in 1% (v/v) NGS in PBS containing 0.01% (v/v) Triton X-100. Monocytes sorted with anti-CD11b/Ly6C (B, F, J) were labeled with anti-CLIC1 (C), anti-CLIC4 (G), and anti-CLIC5 (K, green) antibodies. The nucleus was labeled with DAPI (blue: A, E, I). Cells were mounted with Mowiol. Merged images of A–C, E–G, and I–K are shown in D, H, and L, respectively. Cells in squares in images D, H, and L are shown in D', H', and L', respectively.

Source: Images were acquired with a confocal microscope (Zeiss confocal microscope).

in PBMCs in chronic inflammatory conditions of the central nervous system, such as Alzheimer's disease, and can be considered as a potential biomarker for neurodegenerative disease conditions[149]. The absence of CLIC1 impaired phagosomal acidification and reduced ROS generation in macrophages[150,151]. CLICs also play a role in NLRP3 inflammasome complex formation by macrophages[118,119]. NLRP3 is a multiprotein inflammasome complex formed by the innate immune sensor protein NLRP3, adapter protein ASC, and proteolysis enzyme caspase 1[152,153]. NLRP3 complex formation is required for the secretion of pro-inflammatory cytokines such as IL-1β and IL-18 against stress conditions or upon infection. K+ efflux is known to cause mitochondrial damage, increasing the ROS production by the mitochondria and leading to activation of NLRP3 inflammasome complex[154]. The mitochondrial ROS generated in this process was shown to induce translocation of CLICs (CLIC1, CLIC4, and CLIC5) to the plasma membrane, leading to chloride efflux and thus contributing to inflammasome assembly and IL-1β secretion[118,154]. These studies provide substantial evidence that the CLIC-mediated upstream event is a prerequisite for the regulation of NLRP3 activation, and Cl⁻ flux changes facilitated by them play a key role in activating the innate immune system. Because CLICs are mitochondrial ion channel proteins that affect mitochondrial physiology[117], their specific role in both innate and adaptive immune cell activation via modulating mitochondrial function needs to be addressed. In addition, the increasing evidence implicating the role of chloride flux changes in immune cell activation, development, and function cannot be ignored, and more attention should be given to the molecular identification of other uncharacterized chloride channels in immune cells.

ION CHANNELS OF IMMUNE CELLS IN CARDIAC PHYSIOLOGY AND PATHOPHYSIOLOGY

A clinical study in 1953 demonstrated that 30 out of 40 heart failure (HF) patients showed the presence of C-reactive protein in their blood, indicating the involvement of inflammatory components to the complexity related to HF[155]. Since then, many cardiac pathophysiological conditions such as atherosclerosis, atrial fibrillation (AF), myocarditis, endocarditis, arrhythmia, and myocardial infarction (MI) have also been associated with defects in immune cell function[156,157]. The immune cell populations, including macrophages, mast cells, eosinophils, neutrophils, monocytes, and B and T cells, reside in the heart or infiltrate the cardiac tissue upon a variety of stimuli[158]. The resident immune cells are not distributed homogeneously, as they localize to different locations in the heart[158]. The differential localization of resident immune populations in the heart defines their distinct interaction with the various other cells, including cardiomyocytes, endothelial cells, and fibroblasts. These interactions are important because the non-leukocytes send signals in the form of cytokines, chemokines, and growth factors, to which the leukocytes respond and initiate the inflammatory signaling cascade. Similarly, non-leukocytes contain receptors that are specific to leukocyte products and upon binding activate the downstream signaling pathway. These interactions serve as one of the important regulatory mechanisms that aids in maintaining the structure and function of the heart. Interestingly, there are also studies focused on how the ion channel proteins in immune cells, namely, connexins and

$K_{Ca}3.1$, influence these interactions and regulate cardiac physiology and pathophysiology. The structure-function properties of these channels and their specific role in maintaining cardiac physiology will be discussed briefly in this section.

CONNEXINS

Connexins are ubiquitous, integral membrane proteins present in almost all of the cells of the body. Connexins are known to form cell-cell communication in tissues and between the extracellular environment and cytoplasm by forming gap junctions. In electrically excitable cells like cardiomyocytes, connexins serve as a powerful coordinator for allowing the cell-to-cell passage of ions to facilitate uniform electrical conduction throughout the heart[159–161].

Gap junctions are formed when two opposing hexameric connexons, also called connexin hemichannels, that are present on respective cells dock to each other. Hemichannels can be homomeric (composed of the same connexins) or heteromeric (composed of different connexins)[162]. Gap junctions formed of two homomeric or two heteromeric hemichannels with the same connexin composition are called homotypic gap junctions. Heterotypic gap junctions are formed by two hemichannels, each with a different composition of connexins[163]. Cardiac muscle predominantly expresses connexin 40 (Cx40), connexin 43 (Cx43), connexin 45 (Cx45), and connexin 37 (Cx37) in humans and rodents[159,164]. These connexins are differentially expressed in various regions of the heart. For instance, Cx40 is expressed in atrial cardiomyocytes, and Cx43 is mainly expressed between the atrial and ventricular conduction system[161].

The permeability and size of the pore depend on the permutation and combination of connexins that make up the gap junctions. Several reviews have outlined the biophysical characterization of different gap junctions[165–167]. In general, gap junctions have a pore diameter range of 10–20 Å and are permeable to ions[159,168,169] such as K^+, Ca^{2+}, Na^+, or Cl^-. Gap junctions allow the passage of small metabolites[170,171] of ~1.5 kDa such as glucose, glutamate, glutathione, acetate, and ascorbic acid and second messengers[172–175] such as cAMP, cGMP, ATP, NAD^+, prostaglandins, and IP_3.

Cardiac macrophages have been established to play an important role in cardiac physiology. In the heart, macrophages are found as spindle-shaped structures among the myocytes, fibroblasts, and endothelial cells in both humans and mice[176,177]. The most abundant type of macrophage found in the heart is M2, expressing M2-specific anti-inflammatory markers like Mrc1, CD163, and Lyve-1[177]. These resident macrophages evolve during embryonic development and populate the heart, rather than differentiating via blood monocytes[176]. Hulsmans et al. studied resident macrophages in the AV node, as it acts as a crucial link between the atria and the ventricles[178]. It was discovered that macrophages can electrically couple with cardiomyocytes via connexin 43 (Cx43), which causes macrophage depolarization and modulates AV nodal conduction[178]. By using immunofluorescence and qPCR analysis, researchers established that these macrophages express Cx43, which mediates their interaction with cardiomyocytes. They used optogenetic methods to induce macrophage depolarization and observed better AV nodal conduction. Because Cx43 homozygous knockout mice are lethal and die of heart failure, the researchers used *Cx43⁻/⁻ CX₃CR1⁺* mice

(CX$_3$CR1$^+$ is expressed in cardiac macrophages) and found prolonged PR and AH interval post-telemetry recordings, suggesting improper AV node conduction[178] and, hence, demonstrating that macrophages can directly contribute to cardiac conduction with the help of connexins. The observation made by Hulsmans et al. that macrophages express Cx43 and modulate electrical coupling showed the direct importance of connexins present in macrophages to modulating cardiac physiology[178].

Defects in Cx43 expression in macrophages post-MI were shown to alter the conduction of the heart. For instance, lower levels of Cx43 have been observed in mice with post-MI arrhythmias and those with overall decreased cardiac conduction. The infarcted areas showed increased Cx43 degradation and internalization. These infarcted mice also exhibited increased IL-1β levels, which are secreted by macrophages and tend to disrupt or decrease Cx43 expression[179]. Overall, macrophages tend to have direct and indirect roles in cardiac conduction, which is strongly modulated via gap junction Cx43.

Macrophage connexins also play an important role in the development of atherosclerosis by contributing to adhesion and plaque development[180]. Atherosclerosis is an inflammatory phenomenon of the vascular wall that arises due to a defect in cholesterol metabolism that primes lipid deposition, eventually obstructing blood flow[181]. Vascular lipid deposition activates the innate immune cell macrophages, triggering an inflammatory response[181,182]. However, this response of the macrophages transforms them into foam cells, which eventually contribute to the huge lipid core in the plaque[183,184]. This phenomenon eventually leads to ischemia and increases the prevalence of MI and stroke[185,186]. Following ischemia or an infarct, recruitment of neutrophils accentuates the inflammatory cascade contributing to atherogenesis[187]. Thus, this atherogenic state is prevalent in interactions of multiple cell types, which are regulated by cell-interacting proteins like Cx43 and Cx37[188]. Deleting Cx37 in atherosclerotic mice led to the presence of macrophages in atherosclerotic plaques and enhanced endothelial macrophage adhesion, thus accentuating atherosclerosis. This was validated by staining for lipids in the plaque, which depicted a 58% increase in atherogenic mice with the Cx37 deletion. To understand whether altering the expression of Cx37 in macrophages or endothelium promotes the recruitment and migration of macrophages, Wong et al. injected Cx37-depleted macrophages into Cx37-expressing atherogenic mice[189]. They observed enhanced atherogenic plaques and increased lipid stain in the plaques, a hallmark of atherosclerosis. In contrast, similar results were not observed in Cx37-depleted mice that received CX37-expressing macrophages, suggesting that Cx37 expression in the macrophages and not in the endothelium plays an important role in macrophage adhesion and overall atherogenic pathology. Subsequently, inhibition of Cx37 hemichannel activity by a blocker (gap26 and gap27) in atherogenic mice increased its pathology by twofold, establishing the importance of hemichannel activity in atherosclerosis development[190]. Additionally, macrophage Cx43 has been shown to contribute to atherosclerotic plaques by attracting neutrophils in the plaque itself[187]. Cx43$^{+/-}$ chimeric mice reduced atherosclerosis by altering chemoattractant proteins and, hence, showing reduced neutrophils in the plaque itself, slowing the progression[187]. However, the mechanism by which Cx43 manipulates the chemoattractive properties of macrophages is still unknown. Overall, Cx37 and Cx43 have contradictory roles in atherosclerosis development, wherein Cx37 has the potential to be a "protector" protein while Cx43 could be a target for mitigating the pathology. However, even in their polarizing roles, gap junctions and their subsequent proteins have proven to be important and help to encourage future research for their role in cardiac pathology.

$K_{Ca}3.1$ CHANNEL

Among the three groups of K_{Ca} channels, IK_{Ca} present in immune cells has been shown to contribute to cardiac pathophysiology. In macrophages, $K_{Ca}3.1$ has been shown to transcriptionally regulate their polarization and play a role in atherosclerotic plaque instability[104]. It has been observed that both the channel conductance and the amplitude of $K_{Ca}3.1$ and its expression were increased in M1 and M2 macrophages upon stimulation with LPS, IFN-γ, or IL-4, with M1 macrophages showing a more prominent increase than M2 macrophages[104]. Blockage of these channels with its inhibitor TRAM-34 during stimulation with LPS and IFN-γ abrogated the expression of cell surface markers of M1 macrophages such as CD80 and CD197, as well as pro-inflammatory cytokine and chemokine mRNA expression, suggesting that $K_{Ca}3.1$ plays a role in pro-inflammatory gene expression during macrophage polarization[104]. There was no significant effect on M2 macrophages. In addition, it was demonstrated that $K_{Ca}3.1$ upregulates pro-inflammatory genes via phosphorylation of STAT-1, which is a key pathway mediating M1 polarization[104,191,192], implicating a potential role for $K_{Ca}3.1$ in regulating the function and activation of proinflammatory M1 macrophages and disease conditions mediated by them, such as atherosclerosis. In certain conditions, abrupt rupture of the atherosclerotic plaques or lesions results in the accumulation and activation of platelets that prompts thrombotic vascular occlusion, which sometimes can cause acute coronary syndrome and cardiac death[193]. Treatment of atherosclerotic mice with TRAM-34 abrogated atherosclerotic lesion formation as well as prevented the rupture of atherosclerotic plaque, providing a novel potential role of $K_{Ca}3.1$ for treatment of the disease[194].

Ventricular arrhythmia is observed in patients post-MI injury and is considered a primary cause of cardiac death[195]. It was observed that the number of pro-inflammatory mononuclear cells was significantly higher in patients exhibiting post-MI arrhythmia than in patients post-MI without arrhythmia or in healthy controls[196]. Interestingly, after MI injury in mice, it was shown that the expression of $K_{Ca}3.1$ was more than 60-fold higher in M1 macrophages than in cardiomyocytes or fibroblasts[196]. Further activation and expression of $K_{Ca}3.1$ in macrophages correlated with post-MI arrhythmia observed in mice, suggesting a probable link between $K_{Ca}3.1$ channel activity and post-MI arrhythmia[196]. Additionally, co-culturing of M1 macrophages with cardiomyocytes was shown to prolong the action potential durations of cardiomyocytes via $K_{Ca}3.1$ activation and gap junction proteins *in vitro*. Furthermore, treatment with TRAM34 inhibited the post-MI arrhythmia *in vivo*, suggesting that macrophages impact post-MI arrhythmia via $K_{Ca}3.1$ activation and can be considered as a potential therapeutic target for treating post-MI arrhythmia[196], similar to atherosclerosis.

$K_{Ca}3.1$ and gap junction protein connexin in macrophages have been well studied and determined to impact cardiac physiology and pathophysiology. They have also been considered to be promising potential targets for therapeutics. This further provokes interest in understanding the role of other channels of immune cells in maintaining the physiology of the organs they infiltrate. This is an important area of research and, hence, needs to be pursued further.

CONCLUDING REMARKS

From the time the first ion channel was identified in immune cells, remarkable progress has been made in understanding the specific role of each channel and their interdependence in mediating immune cell activation and function. Interestingly, advancements have also been made in understanding the function of some of the ion channels in immune cells in modulating the function of organs they infiltrate. A large body of evidence also exists pertaining to their consideration as potential novel targets for therapeutics in many disease conditions, including CVDs and stroke. Therefore, a major goal of future research should be focused on uncovering the molecular identity and functional interplay of different ion channels of immune cells in regulating immune cell function as well as their communication with other non-leukocyte cells. Furthermore, effort should be put into evaluating the efficacy and therapeutic potential of small-molecule inhibitors, agonists, or antagonists of ion channels in preclinical trials that can be later translated to clinical studies.

ACKNOWLEDGMENTS

We thank Rachel Rosenzweig for helping with data collection. This work is supported by the National Heart, Lung, and Blood Institute of the National Institutes of Health [HL133050 (HS), HL132123 (SSB)] and American Heart Association Grant [20CDA35310714 (DP)]. DP, SS, and HS contributed to the writing and designing of the book chapter. SSB provided cells for the investigation. The authors declare that there are no conflicts of interest.

ABBREVIATIONS

ADP, adenosine diphosphate; AFDPR, ADP ribose; ASC, apoptosis-associated spec-like proteins; AF, atrial fibrillation; ATP, adenosine triphosphate; AV, atrioventricular; BMDCs, bone marrow-derived dendritic cells; BK, large conductance calcium-activated potassium channel; cAMP, cyclic adenosine monophosphate; cGMP, cyclic guanosine monophosphate; CLIC, chloride intracellular channel; CRAC, calcium release–activated Calcium; CFTR, cystic fibrosis transmembrane conductance regulator; Cx, connexins; CD, cluster of differentiation; CVDs, cardiovascular diseases; CaM, calmodulin; DCs, dendritic cells; ER, endoplasmic reticulum; EAE, encephalomyelitis; $GABA_A$, γ-aminobutyric acid; GST, glutathione S transferase; HF, heart failure; IL, interleukin; Ig, immunoglobulin; IFN, interferon; IAA-94, indanyloxyacetic acid; IP_3, inositol triphosphate; $K_v1.3$, voltage-activated potassium channel; $K_{Ca}3.1$, Ca^{2+}-activated intermediate conductance potassium channel; Kir, inward rectifier K^+ channels; K2P, two-pore K^+ channels; LRRC8A, leucine-rich repeat-containing protein 8A; LPS, lipopolysaccharide; Lyve1, lymphatic vessel endothelial hyaluronan receptor 1; MI, myocardial infarction; MRC1, mannose receptor C type 1; MS, multiple sclerosis; MHC, major histocompatibility complex; NAD, nicotinamide adenine dinucleotide; NADPH, nicotinamide adenine dinucleotide phosphate; NK, natural killer; NLRP3, nucleotide-binding oligomerization domain and leucine-rich repeat-containing receptors family pyrin domain containing 3; NFAT, nuclear factor of activated T cells; PTM, putative transmembrane domain; PBMCs, peripheral blood mononuclear cells; ROS, reactive oxygen species; RyR, ryanodine receptor; SK, small conductance calcium-activated potassium channel; SOCE, store-operated calcium entry; STIM, stromal interaction molecule; SNPs, single nucleotide polymorphisms; STAT, signal transducer and activation of transcription proteins; TCR, T cell receptor; TRPC, transient receptor potential canonical; TRPM, transient receptor potential melastatin; TRPV, transient receptor potential vanilloid; TRPM, transient receptor potential mucolipin; TRPP, transient receptor potential polycystin; TRPA, transient receptor potential ankyrin; T_{EM}, effector memory T cells; VSD, voltage sensor domain; VRAC, volume-regulated anion channel.

BIBLIOGRAPHY

1. Ponnalagu, D. & Singh, H. Insights into the role of mitochondrial ion channels in inflammatory response. *Front Physiol* **11**, 258, doi:10.3389/fphys.2020.00258 (2020).
2. Feske, S., Concepcion, A. R. & Coetzee, W. A. Eye on ion channels in immune cells. *Sci Signal* **12**, doi:10.1126/scisignal.aaw8014 (2019).
3. Feske, S., Skolnik, E. Y. & Prakriya, M. Ion channels and transporters in lymphocyte function and immunity. *Nat Rev Immunol* **12**, 532–547, doi:10.1038/nri3233 (2012).
4. Vig, M. & Kinet, J. P. Calcium signaling in immune cells. *Nat Immunol* **10**, 21–27, doi:10.1038/ni.f.220 (2009).
5. Cahalan, M. D. & Chandy, K. G. The functional network of ion channels in T lymphocytes. *Immunol Rev* **231**, 59–87, doi:10.1111/j.1600-065X.2009.00816.x (2009).
6. Hoth, M. & Penner, R. Depletion of intracellular calcium stores activates a calcium current in mast cells. *Nature* **355**, 353–356, doi:10.1038/355353a0 (1992).
7. Lewis, R. S. & Cahalan, M. D. Mitogen-induced oscillations of cytosolic Ca2+ and transmembrane Ca2+ current in human leukemic T cells. *Cell Regul* **1**, 99–112, doi:10.1091/mbc.1.1.99 (1989).
8. Zweifach, A. & Lewis, R. S. Mitogen-regulated Ca2+ current of T lymphocytes is activated by depletion of intracellular Ca2+ stores. *Proc Natl Acad Sci U S A* **90**, 6295–6299, doi:10.1073/pnas.90.13.6295 (1993).
9. DeCoursey, T. E., Chandy, K. G., Gupta, S. & Cahalan, M. D. Voltage-dependent ion channels in T-lymphocytes. *J Neuroimmunol* **10**, 71–95, doi:10.1016/0165-5728(85)90035-9 (1985).
10. Matteson, D. R. & Deutsch, C. K channels in T lymphocytes: A patch clamp study using monoclonal antibody adhesion. *Nature* **307**, 468–471, doi:10.1038/307468a0 (1984).
11. Launay, P. *et al.* TRPM4 regulates calcium oscillations after T cell activation. *Science* **306**, 1374–1377, doi:10.1126/science.1098845 (2004).
12. Feske, S., Wulff, H. & Skolnik, E. Y. Ion channels in innate and adaptive immunity. *Annu Rev Immunol* **33**, 291–353, doi:10.1146/annurev-immunol-032414-112212 (2015).
13. Mueller, C. *et al.* Lack of cystic fibrosis transmembrane conductance regulator in CD3+ lymphocytes leads to aberrant cytokine secretion and hyperinflammatory adaptive immune responses. *Am J Respir Cell Mol Biol* **44**, 922–929, doi:10.1165/rcmb.2010-0224OC (2011).

14. Cahalan, M. D., Chandy, K. G., DeCoursey, T. E. & Gupta, S. A voltage-gated potassium channel in human T lymphocytes. *J Physiol* **358**, 197–237, doi:10.1113/jphysiol.1985. sp015548 (1985).

15. DeCoursey, T. E., Chandy, K. G., Gupta, S. & Cahalan, M. D. Voltage-gated K+ channels in human T lymphocytes: A role in mitogenesis? *Nature* **307**, 465–468, doi:10.1038/307465a0 (1984).

16. Fukushima, Y., Hagiwara, S. & Henkart, M. Potassium current in clonal cytotoxic T lymphocytes from the mouse. *J Physiol* **351**, 645–656, doi:10.1113/jphysiol.1984.sp015268 (1984).

17. Grissmer, S., Nguyen, A. N. & Cahalan, M. D. Calcium-activated potassium channels in resting and activated human T lymphocytes. Expression levels, calcium dependence, ion selectivity, and pharmacology. *J Gen Physiol* **102**, 601–630, doi:10.1085/jgp.102.4.601 (1993).

18. Kerschbaum, H. H. & Cahalan, M. D. Monovalent permeability, rectification, and ionic block of store-operated calcium channels in Jurkat T lymphocytes. *J Gen Physiol* **111**, 521–537, doi:10.1085/jgp.111.4.521 (1998).

19. Prakriya, M. & Lewis, R. S. Separation and characterization of currents through store-operated CRAC channels and Mg2+-inhibited cation (MIC) channels. *J Gen Physiol* **119**, 487–507, doi:10.1085/jgp.20028551 (2002).

20. Hermosura, M. C., Monteilh-Zoller, M. K., Scharenberg, A. M., Penner, R. & Fleig, A. Dissociation of the store-operated calcium current I(CRAC) and the Mg-nucleotide-regulated metal ion current MagNuM. *J Physiol* **539**, 445–458, doi:10.1113/jphysiol. 2001.013361 (2002).

21. Cahalan, M. D. & Lewis, R. S. Role of potassium and chloride channels in volume regulation by T lymphocytes. *Soc Gen Physiol Ser* **43**, 281–301 (1988).

22. Mahtani, T. & Treanor, B. Beyond the CRAC: Diversification of ion signaling in B cells. *Immunol Rev* **291**, 104–122, doi:10.1111/imr.12770 (2019).

23. Kumar, L. *et al.* Leucine-rich repeat containing 8A (LRRC8A) is essential for T lymphocyte development and function. *J Exp Med* **211**, 929–942, doi:10.1084/jem.20131379 (2014).

24. Krishnamoorthy, M. *et al.* The ion channel TRPM7 is required for B cell lymphopoiesis. *Sci Signal* **11**, doi:10.1126/scisignal.aan2693 (2018).

25. Hobeika, E. *et al.* Testing gene function early in the B cell lineage in mb1-cre mice. *Proc Natl Acad Sci U S A* **103**, 13789–13794, doi:10.1073/pnas.0605944103 (2006).

26. Anzilotti, C. *et al.* An essential role for the Zn(2+) transporter ZIP7 in B cell development. *Nat Immunol* **20**, 350–361, doi:10.1038/s41590-018-0295-8 (2019).

27. Felix, R. *et al.* The Orai-1 and STIM-1 complex controls human dendritic cell maturation. *PLoS ONE* **8**, e61595, doi:10.1371/journal.pone.0061595 (2013).

28. Matzner, N. *et al.* Ion channels modulating mouse dendritic cell functions. *J Immunol* **181**, 6803–6809, doi:10.4049/jimmunol.181.10.6803 (2008).

29. Vukcevic, M., Spagnoli, G. C., Iezzi, G., Zorzato, F. & Treves, S. Ryanodine receptor activation by Ca v 1.2 is involved in dendritic cell major histocompatibility complex class II surface expression. *J Biol Chem* **283**, 34913–34922, doi:10.1074/jbc.M804472200 (2008).

30. Shumilina, E., Huber, S. M. & Lang, F. Ca2+ signaling in the regulation of dendritic cell functions. *Am J Physiol Cell Physiol* **300**, C1205–1214, doi:10.1152/ajpcell.00039.2011 (2011).

31. Redmond, J., O'Rilley, D. & Buchanan, P. Role of ion channels in natural killer cell function towards cancer. *Discov Med* **23**, 353–360 (2017).

32. Prakriya, M. & Lewis, R. S. Store-operated calcium channels. *Physiol Rev* **95**, 1383–1436, doi:10.1152/physrev.00020.2014 (2015).

33. Lewis, R. S. The molecular choreography of a store-operated calcium channel. *Nature* **446**, 284–287, doi:10.1038/nature05637 (2007).

34. Hogan, P. G., Lewis, R. S. & Rao, A. Molecular basis of calcium signaling in lymphocytes: STIM and ORAI. *Annu Rev Immunol* **28**, 491–533, doi:10.1146/annurev. immunol.021908.132550 (2010).

35. Hoth, M. & Penner, R. Calcium release-activated calcium current in rat mast cells. *J Physiol* **465**, 359–386, doi:10.1113/jphysiol.1993.sp019681 (1993).

36. Prakriya, M. The molecular physiology of CRAC channels. *Immunol Rev* **231**, 88–98, doi:10.1111/j.1600-065X.2009.00820.x (2009).

37. Liou, J. *et al.* STIM is a Ca2+ sensor essential for Ca2+-store-depletion-triggered Ca2+ influx. *Curr Biol* **15**, 1235–1241, doi:10.1016/j.cub.2005.05.055 (2005).

38. Zhang, S. L. *et al.* STIM1 is a Ca2+ sensor that activates CRAC channels and migrates from the Ca2+ store to the plasma membrane. *Nature* **437**, 902–905, doi:10.1038/ nature04147 (2005).

39. Park, C. Y. *et al.* STIM1 clusters and activates CRAC channels via direct binding of a cytosolic domain to Orai1. *Cell* **136**, 876–890, doi:10.1016/j.cell.2009.02.014 (2009).

40. Byun, M. *et al.* Whole-exome sequencing-based discovery of STIM1 deficiency in a child with fatal classic Kaposi sarcoma. *J Exp Med* **207**, 2307–2312, doi:10.1084/jem.20101597 (2010).

41. McCarl, C. A. *et al.* ORAI1 deficiency and lack of store-operated Ca2+ entry cause immunodeficiency, myopathy, and ectodermal dysplasia. *J Allergy Clin Immunol* **124**, 1311–1318, e1317, doi:10.1016/j.jaci.2009.10.007 (2009).

42. Feske, S., Giltnane, J., Dolmetsch, R., Staudt, L. M. & Rao, A. Gene regulation mediated by calcium signals in T lymphocytes. *Nat Immunol* **2**, 316–324, doi:10.1038/86318 (2001).

43. Feske, S. ORAI1 and STIM1 deficiency in human and mice: Roles of store-operated Ca2+ entry in the immune system and beyond. *Immunol Rev* **231**, 189–209, doi:10.1111/ j.1600-065X.2009.00818.x (2009).

44. Maul-Pavicic, A. *et al.* ORAI1-mediated calcium influx is required for human cytotoxic lymphocyte degranulation and target cell lysis. *Proc Natl Acad Sci U S A* **108**, 3324–3329, doi:10.1073/pnas.1013285108 (2011).

45. Gwack, Y. *et al.* Hair loss and defective T- and B-cell function in mice lacking ORAI1. *Mol Cell Biol* **28**, 5209–5222, doi:10.1128/MCB.00360-08 (2008).

46. Fenninger, F. & Jefferies, W. A. What's bred in the bone: Calcium channels in lymphocytes. *J Immunol* **202**, 1021–1030, doi:10.4049/jimmunol.1800837 (2019).

47. Hartzell, C. A., Jankowska, K. I., Burkhardt, J. K. & Lewis, R. S. Calcium influx through CRAC channels controls actin organization and dynamics at the immune synapse. *Elife* **5**, doi:10.7554/eLife.14850 (2016).

48. Matsumoto, M. *et al.* The calcium sensors STIM1 and STIM2 control B cell regulatory function through interleukin-10 production. *Immunity* **34**, 703–714, doi:10.1016/j. immuni.2011.03.016 (2011).

49. Picard, C. *et al.* STIM1 mutation associated with a syndrome of immunodeficiency and autoimmunity. *N Engl J Med* **360**, 1971–1980, doi:10.1056/NEJMoa0900082 (2009).

50. Clemens, R. A. & Lowell, C. A. CRAC channel regulation of innate immune cells in health and disease. *Cell Calcium* **78**, 56–65, doi:10.1016/j.ceca.2019.01.003 (2019).

51. Clemens, R. A., Chong, J., Grimes, D., Hu, Y. & Lowell, C. A. STIM1 and STIM2 cooperatively regulate mouse neutrophil store-operated calcium entry and cytokine production. *Blood* **130**, 1565–1577, doi:10.1182/blood-2016-11-751230 (2017).

52. Zhang, H. *et al.* STIM1 calcium sensor is required for activation of the phagocyte oxidase during inflammation and host defense. *Blood* **123**, 2238–2249, doi:10.1182/blood-2012-08-450403 (2014).

53. Nunes, P. *et al.* STIM1 juxtaposes ER to phagosomes, generating Ca(2)(+) hotspots that boost phagocytosis. *Curr Biol* **22**, 1990–1997, doi:10.1016/j.cub.2012.08.049 (2012).

54. Ashmole, I. *et al.* CRACM/Orai ion channel expression and function in human lung mast cells. *J Allergy Clin Immunol* **129**, 1628–1635, e1622, doi:10.1016/j.jaci.2012.01.070 (2012).

55. Wajdner, H. E. *et al.* Orai and TRPC channel characterization in FcepsilonRI-mediated calcium signaling and mediator secretion in human mast cells. *Physiol Rep* **5**, doi:10.14814/phy2.13166 (2017).

56. Vig, M. *et al.* Defective mast cell effector functions in mice lacking the CRACM1 pore subunit of store-operated calcium release-activated calcium channels. *Nat Immunol* **9**, 89–96, doi:10.1038/ni1550 (2008).

57. Samanta, A., Hughes, T. E. T. & Moiseenkova-Bell, V. Y. Transient receptor potential (TRP) channels. *Subcell Biochem* **87**, 141–165, doi:10.1007/978-981-10-7757-9_6 (2018).

58. Clapham, D. E. TRP channels as cellular sensors. *Nature* **426**, 517–524, doi:10.1038/nature02196 (2003).

59. Wenning, A. S. *et al.* TRP expression pattern and the functional importance of TRPC3 in primary human T-cells. *Biochim Biophys Acta* **1813**, 412–423, doi:10.1016/j.bbamcr.2010.12.022 (2011).

60. Parenti, A., De Logu, F., Geppetti, P. & Benemei, S. What is the evidence for the role of TRP channels in inflammatory and immune cells? *Br J Pharmacol* **173**, 953–969, doi:10.1111/bph.13392 (2016).

61. Melzer, N., Hicking, G., Gobel, K. & Wiendl, H. TRPM2 cation channels modulate T cell effector functions and contribute to autoimmune CNS inflammation. *PLoS One* **7**, e47617, doi:10.1371/journal.pone.0047617 (2012).

62. Sumoza-Toledo, A. *et al.* Dendritic cell maturation and chemotaxis is regulated by TRPM2-mediated lysosomal Ca2+ release. *FASEB J* **25**, 3529–3542, doi:10.1096/fj.10-178483 (2011).

63. Bachmann, M. *et al.* Voltage-gated potassium channels as regulators of cell death. *Front Cell Dev Biol* **8**, 611853, doi:10.3389/fcell.2020.611853 (2020).

64. Gutman, G. A. *et al.* International Union of Pharmacology. LIII. Nomenclature and molecular relationships of voltage-gated potassium channels. *Pharmacol Rev* **57**, 473–508, doi:10.1124/pr.57.4.10 (2005).

65. Kaczmarek, L. K. *et al.* International union of basic and clinical pharmacology. C. Nomenclature and properties of calcium-activated and sodium-activated potassium channels. *Pharmacol Rev* **69**, 1–11, doi:10.1124/pr.116.012864 (2017).

66. Hibino, H. *et al.* Inwardly rectifying potassium channels: Their structure, function, and physiological roles. *Physiol Rev* **90**, 291–366, doi:10.1152/physrev.00021.2009 (2010).

67. Isomoto, S., Kondo, C. & Kurachi, Y. Inwardly rectifying potassium channels: Their molecular heterogeneity and function. *Jpn J Physiol* **47**, 11–39, doi:10.2170/jjphysiol.47.11 (1997).

68. Enyedi, P. & Czirjak, G. Molecular background of leak K+ currents: Two-pore domain potassium channels. *Physiol Rev* **90**, 559–605, doi:10.1152/physrev.00029.2009 (2010).

69. Chandy, K. G., DeCoursey, T. E., Cahalan, M. D., McLaughlin, C. & Gupta, S. Voltage-gated potassium channels are required for human T lymphocyte activation. *J Exp Med* **160**, 369–385, doi:10.1084/jem.160.2.369 (1984).

70. Vicente, R. *et al.* Association of Kv1.5 and Kv1.3 contributes to the major voltage-dependent K+ channel in macrophages. *J Biol Chem* **281**, 37675–37685, doi:10.1074/jbc.M605617200 (2006).

71. Gonzalez, C. *et al.* K(+) channels: Function-structural overview. *Compr Physiol* **2**, 2087–2149, doi:10.1002/cphy.c110047 (2012).

72. Attali, B. *et al.* Cloning, functional expression, and regulation of two K+ channels in human T lymphocytes. *J Biol Chem* **267**, 8650–8657 (1992).

73. Douglass, J. *et al.* Characterization and functional expression of a rat genomic DNA clone encoding a lymphocyte potassium channel. *J Immunol* **144**, 4841–4850 (1990).

74. Szabo, I. *et al.* A novel potassium channel in lymphocyte mitochondria. *J Biol Chem* **280**, 12790–12798, doi:10.1074/jbc.M413548200 (2005).

75. Szabo, I. *et al.* Mitochondrial potassium channel Kv1.3 mediates Bax-induced apoptosis in lymphocytes. *Proc Natl Acad Sci U S A* **105**, 14861–14866, doi:10.1073/pnas.0804236105 (2008).

76. Perez-Garcia, M. T., Cidad, P. & Lopez-Lopez, J. R. The secret life of ion channels: Kv1.3 potassium channels and proliferation. *Am J Physiol Cell Physiol* **314**, C27–C42, doi:10.1152/ajpcell.00136.2017 (2018).

77. Decoursey, T. E., Chandy, K. G., Gupta, S. & Cahalan, M. D. Two types of potassium channels in murine T lymphocytes. *J Gen Physiol* **89**, 379–404, doi:10.1085/jgp.89.3.379 (1987).

78. Gelfand, E. W., Cheung, R. K., Mills, G. B. & Grinstein, S. Role of membrane potential in the response of human T lymphocytes to phytohemagglutinin. *J Immunol* **138**, 527–531 (1987).

79. Hu, L. *et al.* Blockade of Kv1.3 potassium channels inhibits differentiation and granzyme B secretion of human CD8+ T effector memory lymphocytes. *PLoS ONE* **8**, e54267, doi:10.1371/journal.pone.0054267 (2013).

80. Kitagawa, S. & Johnston, R. B., Jr. Relationship between membrane potential changes and superoxide-releasing capacity in resident and activated mouse peritoneal macrophages. *J Immunol* **135**, 3417–3423 (1985).

81. Sutro, J. B., Vayuvegula, B. S., Gupta, S. & Cahalan, M. D. Voltage-sensitive ion channels in human B lymphocytes. *Adv Exp Med Biol* **254**, 113–122, doi:10.1007/978-1-4757-5803-0_14 (1989).

82. Panyi, G. *et al.* Kv1.3 potassium channels are localized in the immunological synapse formed between cytotoxic and target cells. *Proc Natl Acad Sci U S A* **101**, 1285–1290, doi:10.1073/pnas.0307421100 (2004).

83. Solovera, J. J., Alvarez-Mon, M., Casas, J., Carballido, J. & Durantez, A. Inhibition of human natural killer (NK) activity by calcium channel modulators and a calmodulin antagonist. *J Immunol* **139**, 876–880 (1987).

84. Rah, S. Y., Kwak, J. Y., Chung, Y. J. & Kim, U. H. ADP-ribose/TRPM2-mediated Ca2+ signaling is essential for cytolytic degranulation and antitumor activity of natural killer cells. *Sci Rep* **5**, 9482, doi:10.1038/srep09482 (2015).

85. Schlichter, L., Sidell, N. & Hagiwara, S. Potassium channels mediate killing by human natural killer cells. *Proc Natl Acad Sci U S A* **83**, 451–455, doi:10.1073/pnas.83.2.451 (1986).

86. Schulte-Mecklenbeck, A. *et al.* The two-pore domain K2 P channel TASK2 drives human NK-cell proliferation and cytolytic function. *Eur J Immunol* **45**, 2602–2614, doi:10.1002/eji.201445208 (2015).

87. Koshy, S. *et al.* Blocking KCa3.1 channels increases tumor cell killing by a subpopulation of human natural killer lymphocytes. *PLoS ONE* **8**, e76740, doi:10.1371/journal.pone.0076740 (2013).

88. Wulff, H. *et al.* The voltage-gated Kv1.3 K(+) channel in effector memory T cells as new target for MS. *J Clin Invest* **111**, 1703–1713, doi:10.1172/JCI16921 (2003).

89. Beeton, C. *et al.* Kv1.3 channels are a therapeutic target for T cell-mediated autoimmune diseases. *Proc Natl Acad Sci U S A* **103**, 17414–17419, doi:10.1073/pnas.0605136103 (2006).

90. Beeton, C. *et al.* Targeting effector memory T cells with a selective peptide inhibitor of Kv1.3 channels for therapy of autoimmune diseases. *Mol Pharmacol* **67**, 1369–1381, doi:10.1124/mol.104.008193 (2005).

91. Panyi, G., Beeton, C. & Felipe, A. Ion channels and anti-cancer immunity. *Philos Trans R Soc Lond B Biol Sci* **369**, 20130106, doi:10.1098/rstb.2013.0106 (2014).

92. Wang, L. H. *et al.* Rituximab inhibits Kv1.3 channels in human B lymphoma cells via activation of FcgammaRIIB receptors. *Biochim Biophys Acta* **1823**, 505–513, doi:10.1016/j.bbamcr.2011.11.012 (2012).

93. Brown, B. M., Shim, H., Christophersen, P. & Wulff, H. Pharmacology of small- and intermediate-conductance calcium-activated potassium channels. *Annu Rev Pharmacol Toxicol* **60**, 219–240, doi:10.1146/annurev-pharmtox-010919-023420 (2020).

94. Hoffman, J. F. *et al.* The hSK4 (KCNN4) isoform is the Ca2+-activated K+ channel (Gardos channel) in human red blood cells. *Proc Natl Acad Sci U S A* **100**, 7366–7371, doi:10.1073/pnas.1232342100 (2003).

95. Ghanshani, S. *et al.* Up-regulation of the IKCa1 potassium channel during T-cell activation. Molecular mechanism and functional consequences. *J Biol Chem* **275**, 37137–37149, doi:10.1074/jbc.M003941200 (2000).

96. Shumilina, E. *et al.* Blunted IgE-mediated activation of mast cells in mice lacking the Ca2+-activated K+ channel KCa3.1. *J Immunol* **180**, 8040–8047, doi:10.4049/jimmunol.180.12.8040 (2008).

97. Kaushal, V., Koeberle, P. D., Wang, Y. & Schlichter, L. C. The Ca2+-activated K+ channel KCNN4/KCa3.1 contributes to microglia activation and nitric oxide-dependent neurodegeneration. *J Neurosci* **27**, 234–244, doi:10.1523/JNEUROSCI.3593-06.2007 (2007).

98. Szteyn, K. & Singh, H. BKCa channels as targets for cardioprotection. *Antioxidants (Basel)* **9**, doi:10.3390/antiox9080760 (2020).

99. Lee, C. H. & MacKinnon, R. Activation mechanism of a human SK-calmodulin channel complex elucidated by cryo-EM structures. *Science* **360**, 508–513, doi:10.1126/science.aas9466 (2018).

100. Kohler, M. *et al.* Small-conductance, calcium-activated potassium channels from mammalian brain. *Science* **273**, 1709–1714, doi:10.1126/science.273.5282.1709 (1996).

101. Khanna, R., Chang, M. C., Joiner, W. J., Kaczmarek, L. K. & Schlichter, L. C. hSK4/hIK1, a calmodulin-binding KCa channel in human T lymphocytes. Roles in proliferation and volume regulation. *J Biol Chem* **274**, 14838–14849, doi:10.1074/jbc.274.21.14838 (1999).

102. Xia, X. M. *et al.* Mechanism of calcium gating in small-conductance calcium-activated potassium channels. *Nature* **395**, 503–507, doi:10.1038/26758 (1998).

103. Fanger, C. M. *et al.* Calmodulin mediates calcium-dependent activation of the intermediate conductance KCa channel, IKCa1. *J Biol Chem* **274**, 5746–5754, doi:10.1074/jbc.274.9.5746 (1999).

104. Xu, R. *et al.* Role of KCa3.1 channels in macrophage polarization and its relevance in atherosclerotic plaque instability. *Arterioscler Thromb Vasc Biol* **37**, 226–236, doi:10.1161/ATVBAHA.116.308461 (2017).

105. Di, L. *et al.* Inhibition of the K+ channel KCa3.1 ameliorates T cell-mediated colitis. *Proc Natl Acad Sci U S A* **107**, 1541–1546, doi:10.1073/pnas.0910133107 (2010).

106. Ma, X. Z. *et al.* The role and mechanism of KCa3.1 channels in human monocyte migration induced by palmitic acid. *Exp Cell Res* **369**, 208–217, doi:10.1016/j.yexcr.2018.05.020 (2018).

107. Mitolo, M. [Studies on physical training. X. Weight curve during training in man]. *Boll Soc Ital Biol Sper* **26**, 456–458 (1950).

108. Behe, P. *et al.* The LRRC8A mediated "swell activated" chloride conductance is dispensable for vacuolar homeostasis in neutrophils. *Front Pharmacol* **8**, 262, doi:10.3389/fphar.2017.00262 (2017).

109. Voss, F. K. *et al.* Identification of LRRC8 heteromers as an essential component of the volume-regulated anion channel VRAC. *Science* **344**, 634–638, doi:10.1126/science.1252826 (2014).

110. Qiu, Z. *et al.* SWELL1, a plasma membrane protein, is an essential component of volume-regulated anion channel. *Cell* **157**, 447–458, doi:10.1016/j.cell.2014.03.024 (2014).

111. Tian, J. *et al.* Gamma-aminobutyric acid inhibits T cell autoimmunity and the development of inflammatory responses in a mouse type 1 diabetes model. *J Immunol* **173**, 5298–5304, doi:10.4049/jimmunol.173.8.5298 (2004).

112. Mendu, S. K. *et al.* Increased GABA(A) channel subunits expression in CD8(+) but not in CD4(+) T cells in BB rats developing diabetes compared to their congenic littermates. *Mol Immunol* **48**, 399–407, doi:10.1016/j.molimm.2010.08.005 (2011).

113. Moss, R. B. *et al.* Reduced IL-10 secretion by CD4+ T lymphocytes expressing mutant cystic fibrosis transmembrane conductance regulator (CFTR). *Clin Exp Immunol* **106**, 374–388, doi:10.1046/j.1365-2249.1996.d01-826.x (1996).

114. Chen, J. H., Schulman, H. & Gardner, P. A cAMP-regulated chloride channel in lymphocytes that is affected in cystic fibrosis. *Science* **243**, 657–660, doi:10.1126/science.2464852 (1989).

115. Cheng, G., Ramanathan, A., Shao, Z. & Agrawal, D. K. Chloride channel expression and functional diversity in the immune cells of allergic diseases. *Curr Mol Med* **8**, 401–407, doi:10.2174/156652408785160934 (2008).

116. Sawada, A. *et al.* A congenital mutation of the novel gene LRRC8 causes agammaglobulinemia in humans. *J Clin Invest* **112**, 1707–1713, doi:10.1172/JCI18937 (2003).

117. Ponnalagu, D. *et al.* Molecular identity of cardiac mitochondrial chloride intracellular channel proteins. *Mitochondrion* **27**, 6–14, doi:10.1016/j.mito.2016.01.001 (2016).

118. Domingo-Fernandez, R., Coll, R. C., Kearney, J., Breit, S. & O'Neill, L. A. J. The intracellular chloride channel proteins CLIC1 and CLIC4 induce IL-1beta transcription and activate the NLRP3 inflammasome. *J Biol Chem* **292**, 12077–12087, doi:10.1074/jbc.M117.797126 (2017).

119. Tang, T. *et al.* CLICs-dependent chloride efflux is an essential and proximal upstream event for NLRP3 inflammasome activation. *Nat Commun* **8**, 202, doi:10.1038/s41467-017-00227-x (2017).

120. He, G. *et al.* Role of CLIC4 in the host innate responses to bacterial lipopolysaccharide. *Eur J Immunol* **41**, 1221–1230, doi:10.1002/eji.201041266 (2011).

121. Harrop, S. J. *et al.* Crystal structure of a soluble form of the intracellular chloride ion channel CLIC1 (NCC27) at 1.4-A resolution. *J Biol Chem* **276**, 44993–45000, doi:10.1074/jbc.M107804200 (2001).

122. Al Khamici, H. *et al.* Members of the chloride intracellular ion channel protein family demonstrate glutaredoxin-like enzymatic activity. *PLoS ONE* **10**, e115699, doi:10.1371/journal.pone.0115699 (2015).

123. Ponnalagu, D. & Singh, H. Anion channels of mitochondria. *Handb Exp Pharmacol* **240**, 71–101, doi:10.1007/164_2016_39 (2017).

124. Singh, H. Two decades with dimorphic Chloride Intracellular Channels (CLICs). *FEBS letters* **584**, 2112–2121, doi:10.1016/j.febslet.2010.03.013 (2010).

125. Gururaja Rao, S., Ponnalagu, D., Patel, N. J. & Singh, H. Three decades of chloride intracellular channel proteins: From organelle to organ physiology. *Curr Protoc Pharmacol* **80**, 11.21.11–11.21.17, doi:10.1002/cpph.36 (2018).

126. Littler, D. R. *et al.* The enigma of the CLIC proteins: Ion channels, redox proteins, enzymes, scaffolding proteins? *FEBS Lett* **584**, 2093–2101, doi:10.1016/j.febslet.2010.01.027 (2010).

127. Valenzuela, S. M. *et al.* Molecular cloning and expression of a chloride ion channel of cell nuclei. *J Biol Chem* **272**, 12575–12582, doi:10.1074/jbc.272.19.12575 (1997).

128. Heiss, N. S. & Poustka, A. Genomic structure of a novel chloride channel gene, CLIC2, in Xq28. *Genomics* **45**, 224–228, doi:10.1006/geno.1997.4922 (1997).

129. Qian, Z., Okuhara, D., Abe, M. K. & Rosner, M. R. Molecular cloning and characterization of a mitogen-activated protein kinase-associated intracellular chloride channel. *J Biol Chem* **274**, 1621–1627, doi:10.1074/jbc.274.3.1621 (1999).

130. Landry, D. *et al.* Molecular cloning and characterization of p64, a chloride channel protein from kidney microsomes. *J Biol Chem* **268**, 14948–14955 (1993).

131. Berryman, M. & Bretscher, A. Identification of a novel member of the chloride intracellular channel gene family (CLIC5) that associates with the actin cytoskeleton of placental microvilli. *Mol Biol Cell* **11**, 1509–1521, doi:10.1091/mbc.11.5.1509 (2000).

132. Landry, D. W., Reitman, M., Cragoe, E. J., Jr. & Al-Awqati, Q. Epithelial chloride channel. Development of inhibitory ligands. *J Gen Physiol* **90**, 779–798, doi:10.1085/jgp.90.6.779 (1987).

133. Landry, D. W. *et al.* Purification and reconstitution of chloride channels from kidney and trachea. *Science* **244**, 1469–1472, doi:10.1126/science.2472007 (1989).

134. Landry, D. W., Akabas, M. A., Redhead, C. & al-Awqati, Q. Purification and reconstitution of epithelial chloride channels. *Methods Enzymol* **191**, 572–583, doi:10.1016/0076-6879(90)91036-6 (1990).

135. Friedli, M. *et al.* Identification of a novel member of the CLIC family, CLIC6, mapping to 21q22.12. *Gene* **320**, 31–40, doi:10.1016/s0378-1119(03)00830-8 (2003).

136. Dixon, D. P., Davis, B. G. & Edwards, R. Functional divergence in the glutathione transferase superfamily in plants. Identification of two classes with putative functions in redox homeostasis in Arabidopsis thaliana. *J Biol Chem* **277**, 30859–30869, doi:10.1074/jbc.M202919200 (2002).

137. Littler, D. R. *et al.* Comparison of vertebrate and invertebrate CLIC proteins: The crystal structures of Caenorhabditis elegans EXC-4 and Drosophila melanogaster DmCLIC. *Proteins* **71**, 364–378, doi:10.1002/prot.21704 (2008).

138. Berry, K. L., Bulow, H. E., Hall, D. H. & Hobert, O. A C. Elegans CLIC-like protein required for intracellular tube formation and maintenance. *Science* **302**, 2134–2137, doi:10.1126/science.1087667 (2003).

139. Gururaja Rao, S. *et al.* Identification and characterization of a bacterial homolog of chloride intracellular channel (CLIC) protein. *Sci Rep* **7**, 8500, doi:10.1038/s41598-017-08742-z (2017).

140. Elter, A. *et al.* A plant homolog of animal chloride intracellular channels (CLICs) generates an ion conductance in heterologous systems. *J Biol Chem* **282**, 8786–8792, doi:10.1074/jbc.M607241200 (2007).

141. Gururaja Rao, S., Patel, N. J. & Singh, H. Intracellular chloride channels: Novel biomarkers in diseases. *Front Physiol* **11**, 96, doi:10.3389/fphys.2020.00096 (2020).

142. Hare, J. E., Goodchild, S. C., Breit, S. N., Curmi, P. M. & Brown, L. J. Interaction of human chloride intracellular channel protein 1 (CLIC1) with lipid bilayers: A fluorescence study. *Biochemistry* **55**, 3825–3833, doi:10.1021/acs.biochem.6b00080 (2016).

143. Ashley, R. H. Challenging accepted ion channel biology: P64 and the CLIC family of putative intracellular anion channel proteins (Review). *Mol Membr Biol* **20**, 1–11, doi:10.1080/09687680210042746 (2003).

144. Warton, K. *et al.* Recombinant CLIC1 (NCC27) assembles in lipid bilayers via a pH-dependent two-state process to form chloride ion channels with identical characteristics

to those observed in Chinese hamster ovary cells expressing CLIC1. *J Biol Chem* **277**, 26003–26011, doi:10.1074/jbc.M203666200 (2002).

145. Tulk, B. M., Kapadia, S. & Edwards, J. C. CLIC1 inserts from the aqueous phase into phospholipid membranes, where it functions as an anion channel. *Am J Physiol Cell Physiol* **282**, C1103–1112, doi:10.1152/ajpcell.00402.2001 (2002).

146. Fanucchi, S., Adamson, R. J. & Dirr, H. W. Formation of an unfolding intermediate state of soluble chloride intracellular channel protein CLIC1 at acidic pH. *Biochemistry* **47**, 11674–11681, doi:10.1021/bi801147r (2008).

147. Singh, H. & Ashley, R. H. Redox regulation of CLIC1 by cysteine residues associated with the putative channel pore. *Biophys J* **90**, 1628–1638, doi:10.1529/biophysj.105.072678 (2006).

148. Salao, K. *et al.* CLIC1 regulates dendritic cell antigen processing and presentation by modulating phagosome acidification and proteolysis. *Biol Open* **5**, 620–630, doi:10.1242/bio.018119 (2016).

149. Carlini, V. *et al.* CLIC1 protein accumulates in circulating monocyte membrane during neurodegeneration. *Int J Mol Sci* **21**, doi:10.3390/ijms21041484 (2020).

150. Jiang, L. *et al.* Intracellular chloride channel protein CLIC1 regulates macrophage function through modulation of phagosomal acidification. *J Cell Sci* **125**, 5479–5488, doi:10.1242/jcs.110072 (2012).

151. Ulmasov, B. *et al.* CLIC1 null mice demonstrate a role for CLIC1 in macrophage super-oxide production and tissue injury. *Physiol Rep* **5**, doi:10.14814/phy2.13169 (2017).

152. Davis, B. K., Wen, H. & Ting, J. P. The inflammasome NLRs in immunity, inflammation, and associated diseases. *Annu Rev Immunol* **29**, 707–735, doi:10.1146/annurev-immunol-031210-101405 (2011).

153. Lamkanfi, M. & Dixit, V. M. Inflammasomes and their roles in health and disease. *Annu Rev Cell Dev Biol* **28**, 137–161, doi:10.1146/annurev-cellbio-101011-155745 (2012).

154. Munoz-Planillo, R. *et al.* K(+) efflux is the common trigger of NLRP3 inflammasome activation by bacterial toxins and particulate matter. *Immunity* **38**, 1142–1153, doi:10.1016/j.immuni.2013.05.016 (2013).

155. Elster, S. K., Braunwald, E. & Wood, H. F. A study of C-reactive protein in the serum of patients with congestive heart failure. *Am Heart J* **51**, 533–541, doi:10.1016/0002-8703(56)90099-0 (1956).

156. Fani, L. *et al.* The association of innate and adaptive immunity, subclinical atherosclerosis, and cardiovascular disease in the Rotterdam Study: A prospective cohort study. *PLoS Med* **17**, e1003115, doi:10.1371/journal.pmed.1003115 (2020).

157. Torre-Amione, G. Immune activation in chronic heart failure. *Am J Cardiol* **95**, 3C–8C; discussion 38C–40C, doi:10.1016/j.amjcard.2005.03.006 (2005).

158. Swirski, F. K. & Nahrendorf, M. Cardioimmunology: The immune system in cardiac homeostasis and disease. *Nat Rev Immunol* **18**, 733–744, doi:10.1038/s41577-018-0065-8 (2018).

159. Leybaert, L. *et al.* Connexins in cardiovascular and neurovascular health and disease: Pharmacological implications. *Pharmacol Rev* **69**, 396–478, doi:10.1124/pr.115.012062 (2017).

160. Sheikh, F., Ross, R. S. & Chen, J. Cell-cell connection to cardiac disease. *Trends Cardiovasc Med* **19**, 182–190, doi:10.1016/j.tcm.2009.12.001 (2009).

161. Jansen, J. A., van Veen, T. A., de Bakker, J. M. & van Rijen, H. V. Cardiac connexins and impulse propagation. *J Mol Cell Cardiol* **48**, 76–82, doi:10.1016/j.yjmcc.2009.08.018 (2010).

162. Jongsma, H. J. & Wilders, R. Gap junctions in cardiovascular disease. *Circ Res* **86**, 1193–1197, doi:10.1161/01.res.86.12.1193 (2000).

163. Koval, M., Molina, S. A. & Burt, J. M. Mix and match: Investigating heteromeric and heterotypic gap junction channels in model systems and native tissues. *FEBS Lett* **588**, 1193–1204, doi:10.1016/j.febslet.2014.02.025 (2014).

164. Verheule, S. & Kaese, S. Connexin diversity in the heart: Insights from transgenic mouse models. *Front Pharmacol* **4**, 81, doi:10.3389/fphar.2013.00081 (2013).

165. Juszczak, G. R. & Swiergiel, A. H. Properties of gap junction blockers and their behavioural, cognitive and electrophysiological effects: Animal and human studies. *Prog Neuropsychopharmacol Biol Psychiatry* **33**, 181–198, doi:10.1016/j.pnpbp.2008.12.014 (2009).

166. Rohr, S. Role of gap junctions in the propagation of the cardiac action potential. *Cardiovasc Res* **62**, 309–322, doi:10.1016/j.cardiores.2003.11.035 (2004).

167. Moreno, A. P. Biophysical properties of homomeric and heteromultimeric channels formed by cardiac connexins. *Cardiovasc Res* **62**, 276–286, doi:10.1016/j.cardiores.2004.03.003 (2004).

168. Schalper, K. A. *et al.* Connexin 43 hemichannels mediate the Ca2+ influx induced by extracellular alkalinization. *Am J Physiol Cell Physiol* **299**, C1504–1515, doi:10.1152/ajpcell.00015.2010 (2010).

169. Saez, J. C., Berthoud, V. M., Branes, M. C., Martinez, A. D. & Beyer, E. C. Plasma membrane channels formed by connexins: Their regulation and functions. *Physiol Rev* **83**, 1359–1400, doi:10.1152/physrev.00007.2003 (2003).

170. Ye, Z. C., Wyeth, M. S., Baltan-Tekkok, S. & Ransom, B. R. Functional hemichannels in astrocytes: A novel mechanism of glutamate release. *J Neurosci* **23**, 3588–3596 (2003).

171. Karagiannis, A. *et al.* Hemichannel-mediated release of lactate. *J Cereb Blood Flow Metab* **36**, 1202–1211, doi:10.1177/0271678X15611912 (2016).

172. Eltzschig, H. K. *et al.* ATP release from activated neutrophils occurs via connexin 43 and modulates adenosine-dependent endothelial cell function. *Circ Res* **99**, 1100–1108, doi:10.1161/01.RES.0000250174.31269.70 (2006).

173. Bruzzone, S., Guida, L., Zocchi, E., Franco, L. & De Flora, A. Connexin 43 hemi channels mediate Ca2+-regulated transmembrane NAD+ fluxes in intact cells. *FASEB J* **15**, 10–12, doi:10.1096/fj.00-0566fje (2001).

174. Cherian, P. P. *et al.* Mechanical strain opens connexin 43 hemichannels in osteocytes: A novel mechanism for the release of prostaglandin. *Mol Biol Cell* **16**, 3100–3106, doi:10.1091/mbc.e04-10-0912 (2005).

175. Gossman, D. G. & Zhao, H. B. Hemichannel-mediated inositol 1,4,5-trisphosphate (IP3) release in the cochlea: A novel mechanism of IP3 intercellular signaling. *Cell Commun Adhes* **15**, 305–315, doi:10.1080/15419060802357217 (2008).

176. Epelman, S. *et al.* Embryonic and adult-derived resident cardiac macrophages are maintained through distinct mechanisms at steady state and during inflammation. *Immunity* **40**, 91–104, doi:10.1016/j.immuni.2013.11.019 (2014).

177. Pinto, A. R. *et al.* An abundant tissue macrophage population in the adult murine heart with a distinct alternatively-activated macrophage profile. *PLoS ONE* **7**, e36814, doi:10.1371/journal.pone.0036814 (2012).

178. Hulsmans, M. *et al.* Macrophages facilitate electrical conduction in the heart. *Cell* **169**, 510–522, e520, doi:10.1016/j.cell.2017.03.050 (2017).

179. De Jesus, N. M. *et al.* Atherosclerosis exacerbates arrhythmia following myocardial infarction: Role of myocardial inflammation. *Heart Rhythm* **12**, 169–178, doi:10.1016/j.hrthm.2014.10.007 (2015).

180. Frangogiannis, N. G. Regulation of the inflammatory response in cardiac repair. *Circ Res* **110**, 159–173, doi:10.1161/CIRCRESAHA.111.243162 (2012).

181. Schulz, C. & Massberg, S. Atherosclerosis—multiple pathways to lesional macrophages. *Sci Transl Med* **6**, 239ps232, doi:10.1126/scitranslmed.3008922 (2014).
182. Witztum, J. L. & Lichtman, A. H. The influence of innate and adaptive immune responses on atherosclerosis. *Annu Rev Pathol* **9**, 73–102, doi:10.1146/annurev-pathol-020712-163936 (2014).
183. Hansson, G. K. & Libby, P. The immune response in atherosclerosis: A double-edged sword. *Nat Rev Immunol* **6**, 508–519, doi:10.1038/nri1882 (2006).
184. Gerrity, R. G. The role of the monocyte in atherogenesis: I. Transition of blood-borne monocytes into foam cells in fatty lesions. *Am J Pathol* **103**, 181–190 (1981).
185. Tabas, I., Williams, K. J. & Boren, J. Subendothelial lipoprotein retention as the initiating process in atherosclerosis: Update and therapeutic implications. *Circulation* **116**, 1832–1844, doi:10.1161/CIRCULATIONAHA.106.676890 (2007).
186. Swirski, F. K. & Nahrendorf, M. Leukocyte behavior in atherosclerosis, myocardial infarction, and heart failure. *Science* **339**, 161–166, doi:10.1126/science.1230719 (2013).
187. Morel, S. *et al.* Titration of the gap junction protein Connexin43 reduces atherogenesis. *Thromb Haemost* **112**, 390–401, doi:10.1160/TH13-09-0773 (2014).
188. Pfenniger, A., Chanson, M. & Kwak, B. R. Connexins in atherosclerosis. *Biochim Biophys Acta* **1828**, 157–166, doi:10.1016/j.bbamem.2012.05.011 (2013).
189. Wong, C. W. *et al.* Connexin37 protects against atherosclerosis by regulating monocyte adhesion. *Nat Med* **12**, 950–954, doi:10.1038/nm1441 (2006).
190. Mellow, M. H., Simpson, A. G., Watt, L., Schoolmeester, L. & Haye, O. L. Esophageal acid perfusion in coronary artery disease. Induction of myocardial ischemia. *Gastroenterology* **85**, 306–312 (1983).
191. Lawrence, T. & Natoli, G. Transcriptional regulation of macrophage polarization: Enabling diversity with identity. *Nat Rev Immunol* **11**, 750–761, doi:10.1038/nri3088 (2011).
192. Biswas, S. K. & Mantovani, A. Macrophage plasticity and interaction with lymphocyte subsets: Cancer as a paradigm. *Nat Immunol* **11**, 889–896, doi:10.1038/ni.1937 (2010).
193. Silvestre-Roig, C. *et al.* Atherosclerotic plaque destabilization: Mechanisms, models, and therapeutic strategies. *Circ Res* **114**, 214–226, doi:10.1161/CIRCRESAHA.114.302355 (2014).
194. Toyama, K. *et al.* The intermediate-conductance calcium-activated potassium channel KCa3.1 contributes to atherogenesis in mice and humans. *J Clin Invest* **118**, 3025–3037, doi:10.1172/JCI30836 (2008).
195. Israel, C. W. Mechanisms of sudden cardiac death. *Indian Heart J* **66 Suppl 1**, S10–17, doi:10.1016/j.ihj.2014.01.005 (2014).
196. Fei, Y. D. *et al.* Macrophages facilitate post myocardial infarction arrhythmias: Roles of gap junction and KCa3.1. *Theranostics* **9**, 6396–6411, doi:10.7150/thno.34801 (2019).

Index

Page numbers in *italics* indicate a figure and page numbers in **bold** indicate a table on the corresponding page.

Methods in Signal Transduction (Continued)

For more information about this series, please visit: https://www.crcpress.com/ Methods-in-Signal-Transduction-Series/book-series/CRCMETSIGTRA?page=&or der=pubdate&size=12&view=list&status=published,forthcoming

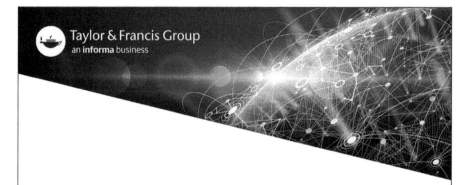

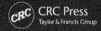

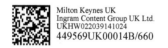